Assessing Medical Rehabilitation Practices

This book is printed on recycled paper. ♻

Assessing Medical Rehabilitation Practices

The Promise of Outcomes Research

edited by

Marcus J. Fuhrer, Ph.D.
National Center for Medical Rehabilitation Research
National Institute of Child Health and Human Development
National Institutes of Health
Rockville, Maryland

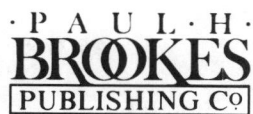
·P·A·U·L·H·
BROOKES
PUBLISHING CO

Baltimore • London • Toronto • Sydney

Paul H. Brookes Publishing Co.
Post Office Box 10624
Baltimore, Maryland 21285-0624

Typeset by PRO-IMAGE Corp., York, Pennsylvania.
Manufactured in the United States of America by
Thomson-Shore, Inc., Dexter, Michigan.

This work may be reproduced in whole or in part for the official use of the U.S. government or any authorized agency thereof.

The conference on which this book is based, "An Agenda for Medical Rehabilitation Outcomes Research," was supported by the National Center for Medical Rehabilitation Research, the National Institute of Child Health and Human Development, the National Institutes of Health, and the Agency for Health Care Policy and Research.

FIM[SM] is a service mark of the Uniform Data System for Medical Rehabilitation (UDSMR[SM]), a division of UB Foundation Activities, Inc.

Library of Congress Cataloging-in-Publication Data

Assessing medical rehabilitation practices : the promise of outcomes
  research / edited by Marcus J. Fuhrer.
     p. cm.
  Includes bibliographical references and index.
  ISBN 1-55766-274-6
  1. Medical rehabilitation.   2. Outcomes assessment (Medical care)
I. Fuhrer, Marcus J., 1933–
  [DNLM: 1. Outcome and Process Assessment (Health Care)
2. Rehabilitation.   3. Disability Evaluation.   WB   320   A847   1996]
RM930.A87   1997
617′.03—DC20
DNLM/DLC
for Library of Congress   96-31051
                                                                                  CIP

British Cataloguing in Publication data are available from the British Library.

Assessing medical
rehabilitation practices

Contents

Contributors

THE EDITOR

Marcus J. Fuhrer, Ph.D., Director, National Center for Medical Rehabilitation Research, National Institute of Child Health and Human Development, National Institutes of Health, 6100 Building, Room 2A03, 6100 Executive Boulevard MSC 7510, Rockville, Maryland 20852. Prior to his appointment as the first director of the National Center for Medical Rehabilitation Research in April 1993, Dr. Fuhrer was Professor in the Departments of Physical Medicine and Rehabilitation and of Psychiatry and Behavioral Sciences at Baylor College of Medicine. He also served as Vice President for Research of The Institute for Rehabilitation and Research in Houston, Texas. He is a past president of the American Congress of Rehabilitation Medicine and of the National Association of Rehabilitation Research and Training Centers. He coedited *Functional Assessment in Rehabilitation* and edited *Selected Research Topics in Spinal Cord Injury* and *Rehabilitation Outcomes: Analysis and Measurement.* His research and writing have been concerned predominantly with medical rehabilitation outcomes research, factors affecting the life status of people with spinal cord injury, cognitive processes in the Pavlovian conditioning of human autonomic responses, and the characteristics of peripheral sympathetic activity following transection of the human spinal cord.

THE CONTRIBUTORS

Jennifer Button, M.A., Coordinator of Research, Ontario Brain Injury Association, P.O. Box 2338, Station B, St. Catharines, Ontario, L2M 7M7, CANADA. Ms. Button completed her master's degree in experimental psychology and did graduate course work in mathematical statistics. Her position at the Ontario Brain Injury Association allows her to pursue her interest in statistical analysis and research design.

John D. Corrigan, Ph.D., Associate Professor, Division of Rehabilitation Psychology, Department of Physical Medicine and Rehabilitation, Ohio State University, 480 West 9th Avenue, Columbus, Ohio 43210. In addition to being an associate professor at Ohio State University, Dr. Corrigan is a psychologist and is Director of the Ohio Valley Center for Brain Injury Prevention and Rehabilitation and chairs its Division of Rehabilitation Psychology. His research interests include measurement and treatment of agitation, substance abuse following acquired brain injury, and long-term outcomes from brain injury.

Gerben DeJong, Ph.D., Director, National Rehabilitation Hospital Research Center, Director, Research and Training Center in Medical Rehabilitation and Health Policy, NRH Research Center, 102 Irving Street, N.W., Washington, D.C. 20010-2949. Dr. DeJong is also a professor in the Department of Family Medicine and an adjunct professor in the Graduate Public Policy Program at Georgetown University, Washington, D.C. His academic training is in economics and public policy studies. His main research interests are in health, disability, and long-term care policies, including issues related to financing, access, utilization, costs, outcomes, and biomedical ethics. Dr. DeJong is the author or coauthor of more than 150 papers on health and disability issues. He is perhaps best known for his seminal work on disability and health policy and the independent living movement. He is a frequently invited speaker, both in the United States and abroad. In 1984, he was a Fulbright Scholar in the Netherlands, serving with the research staff of the Social Security Council. Dr. DeJong is an ardent student of health care reform and the managed care revolution. He is especially interested in managed care's probable impact on medical rehabilitation, on people with disabilities, and on other vulnerable populations.

Marcel Dijkers, Ph.D., Director of Research, Rehabilitation Institute of Michigan, Wayne State University, 261 Mack Avenue, Detroit, Michigan 48201. Dr. Dijkers received his training in the social sciences in the Netherlands and the United States and received his doctoral degree in sociology from Wayne State University in 1978. He is Director of Research at the Rehabilitation Institute of Michigan in Detroit and an associate professor of physical medicine and rehabilitation at Wayne State University. His research involves the sociology and social psychology of disablement and rehabilitation, with a special focus on issues related to service delivery, measurement of disability and handicap, and quality of life. Several grant-supported projects, most focusing on spinal cord injury, have been the basis for most of his papers and chapters.

Pamela W. Duncan, Ph.D., PT, Director of Research, Center on Aging, University of Kansas Medical Center, Wescoe Pavilion, Room 5026, 3901 Rainbow Boulevard, Kansas City, Kansas 66160-7117. In addition to her post as Director of the Center on Aging, Dr. Duncan is an associate professor in the Health Services Administration, Department of Pharmacy, at the University of Kansas, Lawrence. She also serves as Program Director for Health Services Research at the Kansas City and Leavenworth Veterans Administration Medical Center. She was co-chair of the consensus panel on establishing the guidelines for rehabilitation for the Agency for Health Care Policy Research Education. Dr. Duncan is Principal Investigator of the Kansas City Stroke Study, a community study to evaluate measures of motor recovery following stroke. Her primary research areas are the measurement of recovery of function following stroke, imbalance in older adults, and the efficacy of physical intervention for frail older adults and stroke victims. She is a national and international consultant on assessment and rehabilitation of motor control deficits following stroke and on balance deficits in the elderly. She served as President of the Neurology Section of the American Physical Therapy Association and was also selected as Fellow of the American Heart Association in 1993. Dr. Duncan serves on the editorial board of the journal *Stroke*.

Pennifer Erickson, Ph.D., Principal Developer, OLGA: The On-Line Guide to Quality of Life Assessment, 1222 Deerfield Drive, State College, Pennsylvania 16803. Dr. Erickson has designed two information systems specific to health-related quality of life: the Clearinghouse on Health Indexes, at the National Center for Health Statistics; and The On-Line Guide to Quality-of-Life Assessment (OLGA). In addition, she has directed two research teams that have analyzed data from the National Health Interview Survey and the NHANES I Epidemiologic Followup Survey to derive and evaluate national estimates of health-related quality of life and years of healthy life.

Roger C. Fiedler, Ph.D., Research Assistant Professor, Center for Functional Assessment Research (CFAR), Department of Rehabilitation Medicine, State University of New York at Buffalo (SUNY/Buffalo), 232 Parker Hall, 3435 Main Street, Buffalo, New York 14214-3007. As Director of Research at the Uniform Data System for Medical Rehabilitation (UDS$_{MR}$^{SM}), Research Assistant Professor, Rehabilitation Medicine Department, SUNY/Buffalo, and Associate Professor, Division of Rehabilitation Sciences, at D'Youville College, Dr. Fiedler has taught courses in research, measurement, and statistics since 1981. He was Director of Research and Data Management, Department of Cardiac Surgery, Buffalo General Hospital, from 1989 to 1992. He accepted an NIH Fellowship in functional assessment research at CFAR, working with Drs. Carl Granger and Byron Hamilton from 1992 to 1994. Subsequently, he was appointed Director of Research for UDS$_{MR}$ at CFAR, working on projects involving measurement issues and rehabilitation outcomes. He has published articles related to health, cardiac surgery, functional status, measurement, and statistics, and has served as Principal Investigator, Project Director, or Consultant on research projects in medical rehabilitation, physical and occupational therapy, nursing, cancer research, cardiac surgery, psychology, and education, using multivariate statistical methods, including advanced repeated measures and designs, linear stuctural modeling using LISREL, and both traditional and latent trait theory models of measurement.

Patrick Fougeyrollas, Ph.D., Director of Professional Services, Centre Francois-Charon, 525 Boulevard Wilfred Hamel East, Québec, Québec, G1M 2S8, CANADA. Dr. Fougeyrollas is Associate Professor in the Department of Occupational Therapy and Director of Professional and Scientific Services at the University Institute of Rehabilitation and Social Integration Centre, Laval University. He has been President of the Canadian Society on the Classification of Impairments, Disabilities, and Handicaps since 1989 and is an active member of committees on classification of disablement for the World Health Organization, the United Nations, and the Council of Europe. Dr. Fougeyrollas is a founding member of the Research Network of Social Participation. His research focuses on the analysis of the interactive process between the individual and the environment in the realm of social participation of people with disabilities.

Kenneth A. Gerhart, M.S., Research Associate, Craig Hospital, 3425 South Clarkson Street, Englewood, Colorado 80110. In addition to being a research associate,

Mr. Gerhart served as a physical therapist and staff supervisor at Craig Hospital. He helped establish the Colorado Spinal Cord Injury Surveillance Program and its nationally distributed quarterly newsletter *SCI Update*. He has worked with individuals with physical disabilities since the late 1970s and has authored numerous articles in a range of refereed journals and two chapters in *Aging with Spinal Cord Injury*, which he coedited. He is presently involved in the gathering and dissemination of longitudinal research of long-term spinal cord injury survivors.

Carl V. Granger, M.D., Professor of Rehabilitation Medicine, Director, Center for Functional Assessment Research, Department of Rehabilitation Medicine, School of Medicine and Biomedical Sciences, State University of New York at Buffalo, Erie Medical Center, 232 Parker Hall, 3435 Main Street, Buffalo, New York 14214-3007. Dr. Granger is a graduate of Dartmouth College and New York University School of Medicine. He is certified in physical medicine and rehabilitation and electrodiagnostic medicine. His academic and administrative appointments have included Professor and Chairman of Physical and Rehabilitation Medicine and Project Center at Tufts University and Professor of Family Medicine and Community Medicine and Director of the Center for Parkinson Disease Association Information and Referral Center at Brown University. Dr. Granger is a past president of the American Academy of Physical Medicine and Rehabilitation and of the International Federation of Physical Medicine and Rehabilitation and served on the Advisory Committee of the National Center for Medical Rehabilitation Research, National Institute of Child Health and Human Development, National Institutes of Health. He has more than 100 publications. His interests and research are in development and use of measures of disablement and quality of daily living, which include physical, mental/emotional, and social functioning in order to evaluate outcomes of medical rehabilitation. He was one of the developers of the Functional Independence Measure (FIM^{SM}) and the Uniform Data System for Medical Rehabilitation (UDS$_{MR}$). He was awarded the Krusen Award by the American Academy of Physical Medicine and Rehabilitation. Dr. Granger is a member of the executive committee of the RRTC on Functional Assessment and Evaluation of Rehabilitation Outcomes.

Byron Hamilton, M.D., Ph.D., Director, Rehabilitation Services Research and Development Unit, Department of Veterans Affairs Medical Center, 2424 Erwin Road, Room 200, Durham, North Carolina 27705. Since 1994, Dr. Hamilton has been an associate clinical professor of medicine in the Division of Geriatrics at Duke University Medical Center and Director of the Rehabilitation Services Research and Development Unit at the Department of Veterans Affairs Medical Center, Durham, North Carolina. He received medical and doctoral degrees from the State University of New York (SUNY) Health Sciences Center, Syracuse. He was on the faculty of the Department of Rehabilitation Medicine at Northwestern University Medical School and was Director of Research at the Rehabilitation Institute of Chicago from 1970 to 1984. While at Northwestern University Medical School, he was also Director of Research for the Medical Rehabilitation Research and Training Center, sponsored by the National Institute on Disability and Rehabilitation Research (NIDRR). From 1984 to 1994 at the Department of Rehabilitation Medicine at

SUNY/Buffalo, he was codeveloper of the Uniform Data System for Medical Rehabilitation (UDSMR) and the Functional Independence Measure (FIM), which are broadly used by rehabilitation facilities in the United States and other countries for measurement of disability and rehabilitation outcomes. While at SUNY/Buffalo, he was also Principal Investigator of the NIDRR-funded Rehabilitation Research and Training Center on Functional Assessment and Evaluation of Rehabilitation Outcomes (1993–1994), Co-Director of the Center for Functional Assessment Research (1989–1990), and Director of the NIDRR-sponsored National Traumatic Brain Injury Model Systems Data Center (1988–1993).

Helen Hoenig, M.D., M.P.H., O.T., Assistant Professor of Medicine/Geriatrics, Duke University Medical Center, and Chief, Physical Medicine and Rehabilitation Service, Department of Veterans Affairs Medical Center, 508 Fulton Street, Durham, North Carolina 27514. Dr. Hoenig's research and writing are concerned with outcomes research in geriatric rehabilitation, particularly how rehabilitation is provided for older patients and which patterns of use are associated with better outcomes. She is particularly interested in defining rehabilitation interventions and their role in the prevention of excess disability among older adults with disabilities. She has examined the use of rehabilitation after acute hip fracture and for geriatric patients who are functionally impaired. She was co–principal investigator of a project to develop and implement a comprehensive registry of veterans with spinal cord injury, including obtaining primary data on their functional status, data that is currently under analysis. She is Principal Investigator on a national study of the structure and organization of stroke rehabilitation services in the Veterans Administration and the relationship of this to patient outcomes.

W.T. Jackson, Ph.D., Assistant Professor, Department of Psychiatry and Behavioral Neurobiology, Adult Division, University of Alabama at Birmingham School of Medicine, 530 Spain Rehabilitation Center, 1717 Sixth Avenue South, Birmingham, Alabama 35233-7330. Dr. Jackson is a clinical neuropsychologist and an assistant professor in the Department of Psychiatry and Behavioral Neurobiology, Adult Division, University of Alabama, Birmingham (UAB). He received his doctoral degree from Louisiana State University and completed a 2-year NIH postdoctoral fellowship in medical rehabilitation research and clinical neuropsychology in the UAB Department of Physical Medicine and Rehabilitation under the auspices of the National Center for Medical Rehabilitation Research. Dr. Jackson specializes in outcomes-oriented research and treatment of people with severe behavior disorders related to neurologic injury or disease.

Alan M. Jette, Ph.D., PT, Professor and Dean, Sargent College, Boston University, 635 Commonwealth Avenue, Boston, Massachusetts 02215. Dr. Jette has a bachelor's degree in physical therapy from the State University of New York at Buffalo and master's and doctoral degrees in public health from the University of Michigan. His research has focused on the measurement, epidemiology, and prevention of disability. He has published widely in health journals in the United States and abroad.

Diane U. Jette, D.Sc., PT, Program Director and Associate Professor, Graduate Program in Physical Therapy, Graduate School of Health Sciences, Simmons College, 300 The Fenway, Boston, Massachusetts 02115-5898. Dr. Jette is also a clinician providing care to patients with cardiopulmonary diseases at Boston's Beth Israel Hospital. She received a bachelor's degree in physical therapy from Simmons College, a master's degree in physical therapy from Boston University, and a doctoral degree in epidemiology and biostatistics from Boston University. In 1996, she completed a Mary Switzer Research Fellowship granted by the National Institute on Disability and Rehabilitation Research to research outcomes in physcial therapy practice.

Mark V. Johnston, Ph.D., Director of Outcomes Research, Kessler Institute for Rehabilitation, Inc., University of Medicine and Dentistry of New Jersey, Research East, 240 East Central Avenue, East Orange, New Jersey 07018. In addition to his affiliation with the Kessler Institute, Dr. Johnston is an associate professor in the Department of Physical Medicine and Rehabilitation at the University of Medicine and Dentistry of New Jersey. Since the late 1970s, his research has addressed issues of the effectiveness and cost-effectiveness of rehabilitation for people with stroke, acquired brain injury, spinal cord injury, and a variety of other severe, chronic conditions. His doctoral degree is from a department of psychology specializing in program evaluation, and his bachelor's degree is in economics. Dr. Johnston has been Chairman of the Measurement and Evaluation Task Force of the American Congress of Rehabilitation Medicine since 1986 and is also a past chairman of the Committee on TBI Outcomes and Treatment Effectiveness. He has published more than 40 papers on various aspects of rehabilitation outcomes. Topics of his continuing work include research design, measurement of function, objective quality improvement and program evaluation systems, family factors, orthotic device utilization, minority/access issues, and the effectiveness and cost-effectiveness of interventions for people with stroke, acquired brain injury, spinal cord injury, and hip fracture.

Robert Allen Keith, Ph.D., Research Consultant, Casa Colina Hospital, 2850 North Garey Avenue, Pomona, California 91767. After serving for 27 years as Director of the Center for Research and Planning at Casa Colina Hospital, Dr. Keith is a research consultant to that institution. He is also Professor of Psychology Emeritus at Claremont Graduate School, Pomona, California. His academic training included a doctoral degree in clinical psychology from the University of California at Los Angeles. Additional appointments have included Visiting Scholar, Department of Child Development, University of London; Research Fellow, Department of Nutrition, Harvard School of Public Health; and Fellow, International Exchange of Experts and Information in Rehabilitation, a program of the World Rehabilitation Fund. Dr. Keith is a Diplomate in Clinical Psychology of the American Psychological Association. Publications in rehabilitation medicine have included works on functional status measurement, program evaluation, data systems for medical rehabilitation, the organization of treatment delivery, the conceptual basis of treatment and outcomes, and research on a variety of clinical populations. Dr. Keith was a member of the task force that developed the Uniform Data System for Medical Rehabilitation (UDSMR) and served on the national advisory board for that organization.

Bryan Kemp, Ph.D., Director, Rehabilitation Research and Training Center on Aging with Disability, Rancho Los Amigos Medical Center, University of Southern California, P.O. Box 3500, Los Amigos Station, 7601 East Imperial Highway, Downey, California 90242-8202. In addition to his positions as Director of the Rehabilitation Research and Training Centers on Aging with Disability at Rancho Los Amigos Medical Center and the University of Southern California (USC), Dr. Kemp is Director of the Gerontology Program at Rancho Los Amigos and Clinical Associate Professor of Family Medicine and of Psychiatry, as well as Associate Research Professor of Gerontology, at USC.

Laura Mosqueda, M.D., Rancho Los Amigos Medical Center, University of Southern California, 7601 East Imperial Highway, Downey, California 90242-8202. Dr. Mosqueda is board-certified in family medicine and geriatrics. She is Medical Director of Geriatrics for St. Luke Medical Center in Pasadena, California. Dr. Mosqueda is also the Training Director of the Rehabilitation Research and Training Centers on Aging with Disability. At the University of Southern California, she is Assistant Professor of Gerontology.

T.N. Novack, Ph.D., Department of Rehabilitation Medicine, University of Alabama at Birmingham School of Medicine, 530 Spain Rehabilitation Center, 1717 Sixth Avenue South, Birmingham, Alabama 35233-7330. Dr. Novack specializes in rehabilitation of individuals with traumatic brain injury. He has been certified by the American Board of Clinical Neuropsychology.

Kenneth J. Ottenbacher, Ph.D., Professor and Vice Dean, The University of Texas Medical Branch at Galveston, School of Allied Health Sciences, 301 University Boulevard, Galveston, Texas 77555-1028. Dr. Ottenbacher is Professor and Vice Dean in the School of Allied Health Sciences at the University of Texas Medical Branch at Galveston. He was Associate Director of the Center for Functional Assessment Research in the Department of Rehabilitation Medicine at the State University of New York at Buffalo when his chapter was written. Dr. Ottenbacher's research interests include the development and application of design and measurement strategies appropriate for use in clinical environments. He has published more than 100 scientific/technical articles in refereed journals and is the author, coauthor, or editor of four texts. He has served as the Principal Investigator or Co–Principal Investigator on more than a dozen federally funded grants and is a past editor of the *Occupational Therapy Journal of Research* and a member of several editorial boards. He is serving as the Statistical Consulting Editor for the *American Journal of Physical Medicine and Rehabilitation.*

Jacquelin Perry, M.D., Orthopaedic Surgeon, Chief, Pathkinesiology Service, Rancho Los Amigos Medical Center, 7601 East Imperial Highway, Building 304, Downey, California 90242. Dr. Perry is Professor of Orthopaedics at the University of Southern California (USC). She received her bachelor's degree in physical education from the University of California at Los Angeles, a physical therapy certificate from the U.S. Army, and her medical degree from the University of California at San Francisco. She is affiliated with Rancho Los Amigos Medical Center. Her medical practice began with polio patient reconstructive surgery, as well as rehabilitation of people with severe disabilities with clinical programs in stroke, spinal cord injury, arthritis, head trauma, rehabilitation, and gait analysis. Dr. Perry developed a systematic approach for analyzing gait that is accepted worldwide, as well as an instrumented laboratory system with dynamic electromyography to determine the precise timing and intensity of muscle function during walking to assist surgical planning. Her areas of research interest are gait analysis for the spastic, arthritic, and polio patients, and amputees. Her honors and awards include Woman of the Year in Medicine, Southern California, Los Angeles Times Award, 1959; Kappa Delta Award, Orthopedic Research Society, 1976; Isabelle and Leonard H. Goldenson Award in Technology, United Cerebral Palsy Research and Education Foundations, Inc., 1981; Joseph F. Dowling Distinguished Service Award, Rancho Los Amigos Medical Center, June 1985; UCLA Professional Achievement Award, June 1988; Amistad Award, Rancho Los Amigos Medical Center, March 1990; Milton Cohen Distinguished Service Award, National Association of Rehabilitation Facilities, June 1993; Physician of the Year, California Governor's Committee, EDD State of California, October 1994; and Honorary Doctorate in Science, USC, May 1996.

J. Scott Richards, Ph.D., Professor and Director of Research, University of Alabama, Birmingham, Spain Rehabilitation Center, 1717 Sixth Avenue South, Birmingham, Alabama 35233-7330. Dr. Richards received his doctoral degree in clinical psychology from Kent State University in 1977. Since then, he has been on the faculty of the Department of Physical Medicine and Rehabilitation, University of Alabama, Birmingham, and is a full professor. He has been Director of Psychology since 1977 and Director of Research for the Department of Physical Medicine and Rehabilitation since 1987. His areas of research interest have included, among others, psychosocial correlates of coping and adjustment in spinal cord injury, pain in spinal cord injury, and predictors or correlates of outcomes in the treatment of chronic pain.

Gregory Samsa, Ph.D., Associate Director, Center for Health Policy and Education, Duke University, Box 90527, Durham, North Carolina 27705. Dr. Samsa is an assistant professor with appointments in Duke University's Center for Health Policy Research and Education, Department of Medicine, and Department of Community and Family Medicine. He has authored more than 90 peer-reviewed scientific articles. As an applied statistician specializing in health services research clinical epidemiology, his research interests include epidemiology of stroke, epidemiology of spinal cord injury, and statistical education. Dr. Samsa is the Senior Statistician and Director of the Patient Outcomes Research Team (PORT) for the Secondary and Tertiary Prevention of Stroke and was the Principal Investigator of a project to develop a comprehensive national registry of veterans with spinal cord injury.

Margaret Stineman, M.D., Associate Professor, Department of Rehabilitation Medicine, University of Pennsylvania Medical Center, 101 Ralston-Penn Center, 3615 Chestnut Street, Philadelphia, Pennsylvania 19104-2676. At the University of Pennsylvania, Dr. Stineman is Associate Professor, Department of Rehabilitation Medicine; Senior Fellow of the Leonard Davis Institute of Health Economics; and

Associate Scholar in the Clinical Epidemiology Unit of the Department of Biostatistics and Clinical Epidemiology. Her research interests include establishing the relationships among qualitative and quantitative measurement, medical ethics, disability staging, resource use allocation, and the measurement of quality of life, social integration, and functional independence. She is the Principal Investigator on several projects funded through the National Center for Medical Rehabilitation Research of the National Institutes of Health/National Institute of Child Health and Human Development. One of these projects involves the development of a major staging system to establish the likelihood of people with disabling medical conditions recovering to specific levels of functions. Dr. Stineman was the Principal Investigator on the project that led to development of the Functional Independence Measure–Function Related Groups (FIM–FRGs), which are being considered by the Health Care Financing Administration for possible incorporation into a new Medicare prospective payment system. She practices with the University of Pennsylvania Health System and is a guest examiner for the American Board of Physical Medicine and Rehabilitation.

Margaret A. Turk, M.D., Associate Professor of Physical Medicine and Rehabilitation, Department of Pediatrics (joint appointment), State University of New York (SUNY) Health Science Center at Syracuse, 750 East Adams Street, Syracuse, New York 13210. Dr. Turk is also Medical Director of the Brain Injury Rehabilitation Program at St. Camillus Health and Rehabilitation Center in Syracuse and the Prinicipal Investigator on a study of secondary conditions of cerebral palsy in adults. She is the coauthor of several monographs and curricula on secondary conditions and aging with a disability. Dr. Turk sits on the editorial board of *Muscle & Nerve* and was coeditor of *Women with Physical Disabilities: Achieving and Maintaining Health and Well-Being* (Paul H. Brookes Publishing Co., 1996) with Danuta M. Krotoski and Margaret A. Nosek. Dr. Turk serves on a number of advisory boards of national advocacy organizations, including Spina Bifida Association of America, Paralyzed Veterans Association, and the National Osteoporosis Foundation. She belongs to numerous state and national committees directed at the development of practice guidelines and outcomes measurement in rehabilitation. Dr. Turk is a director of the American Board of Physical Medicine and Rehabilitation and a consultant to the Institute of Medicine's (IOM's) Committee on Assessing Rehabilitation Science and Engineering.

Craig A. Velozo, Ph.D., OTR/L, Associate Professor, Department of Occupational Therapy (M/C 811), College of Associated Health Professions, University of Illinois at Chicago, 1919 West Taylor Street, Chicago, Illinois 60612-7250. Dr. Velozo's research focus since 1988 has been on using innovative designs to investigate outcomes in rehabilitation and also on the development of instruments for monitoring medical rehabilitation outcomes. Dr. Velozo has been the Principal Investigator in the development of the Worker Role Interview and the Occupational Outcomes Scale. Much of his recent research has focused on the use of Rasch measurement for instrument development.

Nanette K. Wenger, M.D., Professor of Medicine, Division of Cardiology, Emory University School of Medicine, Consultant, Emory Heart Center, Director, Cardiac

Clinic, Grady Memorial Hospital, 69 Butler Street, S.E., Atlanta, Georgia 30303. Coronary heart disease in women is one of Dr. Wenger's major clinical and research interests. She chaired the U.S. National Heart, Lung, and Blood Institute Conference on Cardiovascular Health and Disease in Women. She also has expertise in cardiac rehabilitation. She chaired the World Health Organization Expert Committee on Rehabilitation After Cardiovascular Disease and co-chaired the Guideline Panel on Cardiac Rehabilitation for the U.S. Agency for Health Care Policy and Research. She has had a long-standing interest in geriatric cardiology as well and is a past president of the Council on Geriatric Cardiology and editor of the *American Journal of Geriatric Cardiology*. Dr. Wenger received the Outstanding Professional Achievement Award from Hunter College in 1993, the President's Woman in Science Award of the American Medical Women's Association in 1993, the Citation Award of the American College of Sports Medicine in 1994, and the Jan J. Kellermann Memorial Award for Cardiovascular Prevention and Rehabilitation of the International Society of Heart Failure in 1995. She is listed in *Best Doctors in America*. She has authored or coauthored more than 800 scientific and review articles and book chapters.

Gale G. Whiteneck, Ph.D., Director of Research, Craig Hospital, 3425 South Clarkson Street, Englewood, Colorado 80110. Dr. Whiteneck, as Director of Research at the Craig Hospital Rehabilitation facility, is responsible for the coordination of all clinical research and manages projects concerning spinal cord injury and aging and the registry and follow-up of traumatic brain injury, as well as program evaluation, functional assessment, handicap measurement, long-term outcomes, and the cost of lifetime care. Dr. Whiteneck has edited two books on spinal cord injury and has authored numerous articles on disability outcomes.

John Whyte, M.D., Ph.D., Director of Research and Attending Physician, MossRehab Hospital, Associate Professor, Department of Physical Medicine and Rehabilitation, Temple University School of Medicine, 1200 West Tabor Road, Philadelphia, Pennsylvania 19141-3099. Dr. Whyte received his medical degree from the University of Pennsylvania, where he also received a doctoral degree in cognitive psychology. He completed a residency in physical medicine and rehabilitation at the University of Minnesota and a neurotrauma fellowship at Tufts University School of Medicine and New England Medical Center. Currently, Dr. Whyte is an associate professor of physical medicine and rehabilitation at Temple University School of Medicine, an attending physician at MossRehab Hospital's Drucker Brain Injury Center, and the Director of the Moss Rehabilitation Research Institute. Dr. Whyte combines clinical work and research with patients with acquired brain injury. In addition to his research interests in the areas of disorders of attention and recovery from coma after brain injury, he has also been interested in the special research methodologic problems inherent in the field of rehabilitation. He also chairs the research committee of the Association of Academic Physiatrists.

Deborah L. Wilkerson, M.A., CARF . . . The Rehabilitation Accreditation Commission, 4891 East Grant Road, Tucson, Arizona 85712. Ms. Wilkerson conducted work on her chapter in this volume while she was Director of Program Evaluation and Outcome Studies at the National Rehabilitation Hospital, Washington, D.C., and Director of Training at the Rehabilitation Research and Training Center on Medical Rehabilitation Services and Health Policy at the National Rehabilitation Hospital Research Center. Ms. Wilkerson has also served as Administrator in the Department of Rehabilitation Medicine at the University of Washington at Seattle and has worked in the vocational rehabilitation and independent living evaluation arenas. She holds a master's degree in anthropology from Wake Forest University. In 1996, Ms. Wilkerson became Director of Research and Quality Improvement at CARF . . . The Rehabilitation Accreditation Commission in Tucson, Arizona.

Barry Willer, Ph.D., 21 Bowen Road, Fort Erie, Ontario, L2A 2Y5, CANADA. Dr. Willer is a professor in the Departments of Psychiatry and Rehabilitation Medicine at the State University of New York at Buffalo. His research interests focus on the community integration outcomes of individuals with disabilities, particularly those individuals with an acquired brain injury.

Preface

The materialization of this book is intimately connected with the founding and early development of the National Center for Medical Rehabilitation Research (NCMRR) at the National Institutes of Health (NIH), the world's preeminent institution for the support and conduct of health-related research. The legislation creating NCMRR was passed by Congress in the fall of 1990, which, significantly, was the same congressional session in which the Americans with Disabilities Act became law. Creation of the center corrected the long-standing anomaly that, though rehabilitation-related research was being sponsored by many of the institutes and centers composing NIH, no organizational focus existed for the support and planning of that research.

The task of developing a long-range plan for NCMRR was undertaken by the National Advisory Board for Medical Rehabilitation Research, which was established by the same legislation that created NCMRR. The result of a 2-year effort, the *Research Plan for the National Center for Medical Rehabilitation Research* (National Institutes of Health, 1993), emphasized the importance of the center in supporting research in seven topical areas:

1. Improving mobility
2. Enhancing behavioral adaptation to disability
3. Understanding the body's responses to disabling conditions from an integrative standpoint
4. Developing new assistive technology to improve useful functioning
5. Improving measurement tools to assess the consequences of irreversible physical impairments
6. Evaluating the effectiveness of medical rehabilitation practices
7. Training medical rehabilitation scientists

Because the plan was intended to provide a sense of direction and not a detailed road map, each area was formulated very broadly. Subsequent efforts to explicate those areas more concretely used an approach characteristic of NIH. A conference or workshop is conducted in which internationally acknowledged experts develop recommendations for needed research initiatives. Those recommendations are disseminated widely by means of reports, journal articles, and edited volumes in an effort to stimulate investigators to undertake the relevant research. The recommendations also may be drawn upon by organizational components of NIH in formulating solicitations for grant applications.

In August 1994, a conference was conducted to develop research recommendations pertinent to the emphasis area of evaluating the effectiveness of medical rehabilitation practices. Organized by NCMRR and cosponsored with the Agency for Health Care Policy and Research, the conference was entitled "An Agenda for Medical Rehabilitation Outcomes Research." The invited presenters were individuals who have contributed importantly to medical rehabilitation outcomes research and who represented the spectrum of disciplines that collaborate in the conduct of medical rehabilitation services and research. Other participants represented federal agencies interested in medical rehabilitation services or research, professional organizations whose memberships provide rehabilitation services, voluntary health organizations that are advocates for the recipients of medical rehabilitation services, or the membership of the National Advisory Board on Medical Rehabilitation Research.

The format of the 2-day conference called for plenary presentations followed by meetings of working groups charged with developing recommendations for future research. A subset of those recommendations addressing issues that cut across many different disabling conditions was published in three journals with different readerships, all relevant to medical rehabilitation (Fuhrer, 1995). Fulfilling the planning intent of the conference, some of those recommendations later appeared as NCMRR funding priorities in an announcement published in the *NIH Guide for Grants and Contracts* (National Institutes of Health, 1995).

The principal conference speakers and their topics were chosen with this book in mind. The first section of the book (Chapters 1–13) addresses conceptual and methodologic issues with broad applicability to the gamut of interventions and disabling conditions germane to medical rehabilitation. The second section of the book (Chapters 14–18) deals with specific groupings of disabling conditions and with the rehabilitation outcomes research relevant to each of them. The authors were asked to 1) characterize briefly the conditions and applicable rehabilitation practices, 2) summarize available outcomes research bearing on those practices, 3) highlight existing knowledge gaps, and 4) recommend the outcomes research that is needed. Finally, Chapter 19 contains the editor's concluding commentary.

The goal of the book is to promote the astute application of the principles and techniques of outcomes research to assessing the impacts of medical rehabilitation interventions. It is targeted at researchers conducting medical rehabilitation research; medical rehabilitation practitioners, administrators, and payers who want to understand both the promise and the limits of outcomes research; and graduate students preparing for careers as clinicians, administrators, or researchers. Medical rehabilitation professionals are expected to find the book useful as a guide in planning outcomes research or in critiquing the research of others. It also can serve as supplemental reading in graduate courses dealing with rehabilitation program management or research. The numerous disciplines for which the book is relevant include (in cautious alphabetical order) medical social workers, occupational therapists, orthotists, physiatrists and physicians in several other specialities, physical therapists, prosthetists, psychologists, rehabilitation counselors, rehabilitation engineers, rehabilitation nurses, and speech-language therapists, among others.

REFERENCES

Fuhrer, M.J. (1995). Conference report: An agenda for medical rehabilitation outcomes research. *American Journal of Physical Medicine and Rehabilitation, 74,* 243–248; *Journal of Allied Health, 24,* 79–87; *Journal of Prosthetics and Orthotics, 71,* 35–39.

National Institutes of Health. (1993). *Research plan for the National Center for Medical Rehabilitation Research.* Bethesda, MD: National Institute of Child Health and Human Development, National Institutes of Health.

National Institutes of Health. (1995). *NIH Guide for Grants and Contracts, 24,* 1101–1120. Bethesda, MD: NIH Guide Printing and Reproduction Branch.

*With deep appreciation
to the staff of
The Institute for Rehabilitation and Research (TIRR),
who taught me what medical rehabilitation means,
one patient at a time*

Assessing Medical Rehabilitation Practices

CHAPTER 1

Outcomes Research in Medical Rehabilitation

Foundations from the Past and Directions for the Future

*Mark V. Johnston,
Margaret Stineman, and Craig A. Velozo*

Rehabilitation has traditionally been defined as the attempt to develop a person "to the fullest physical, psychological, social, vocational, avocational and educational potential consistent with his or her physiological or anatomic impairment and environmental limitations" (DeLisa, Martin, & Currie, 1993, p. 3). Other definitions of rehabilitation emphasize the goal of restoring or improving health or functional abilities through learning or by other means (e.g., DeJong & Sutton, 1995; National Center for Medical Rehabilitation Research, 1993). Such definitions make rehabilitation a concept that incorporates multiple interventions, all of which are designed to improve the independence and quality of life of the patient. By definition, outcomes are central to medical rehabilitation. Nothing, then, can be more essential to research in medical rehabilitation than outcomes research.

Definitions of *rehabilitation outcomes* begin with actual interventions labeled "rehabilitative." "Rehabilitation outcomes may be defined as changes produced by rehabilitative services in the lives of service recipients and their environment" (Fuhrer, 1987, p. 1). *Outcomes research in medical rehabilitation* may be defined as research intended to discover the sustained

This chapter was supported by Grants H133B30041 (Functional Assessment and Evaluation of Rehabilitation Outcomes) and H133B40025 (Medical Rehabilitation and Health Policy) from the National Institute of Disability and Rehabilitation Research and by Grant GR108 from the Henry Kessler Foundation.

impact of rehabilitative strategies and treatments on the everyday lives of persons with severe and lasting disabilities. Outcomes research in medical rehabilitation is motivated both by concern for persons with pathologies and impairments that produce severe and enduring disabilities and by questions about the relative effectiveness and cost-effectiveness of alternative rehabilitation strategies and treatments.

THESES

This chapter reviews past achievements, explains current priorities, and suggests directions for future rehabilitation outcomes research. Medical rehabilitation involves augmenting recovery and readaptation processes. Rehabilitation outcomes research must control for natural recovery and nontreatment factors that affect outcomes. Randomized controlled trials and the stronger types of quasi-experimental research designs are required.

To increase knowledge of the effectiveness of rehabilitation, at least simple or small theoretical bases need to be explicated. Ideally, treatment theories would be so explicit that they could be stated as a treatment protocol or guideline.

Another theme pertains to meaningful outcomes in everyday life. Outcomes research is concerned with the generalization of clinical effects of rehabilitation to the everyday lives of persons with disabilities in the long term. Measures of impairment and pathology are typically necessary to understand the processes by which outcomes are attained, but these technical measures usually are not sufficient to determine whether a worthwhile effect has been induced.

Other points include the need for improved measurement of outcomes, respect for the self-determination of persons with disabilities and appreciation for their experiences, the importance of costs and cost-effectiveness, and prediction and quantitative modeling of recovery curves as a basis for understanding outcomes.

TERMS AND CONCEPTS

Explicating Rehabilitation and Rehabilitation Outcomes

It is valuable to explain more fully what rehabilitation is and the place of outcomes research because there is recurrent controversy and confusion on these matters. Figure 1 presents a simple visual analog of what rehabilitation is and the role of outcomes research. The figure suggests several features of useful outcomes research in medical rehabilitation: Outcomes research attempts to build a bridge between illness and acute medical interventions and long-term improvements in the lives of persons served as they reenter the community.

Rehabilitation and the study of its outcomes begin with acute illness, impairment, and pathology. At the community level, rehabilitation rests on

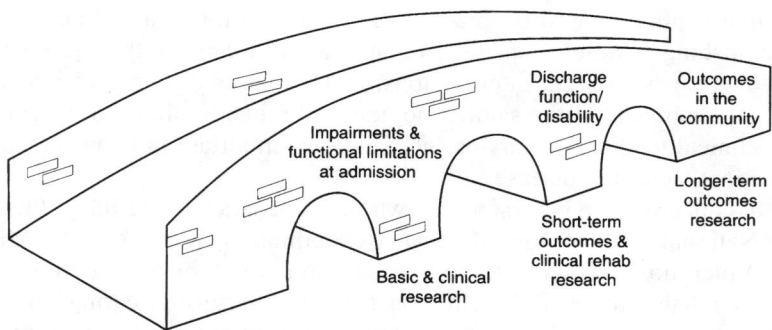

Figure 1. A simple view of rehabilitation: A bridge to a better life.

the art of caring for and maintaining the person in a state of maximal independence and quality of life. It depends largely on augmenting natural healing and adaptation processes. The chasm between the acute illness and the long-term outcome in the community is typically too wide to be spanned without an intermediate foundation; intermediate measures are essential. Basic, clinical, and long-term research on outcomes in the community are all needed.

Definitions of *rehabilitation* are indistinct in that they do not specify any particular content. It is possible to add some substance to the definitions of medical or health-related rehabilitation to a limited degree. *Medical rehabilitation* traditionally concerns severe, long-enduring, or even permanent impairment and disability. *Health-related rehabilitation,* which is the subject of this chapter, concentrates on physical and neurologic disability, usually due to severe accident or disease. Psychiatric rehabilitation and mental health problems, though not our main focus, are also relevant.

Rehabilitation commonly deals with complex cases with multiple comorbidities and complications rather than with single, pure pathologies. Medical rehabilitation is unique in its concern with how to treat such patients with multiple conditions. Many patients with diseases that used to be fatal (e.g., severe spinal cord injury [SCI], acquired brain injury) now survive to enter rehabilitation. As survival improves without full restoration of function, new diseases challenge rehabilitation (e.g., cancer, acquired immunodeficiency syndrome). The rehabilitation literature has not emphasized extension of life per se, but improvement in patient independence and the quality of everyday life.

Improving the functional independence of patients in everyday activities has long been a hallmark of rehabilitation. Medical rehabilitation programs explicitly aim to improve patients' mobility, independence in self-care, ability to communicate, and ability to live independently and engage in productive activities.

Interventions based on practice (i.e., on learning and exercise) are a distinguishing feature of medical rehabilitation. Learning theory, exercise physiology, psychologic interventions, and social-environmental interventions are involved. At the same time, medical rehabilitation can use any of the technical medical or nursing interventions important in management of the patient's chronic disease.

A concern for the person as a whole has characterized rehabilitation. The National Center for Medical Rehabilitation Research (NCMRR) (1993) plan noted that whole body adaptation is one of the core topics of medical rehabilitation. Rehabilitation creates a nurturing, caring environment, synthesizing medical and psychosocial interventions to augment natural healing and adaptation processes. Besides, even with these further descriptors, the field has no essential, unique content in a singular type of treatment (e.g., surgery) or a single class of diseases or organ systems (e.g., neurology). Rather, health-related rehabilitation is eclectic in its content. It is the orchestration of multiple interventions to achieve an improved everyday life for the patient. Outcomes remain essential as the key integrating locus of the field.

Outcomes Research in the History of Medical Care

The history of medicine contains many examples of new treatments being tried and of progress occurring only after the outcomes were carefully measured and compared with alternative interventions (Bender, 1961). The history of medicine also contains numerous examples of advances driven by epidemiologic data, that is, by observations of outcomes subsequently linked to antecedent treatments or events.

Semmelweiss, the 19th-century Viennese physician, studied records of outcomes (mortality) following childbirth and found that women assisted by midwives had a lower mortality rate than did women in a physician-controlled hospital ward. He conducted clinical studies comparing outcomes after altering clinical procedures: hand washing and antiseptic techniques (Bender, 1961). He also conducted basic research to identify underlying causal processes: The pathogen associated with childbirth fever was the same as that found in the cadavers that physicians examined before attending to birth. This story has several lessons:

- Productive medical research involves an interplay between outcomes data and changes in clinical treatment and also between basic research and applied research. It links outcomes to treatment processes and biologic processes. The path to improved treatments may begin, not in the laboratory, but with outcomes data. At the same time, laboratory and more controlled research are essential to develop an understanding of the basic causal processes involved.

- Outcomes research, today as in Semmelweiss's era, rests on a comparative clinical data system. One must do more than record outcomes; one must attempt to link variations in outcomes to variations in treatments.
- Outcomes research is a slow process. It took Semmelweiss most of his lifetime to complete his research. Since the early 1970s Wennberg has studied small area variations in outcomes, and since the mid-1980s he has studied benign prostatic hypertrophy alone (e.g., Barry, Fowler, Mulley, Henderson, & Wennberg, 1995; Wennberg, 1990). Single outcomes studies commonly take years.
- Just as Semmelweiss was opposed by the powers that be, the outcomes researcher today faces recurrent political barriers. Outcomes studies can be worth the time, struggle, and expense, though, because they can direct major improvements to the health care system.

Several changes in approach are needed to apply analogies from the history of medicine to outcomes research today.

- Although relevant, mortality is typically no longer the primary outcome. Primary outcomes of medical rehabilitation are at the level of morbidity, function, or quality of life.
- Single-point outcomes are typically insufficient in the study of ongoing disability and disease. A person's activities can fluctuate from day to day, and level of function in the clinic commonly does not translate fully to the real world. Outcomes need to be measured at several points over time.
- When comparing outcomes, researchers must refine patient groupings and account for case severity.
- Measures of both biologic function (i.e., pathology and impairment) and personal outcomes (i.e., disability or handicap) are needed to understand outcomes.
- Processes in health-related rehabilitation are typically complex; they involve the orchestration of multiple medical and nursing interventions as well as learning- and practice-based therapies and social-environmental interventions.

PAST OUTCOMES RESEARCH

Efficacy and Effectiveness Research

Controlled studies of treatment efficacy, such as randomized clinical trials (RCTs), are essential to establish and test causal relationships. Medical rehabilitation needs well-controlled research involving highly similar or equivalent control groups, that is, efficacy research. Efficacy research is urgently needed because the efficacy of many common rehabilitative interventions has never been clearly determined. This statement may apply to the majority of interventions currently applied in medical rehabilitation. The NCMRR is charged with encouraging research on the efficacy of rehabilitative interventions.

One of the insights from outcomes research in medical care as a whole is the realization that treatment effectiveness in real-world settings can differ substantially from the efficacy reported in controlled studies. Clinical trials are typically conducted on highly selected patients by better-than-average clinicians in university hospitals. The results of such studies may or may not generalize to outcomes experienced by persons with a disability receiving rehabilitation in the general population. Studies of effectiveness in practice are essential to determine whether theoretically efficacious interventions work in practice.

Outcomes researchers have documented substantial variations in the intensity and type of general medical care that are uncorrelated with population morbidity or mortality (Wennberg, 1990). A classic example is Wennberg's comparison of Boston to New Haven, Connecticut, a demographically similar city. Expenditures for inpatient medical care in Boston were found to be twice those of New Haven, but no significant differences in population morbidity or mortality could be found. Variations in intensity of treatment have repeatedly been found to correlate with the availability of hospital beds, specialists, and other treatment resources. The services that persons with disabling conditions receive are highly affected, and can even be controlled, by economic factors. The costs of treatments being studied need to be considered in planning rehabilitation research.

Medical rehabilitation needs research on the effectiveness of the interventions commonly applied to the variety of patients seen in medical rehabilitation programs. Effectiveness research is especially needed in the study of therapies based on learning and practice because the skills of therapists, the dynamics of teams, and the response of patients may differ substantially across programs (e.g., Strasser, Falconer, & Martino-Saltzmann, 1994); thus, results in practice may not resemble those reported in controlled studies. Rehabilitation is accepted as a standard of care throughout most of the United States, making randomized studies involving denial of rehabilitative treatment unethical or infeasible. There are, however, substantial variations in rehabilitative practices across regions of the country and across insurance or payment systems. Therefore, studies comparing the outcomes of similar patients who receive different rehabilitative interventions are possible. Such studies may provide information about which rehabilitative interventions are most effective and cost-effective in practice.

Rehabilitation Outcomes Research

There is a modest body of literature on rehabilitation outcomes. Future research on rehabilitation outcomes will need to have a scholarly grounding; otherwise, it is all too likely that errors of the past will recur or questions that have already been substantially investigated will be revisited.

In brief, rehabilitation outcomes research has seen many case studies and many quantitative descriptive studies. There have been many low-power studies that need replication with adequate sample sizes (Ottenbacher, 1995). There have been many studies of predictive factors or prognosis in major diagnostic groups such as stroke (Johnston, Kirshblum, Zorowitz, & Shiflett, 1992), spinal cord injury (Stover, DeLisa, & Whiteneck, 1995), and other diagnostic groups (e.g., Evans, Baskin, & Yatsu, 1992).

The program evaluation requirement of CARF . . . The Rehabilitation Accreditation Commission has led rehabilitation facilities throughout the United States to collect data on their outcomes since the mid-1970s. This widespread effort has resulted in publications on average expectancies for functional gain in hospital-based rehabilitation (Granger, Ottenbacher, & Fiedler, 1995). That patients routinely and substantially improve in medical rehabilitation hospitals and units has been documented repeatedly. Some work also has been done on determinants of continued improvement or deterioration following discharge and over the long term (e.g., Heinemann, Hamilton, Linacre, Wright, & Granger, 1995; Johnston, Kirshblum, et al., 1992).

However, a close reading of reports on average functional gain reveals that there is great individual variation. Some rehabilitation patients improve enormously; others deteriorate. Moreover, all of this effort to routinely monitor rehabilitation program outcomes has led to little insight into treatment effectiveness or quality improvement. There are several reasons for this. Specific treatments have not been well defined or measured. Improvement has been seen as the result of efforts of a whole team whose interventions were so complex that they cannot be separately identified, but rather must be treated as holistic and uniquely individualized. Mass databases typically have not contained the depth of measurement necessary to clearly understand improvement in any single patient group. The databases and their reports have been based on similar programs (e.g., exempt rehabilitation hospitals), not similar patient groups. Knowledge of treatment effectiveness can be gained only by comparing the outcomes of similar patients who received differing treatments. When treatments or programs are similar, variations in outcomes are most plausibly attributable only to variation in patients selected for admission.

Large longitudinal studies of rehabilitation outcomes have been supported for many years. Prominent examples include the SCI Model Systems Database (Stover et al., 1995), begun in the mid-1970s, and the traumatic brain injury model systems (Dahmer et al., 1993). These longitudinal databases have provided a good amount of knowledge about the recovery that can be expected following a high-quality "system" of acute and rehabilitative medical treatment. Benchmark information on expected improvement, costs, and so forth is available (e.g., Stover et al., 1995). These databases have provided valuable background data for numerous clinical studies. They were set up to demonstrate a "model" system of care. They were not designed to compare the outcomes or effectiveness of major alternative program models. Thus, the yield in terms of knowledge of effectiveness and cost-effectiveness has been modest.

Rehabilitation has developed many clinical theories and approaches that are said to "work" but have never been subject to rigorous scrutiny. It is not known which of these theories and approaches actually produce improvements in patient function or quality of life beyond the effects of natural healing, nor is it known how long these improvements are sustained or for what types of patients. There have been very few well-controlled comparisons of alternative interventions in medical rehabilitation. There has been a reluctance to engage in any comparative, controlled experimental research. Arguments have been made, for instance, that rehabilitation uniquely requires qualitative and ideographic approaches. Many other fields of biomedical research, however, also face enormous qualitative complexities. The chief need in rehabilitation outcomes research is for application of established research methods, especially more rigorously controlled research designs. At the same time, rehabilitation has distinctive populations, interventions, and likely treatment effects to which research designs must be sensitively tailored.

Randomized Clinical Trials in Rehabilitation

Few RCTs have been done in rehabilitation (e.g., Johnston & Granger, 1994; Ottenbacher, 1995; Post-Stroke Rehabilitation Guideline Panel, 1995). This scarcity may reflect in part the general paucity of funding for rehabilitation research. Another factor is that rehabilitation funding agencies have not specified that research designs with control groups are required to obtain grants. More broadly, there is a fear that rehabilitation is too individualized, too complex, and too poorly understood to submit to RCTs. Although there is certainly a danger that some forms of rehabilitation will prove to be relatively ineffective for some patient groups, past RCTs have in fact demonstrated the success of some forms of rehabilitation. The following are some examples:

- Rubenstein's (Rubenstein et al., 1984) randomized study of a "geriatric evaluation unit" combining acute and rehabilitative interventions clearly demonstrated improved patient function, decreased mortality, and decreased long-term cost compared with alternative but previously standard acute medical care in the Veterans Administration system.
- In a randomized trial of a heterogeneous group of 651 acutely ill older patients, Landefeld and colleagues (1995) found that specific rehabili-

tatively oriented changes in acute hospital care improved patients' performance of basic activities of daily living and reduced the frequency of discharge to long-term care institutions.

- Some RCTs have shown the effectiveness of integrated acute stroke units, which involve a number of rehabilitative interventions, in improving functional outcomes and decreasing mortality (Indredavik et al., 1991; Kalra, Dale, & Crome, 1993; Post-Stroke Rehabilitation Guideline Panel, 1995).

Such studies demonstrate that rehabilitation is or *can be* effective, but that the active ingredient in rehabilitation for different patient configurations remains unclear.

Other RCTs, though not reporting the striking effectiveness of rehabilitation, have provided valuable insights, including the following:

- Garraway and colleagues found that a treatment unit involving a somewhat greater rehabilitative emphasis than a control unit resulted in somewhat better functional outcomes at discharge (Garraway, Akhtar, Prescott, & Hockey, 1980); the effect, however, had dissipated by the 1-year follow-up (Garraway, Akhtar, Hockey, & Prescott, 1980).
- Reuben's randomized study, unlike studies that involved more intensive changes in the provision of treatment and follow-up, found no significant effects of comprehensive geriatric assessment by a team of consultants (Reuben et al., 1995).
- Falconer's RCT of inpatient stroke rehabilitation showed that implementation of a particular critical path had no discernible effect on functional or cost outcomes; patient satisfaction, however, was slightly better under traditional care (Falconer, Roth, Sutin, Strasser, & Chang, 1994). One explanation for this finding is that flexibility is needed to tailor rehabilitation to the needs of individuals. Another is that rehabilitation is complex, and initial attempts to explicate or mechanize its processes may not improve the tacit skill of rehabilitation clinicians.

The work of Tinetti and colleagues on falls among older adults provides an example of what productive outcomes research on complex functional problems involves: research on predictive factors (Inouye et al., 1993), highly controlled studies of multifactorial interventions among selected high-risk individuals (Tinetti et al., 1994), and meta-analyses of the literature to obtain an overview (Province et al., 1995).

Beckerman located 400 RCTs relevant to physical therapy in the world literature (Beckerman, Bouter, van der Heijden, de Bie, & Koes, 1993). Although a number of RCTs reported that physical therapy, manipulation, or other interventions were effective for certain conditions, the overall effectiveness of physical therapy was unclear because of methodologic flaws such as small sample sizes and measurement limitations. There are fewer RCTs in occupational therapy and speech-language pathology. The point is neither to doubt nor to affirm the effectiveness of the disciplines involved in rehabilitation. The point is that rehabilitation needs more well-controlled studies to identify highly effective interventions and to distinguish them from ineffective or wasteful efforts.

LINKING PROCESSES AND OUTCOMES

The ultimate aim of outcomes research is to link outcomes to treatment processes so that we can improve the effectiveness of treatment. To do this, research needs to go beyond "black box" models of rehabilitation to explicate key elements of the rehabilitation treatment process. Such research needs to be based on well-grounded theories (i.e., systems of interrelated, carefully considered ideas) regarding recovery, treatment, and community integration processes.

The basis of medical rehabilitation is augmenting natural recovery and, for congenital disabilities, natural growth processes. Recovery is affected by experience, exercise, adequacy of nursing, competency of medical management, and specialized interventions. Recovery may be based on biologic factors and interventions, but psychosocial interventions can also be cost-effective or necessary to enhance adaptation and quality of life. The loving support of family, attendant care, and continuing nursing care are also essential to long-term outcomes in rehabilitation.

Traditional Views of Rehabilitation

Rehabilitation has been described as comprehensive and holistic, a weaving together of many specific interventions (Arokiasamy, 1993; DeLisa et al., 1993). This view is advantageous and sound in that it acknowledges the complexity of rehabilitation and avoids oversimplification and premature specification of what works. The view is also caring, humanistic, flexible, and interdisciplinary. Rehabilitation begins as an ethical commitment that affirms the value of persons with disabilities; its essence can be defined as a blending of caring with elements of science or technique (Arokiasamy, 1993). The holistic approach is vague and often leads to disclaiming the possibility of finding anything in particular that clearly works. Holistic views are a starting place for rehabilitation outcomes research, but people in the field need to elaborate on them to progress.

A Schema for Understanding Outcomes

Rehabilitation outcomes are multiply determined. Outcomes have been associated with both biologic factors and personal and social factors such as the person's strengths, motivations, continuing care, and various environmental factors. The recovery of persons with severe injuries and illnesses is surely due both to the effects of specialized, intensive interventions and to the healing that occurs naturally in unspecialized but warm and caring environments.

The World Health Organization's (WHO's; 1980) taxonomy of impairment, disability, and handicap has become the basis for organizing the complexity of factors associated with health outcomes. A number of works have been devoted to extending the WHO taxonomy (Heerkens, Brandsma, Lakerveld-Hyl, & van Ravensberg, 1994; NCMRR, 1993; Ueda, 1994; Whiteneck, 1992). Figures 2(a) and 2(b) present simplified causal models that can be a useful beginning in understanding rehabilitation outcomes. The figures are not meant to provide causal paths for every circumstance or sample; that is the purpose of controlled research.

Figure 2(a) introduces the following few basic considerations:

- Biologic factors (i.e., structural and functional impairments, cellular or molecular pathology, disease) are essential starting points for health-related rehabilitation research. They are, with some exceptions, powerful factors for determining functional limitations and the experience

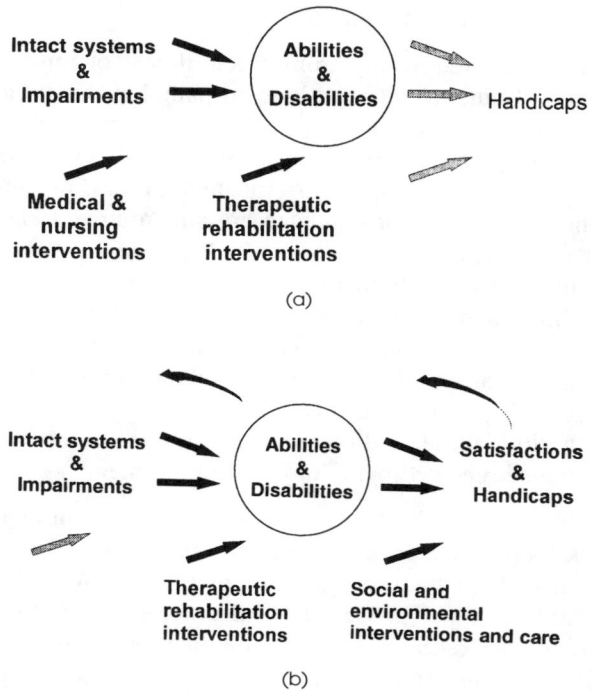

(a)

(b)

Figure 2. Simplistic model of causal relationships: (a) in the physiologic recovery phase after injury or disease onset; (b) over the long term, including readaptation in the community.

of illness. However, pathologies and impairments are not the only factors that typically need to be measured, and they do not necessarily determine the most important or ultimate outcomes, which are at the level of handicap and life satisfaction.

- Disability depends not only on diseases or impairments but also on intact organ systems. For instance, persons with severe musculoskeletal impairments are likely to be more mobile if they have intact cardiovascular systems and are otherwise well conditioned; conversely, general poor conditioning could further reduce the mobility of such persons.
- Handicap, or social disadvantage, depends not only on disability but also on the person's strengths and on the physical, and especially the social, environment.

The last two points are analytic underpinnings of the epigraph "Ask not what disease the person has but rather what person the disease has" (Sachs, 1995).

The most critical processes in the short run during acute and subacute rehabilitation may frequently differ from powerful processes in the long term or in the community (Figure 2[b]).

- When persons are recovering from a new illness or injury, the impact of medical and nursing interventions on pathology or impairment is a key issue. Measures of pathology, impairment, and linked functional limitations are typically most critical. Social and environmental variations are limited while persons are inpatients in an institution. During institutional care, issues of handicap are still routinely encountered in discharge planning.
- In the long term after discharge from inpatient rehabilitation (Figure 2[b]), disability and handicap measures become increasingly pertinent and immediate. Handicap and actual activities become the basic domain for outcomes measures. Social, family, and environmental variation assume increasing prominence. Insufficient or inappropriate care, family breakdown, drug abuse, and other social and environmental factors can and do produce renewed pathology and impairment.

The relationship between biologic and social factors is ultimately a complex feedback loop rather than a unidimensional arrow of causation.

As shown in both figures, measures of the functional limitations or broader disabilities of patients are typically necessary and central in rehabilitation outcomes research. Another implication of the schema underlying both figures is the idea that outcomes research spans the gap between the biologic factors and personal-social factors. Input measures in rehabilitation outcomes research are ideally at the level of pathology or disease stage or severity. The output measure is at the level of disability, handicap, or the quality of everyday living. Rehabilitation outcomes research will benefit from better measurement and modeling of pathologies and impairments and their severity and of social, environmental, and psychologic factors that affect handicap and subjective well-being.

There are advocates of approaches that derogate the importance of physiologic processes and that treat disability as merely a label without basis and treat rehabilitation as a mere placebo undistinguished from other forms of care. These attitudes seem likely to hamper progress and obscure understanding. Likewise, dogmatic beliefs in total biologic determinism will also hamper rehabilitation outcomes research, as measures of pathology or impairment are often poorly coupled with quality of life, and non-biologic factors are clearly linked with such ultimate outcomes (e.g., Adler, Boyce, Chesney, Folkman, & Syme, 1993; Fuhrer, 1994; Ueda, 1994; Whiteneck, 1992).

Family-oriented interventions; many basically educational interventions; adaptive equipment; orthotic and prosthetic devices; and many, perhaps most, therapeutic interventions logically depend on functional or social-environmental factors, and on diagnosis only secondarily. In many rehabilitation studies, diagnosis may be more profitably treated as a categorical moderating variable rather than as the end of the sample universe. If medical rehabilitation research can identify interventions or methods of care that effectively and cost-effectively improve the quality of life of persons across a variety of pathologies or impairments, it will achieve a result of enduring value.

Although the authors' approach is based on the WHO framework, it is useful to augment this framework to clarify specific issues in measurement of rehabilitation processes and outcomes. Measures of cellular pathology and disease stage or severity can be essential in understanding medical outcomes. The term *functional limitation,* often used as a synonym for *disability,* is useful to describe restrictions in specific performances, such as drinking from a straw as opposed to feeding as a whole (Johnston, Hall, Carnevale, & Boake, 1996; Johnston, Keith, & Hinderer, 1992). *Social disadvantage* is a useful near-synonym for *handicap* (NCMRR, 1993), and *objective* or *normative handicap* generally needs to be distinguished from the subjective experience of illness (Ueda, 1994), because the two may correlate highly (Fuhrer, 1994). In summary, both biologic processes in the person and social processes in the environment need to be measured to understand rehabilitation outcomes.

Rehabilitation research has typically used either broad outcomes measures, such as living arrangement, handicap, or physical independence as a whole, or narrow ones, such as strength of an extremity, a specially constructed description of individual behavior, or even range of motion.

The use of broad measures, common in program evaluation systems, risks overstating the generality of effects of rehabilitation interventions. Studies using narrow measures have demonstrated proximal effects but beg the question of whether results generalize to typical patients seen in rehabilitation, are sustained in the long term, or are of sufficient magnitude to justify the expense (cognitive remediation being an example [Ben-Yishay & Diller, 1993]). Rehabilitation outcomes research ideally should assess both proximal short-term outcomes and more general long-term outcomes to trace the causal paths by which outcomes valuable to patients are attained.

Well-Grounded Theory of Recovery and Rehabilitative Interventions

Much rehabilitation outcomes research in the past has been "black box" research (Figure 3, top): Input and outcomes are measured, but what happens in rehabilitation is vaguely defined or even a mystery. Outcomes research in medical rehabilitation needs to open the black box; that is, it needs to articulate a clear theory or model of treatment and test it. Intervening variables, shorter-term effects, and long-term outcomes all need to be assessed (Figure 3, bottom).

Theoretical Bases By *theory* we mean at least a small set of interconnected ideas based on a synthesis of the best-established knowledge. The theory should make specific predictions about the effects of interventions. Often what is needed are fairly prosaic statements and hypotheses about how the rehabilitation program works and how patient problems are generated and prioritized (Glueckauf, 1990).

Items that need to be defined explicitly in even a small or minimal treatment theory include the following (Lipsey, 1990):

1. The problem, its etiology (if possible), its magnitude, and in what persons it occurs
2. The treatment in terms of what are presumed to be specific effect ingredients, including a concept of strength of treatment, and the minimal regime necessary to deliver that treatment at effective strength
3. The mechanisms by which the treatment is supposed to have its effects, including mediating variables or steps between the initial application of the treatment and its longer-term effects
4. The likely desired outcomes, including the minimal magnitude of effect necessary, the maximal magnitude possible, and the time at which effects are likely to occur

Case severity or case selection methods, treatment application, and outcomes need to be explicated with sufficient clarity so that they can be operationalized and measured. To connect rehabilitative treatments to out-

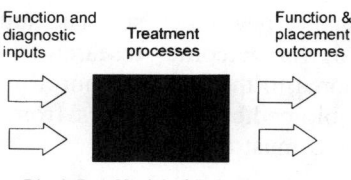

Black Box Model of Rehabilitation

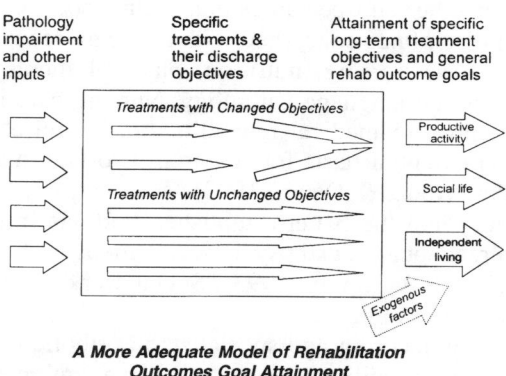

A More Adequate Model of Rehabilitation
Outcomes Goal Attainment

Figure 3. Simple schema for understanding rehabilitation outcomes: The black box and an attempt to open it.

comes, long-term treatment objectives need to be specified, usually in terms of specific aspects of patient function or everyday life. Because panaceas are unlikely, the boundaries of the theory or treatment effect need to be delineated. In general, knowing why the treatment should work implies a connection to established or highly plausible biologic, behavioral, or social processes.

The most plausible alternative explanations to a treatment effect need to be examined logically and tested in research. Well-established or obvious recovery and care processes, not to mention methodologic biases, particularly need to be excluded as explanations for an effect to demonstrate the occurrence of a new process. For instance, claims of an extraordinary new treatment process that is based on weakly controlled research that does not exclude spontaneous recovery or compensatory learning as explanations are unconvincing. Even well-designed correlational or matching studies are likely to lack the degree of control necessary to establish new healing processes and to exclude simpler counterexplanations. Tightly controlled experiments are needed to conclusively establish the efficacy of new treatments or the existence of new processes. The authors argue for a conservative theoretical basis for outcomes research in which the degree of conservatism is proportional to the lack of control in the research.

The following are biomedical disciplines from which rehabilitation outcomes research can and must draw:

- Medical specialties most directly relevant to the pathologies or impairment in question, such as physiatry, neurology, orthopedics, cardiology, internal medicine, psychiatry, pharmacology, rheumatology, urology, or any number of other subspecialties and their associated findings.
- Allied health disciplines concerned with fostering recovery and healing processes, such as nursing, nutrition, physical therapy, occupational therapy, and speech-language pathology. Nursing care is surely fundamental and central to medical rehabilitation. Exercise physiology, for instance, is an essential basis for research involving muscular exercise (Joynt, Findley, Boda, & Daum, 1993).
- Learning theory and the better-established findings in psychology and sociology on readaptation and psychosocial support (Arokiasamy, 1993; Keith, 1995; Keith & Lipsey, 1993). Social work, sociology, and economics are also relevant.
- Rehabilitation engineering and specialists in orthotic devices, prosthetics, environmental modifications, and adaptive equipment

Rehabilitation is also concerned with community reintegration and long-term care in the community. Rehabilitation needs to assess the adequacy of long-term maintenance support. Simple care processes and family training are essential concerns.

There are many controversies in research on basic rehabilitative processes (Fuhrer, 1995; NCMRR, 1993), including the following:

- How do experience and training interact with neural plasticity and enhance recovery from neurotrauma (Bach-y-Rita, 1990)? Do current rehabilitative processes optimize recovery from neurologic injury (Dobkin, 1993)?
- How does rehabilitation enhance whole body system recovery and adaptation from severe or multiple impairments?
- Perhaps the most general question is, What healing and recovery processes can we augment, and on what does rehabilitation have little effect?

Laboratory research and highly controlled randomized experiments are needed to answer questions involving the basic underlying healing processes and the efficacy of treatments.

Although some rehabilitative processes have a relatively rapid effect (e.g., provision of simple adaptive equipment), typical rehabilitative processes take time and involve healing, practice, and activity by the patient, who must be personally involved and motivated. Rehabilitation outcomes research should draw from both biomedical and social-psychological disciplines, especially those dealing with chronic disease management, neurophysiologic recovery, and readaptation processes. Rehabilitation outcomes research faces the challenge of integrating findings from basic research and multiple disciplines to understand their long-term impact on the lives of persons served.

Levels of Certainty Rehabilitation needs to find a middle path between total questioning of all rehabilitation, as expressed by some scientists and skeptics, and the common refusal to question anything (or at least anything established or profitable). Statements such as "Rehab has no scientific basis" are only partially true. Many common practices in health care as a whole also have never been proved to be efficacious in RCTs (Office of Technology Assessment, 1978), but it would be false to state without qualification that medicine has no scientific basis.

Rehabilitation needs to discriminate at least three classes of theories or intervention processes:

1. *Interventions already known to work, or that are so likely to be effective that testing is not a priority.* For example, it is already known that the recovery of persons with severe impairments and disabilities requires a degree of loving care, nutritional support, skin care, movement to lessen contractures, and other basic care. Similarly, research is not needed to investigate whether activity diminishes deconditioning following bed rest or whether wheelchairs and lower-extremity orthoses improve mobility. (Questions at a more detailed level—of grading activities and equipment to different types of patients—remain.)

2. *Important priority controversies for which evidence is mixed.* With processes that basically work, the important issue is not their basic efficacy but their orchestration to meet the needs of varying patient groups, optimal components, intensity, duration, and other more detailed but practical issues. To establish the efficacy of new and unproved rehabilitative interventions, highly controlled (usually randomized) clinical trials are required. The most valuable outcomes studies are likely to be in this middle category.

3. *Long shots.* Open-mindedness is needed regarding entirely new interventions that initially appear to be inexplicable. At the same time, one needs to be realistic regarding the limited scientific basis of many highly controversial treatments and alternative medicine. Research on the efficacy of radically new interventions would need to be tightly controlled to be valuable. Mere demonstration of improvement with

poor control would not establish the efficacy of otherwise inexplicable new interventions.

If a greater degree of consensus can be reached regarding what works in rehabilitation, as opposed to what is controversial and what is a long shot, research efforts can be focused, and rehabilitation, historically a slowly progressing field, can begin to make more rapid progress.

Hierarchical Levels of Theory

Rehabilitation outcomes research needs to address at least two levels of theory. The more basic, specific level may be called *discipline-related theories.* The more embracing but also more abstract and heterogeneous level may be called *systems-related theories.*

Discipline-Related Theories Examples of relatively specific theories include learning theory, exercise physiology, pharmacology, nutrition, biomechanics, and those of other biomedical disciplines. Rehabilitation draws from these. Methodologies are those familiar to controlled research on medical interventions: the study of pure samples, the use of highly controlled interventions, good measures of proximal effects, and tight experimental control. An example of research involving specific theories might be the effect of an antispasticity drug on muscle impairment in multiple sclerosis. Every disease and every discipline in medical rehabilitation has specific questions that only controlled research can answer.

By its very definition, *rehabilitation* also involves the orchestration of multiple disciplines and interventions to improve patients' everyday lives. This systems-level rehabilitation, broader but less clear than discipline-specific theories, also requires investigation. Systems-level rehabilitation concerns the whole organism, its strengths as well as its impairments; it involves the study of whole body system responses (NCMRR, 1993). Rehabilitation specializes in patients with enduring, severe, or multiple impairments. An example of systems-level research is the comparison of the outcomes of an intensive, short-term acute rehabilitation program with a less intensive but longer-term subacute alternative. Outcomes research in medical rehabilitation considers the total system involving multiple impairments or comorbidities and the response of the whole person. Rehabilitation involves the orchestration of multiple interventions for multiple patient problems. Outcomes research consequently needs to encompass the level of rehabilitation planning and strategy. In view of the vast extent of biomedical and psychosocial literature, an understanding of how to better orchestrate established care and healing processes to improve real-world outcomes is a respectable ambition.

Systems-Related Theories Rehabilitation is typically a multiple-objective process. Initially, the concern is to ameliorate pathology and impairment (e.g., to prevent further progression or recurrence of a stroke, to lessen paralysis or augment motor recovery). Clinical concern later shifts to higher systems levels, such as training the person in compensatory strategies. Adaptive equipment may be prescribed. Finally, efforts are made to train the family or caregivers and to modify the home. Throughout, an effort is made to help the person understand his or her changed self, to enable the person to have pleasant experiences, and to communicate good cheer so that the person continues to feel his or her life is valuable and satisfying. Each of these levels of outcomes, from the biologic to the personal and social, is important. Effective rehabilitation can, in principle, fail to achieve one outcome goal but succeed by shifting to another.

Rehabilitation outcomes research needs to deal with the reality of multifaceted intervention systems and the pressing need to determine how effective and how cost-effective they are. Outcomes research at this systems level would study multiple interventions by a rehabilitation team, methods of orchestrating these interventions, and systems for long-term support, including both paid care and unpaid support and the person as a member of a family. It can study prioritization of interventions, that is, when therapists should switch from restorative to compensatory strategies or from compensatory to maintenance strategies. It should study methods of helping the person adapt to his or her changed self and to prioritize life goals and plans. If outcomes research in medical rehabilitation considers complex, systems-level issues, it will be more relevant to the actual practice of rehabilitation.

Substantive Issues

Rehabilitation is replete with unanswered questions regarding the efficacy and effectiveness of treatments, both common and unusual (Fuhrer, 1995; NCMRR, 1993). Does cognitive remediation generalize to valued everyday life activities? How effective are manual medicine and the many manipulative therapies involving human touch, and for whom? What are the long-term effects of therapies on the growth of children with developmental disabilities? What are optimal intervention systems to enhance mobility? Enhancing the mobility of persons with an ongoing disability typically involves multiple interventions: healing of the impairment, compensatory and strengthening therapy, and adaptive equipment.

Rehabilitation frequently involves care and healing processes that can occur in the absence of highly specialized interventions. In these circumstances, the intensity of care and its optimal degree of specialization become a key issue. A typical question for rehabilitation outcomes research is, How much treatment is optimal to speed healing and maximize functional recovery following severe musculoskeletal trauma? The same question holds following neurotrauma. Whether a therapy has some measurable effect on selected patients may be of substantial theoretical importance but may not be a priority issue for outcomes research; for outcomes research, the robustness and practical value of the effect are priority issues. Similarly, exercise "tolerance" is not exactly the issue; the issue is optimal functional gain relative to cost. Cost has become an unavoidable and prominent issue for any rehabilitative treatment that hopes for practical application.

Sustaining effects over the long term is a key, perhaps *the* key, outcomes issue. The expense of medical rehabilitation cannot be justified by outcomes at discharge, unless the outcome at discharge is known to be sustained. Even improvements in function sustained after discharge are not sufficient evidence in patient groups that naturally improve even in the absence of intensive, specialized rehabilitation. Whether the improvement is sustained over time relative to a control group needs to be tested. Furthermore, reported averages mask extensive variations in individuals' outcomes. There are multiple factors to be understood that effect deterioration for some patients and continued improvement by others.

Treatment Protocols

Controlled studies of defined treatment protocols or guidelines are promising in the study of rehabilitative treatment systems. In basic rehabilitation research, a theory of growth processes might provide new insights. For applied outcomes research, however, insight alone is insufficient. Rather, a treatment theory is needed that is sufficiently specified so that it can be implemented in practice. Treatment theories in rehabilitation, when they are sufficiently developed, should have features similar to practice guidelines.

The 1990s have seen a widespread movement to develop clinical practice guidelines (Field & Lohr, 1990). Hundreds of such practice guidelines, practice parameters, or clinical paths have now been developed, including the first official guideline in rehabilitation (Post-Stroke Rehabilitation Guideline Panel, 1995). Practice guidelines focus on what to do to improve outcomes rather than on the processes responsible for better outcomes. However, guidelines do explicate processes to the point that they greatly constrain theorizing. Outcomes research comparing alternative treatment guidelines or protocols will have an impact on clinical practice.

A key feature of practice guidelines is that they can incorporate a degree of multiplicity of patient problems and a contingently associated set of interventions. Guidelines frequently involve multidisciplinary interventions. This is a substantial advantage for applied rehabilitation research because rehabilitative interventions in practice are typically multidisciplinary approaches to multiple patient problems or problems at multiple levels. In principle, it is possible to test an entire guideline or treatment algorithm, rather than a single pure treatment, against another guideline or against usual care. Such research is needed in rehabilitation.

Clinical practice guidelines for poststroke rehabilitation have been published (Post-Stroke Rehabilitation Guideline Panel, 1995) that describe interventions at multiple levels, including exercise-based interventions, orthoses, education, and family-oriented interventions. The authors noted the slim basis of many recommendations in factual data and the necessity of basing many guidelines on expert opinion. The guidelines have not yet been subject to empirical testing. But even the most complex rehabilitation decision and treatment processes can be explicated to some degree. Having been explicated, it becomes possible to test and improve them. Explicit knowledge will improve the future education of clinicians.

There are difficulties with practice guidelines. A guideline may be suboptimal or even dangerous for certain patients, but exceptions may not be definitely specified in the guideline. A guideline may not be clear. When testing a complex treatment algorithm, there is the risk of lumping together effective and ineffective patient–treatment interactions. However, studies of pure patient groups may produce narrow results that are inapplicable to the majority of patients seen in practice. Rehabilitation outcomes research needs to study defined patient groups, but whether these groups can ever be really pure from a rehabilitative standpoint can be questioned. In summary, outcomes research can be oriented toward greater internal validity (efficacy research) or toward greater generalization (effectiveness research), but both internal validity and generalizability are essential to outcomes research.

The private sector is rapidly implementing guidelines and critical paths that are having a major impact on the practice of rehabilitation. These are largely oriented toward cost savings and rapid patient processing. The effects on patient health and independence are undocumented. However, their impact in rehabilitation probably will be similar to that in psychiatric care: They will constrain treatment toward minimal, short-term objectives (Jellinek & Nurcombe, 1993). Cost-saving guidelines could eliminate long-term rehabilitative strategies that yield small functional gains (e.g., intensive long-term therapy to foster difficult-to-detect restoration of neuromuscular systems in a limb). The study of processes underlying such recovery may still be of theoretical interest; but if the corresponding treatment is highly expensive, results will have virtually no practical impact. Studies of methods of decreasing costs without significantly affecting long-term patient outcomes are urgently needed and will have a real impact on the practice of rehabilitation.

Treatment Objectives and Intermediate Outcomes

To link rehabilitative processes to outcomes, the recovery processes over time need to be traced. Direct or proximal short-term outcomes need to be measured to clearly assess the response to treatment and to understand key aspects of the underlying recovery processes (cf. Whyte, 1994). Long-term outcomes in the community are essential to determine whether treatment effects are sustained and are of sufficient value to justify the expense. At the same time, long-term outcomes in the community are affected by factors that clinical rehabilitation usually cannot control, such as the adequacy of continuing care after discharge, family support, unpredictable medical events, polydrug abuse, and patient choices.

Intermediate outcome measures are a needed support in the long bridge between the treatment and the ultimate outcome. The best intermediate outcome to measure depends on the treatment and the research question. The authors would like to emphasize measurement of *long-term treatment objectives* (Haffey & Johnston, 1989, 1990; Johnston & Wilkerson, 1992). Treatment objectives have two key validity characteristics: 1) logical and empirical linkage to rehabilitative treatments, and 2) validation against socially and individually valued real-world outcomes. They should also be clinically practical, so that clinical professionals can use them in specifying the chief functional results of the treatment. A key practical time for measurement of the achievement of treatment objectives is at or close to termination of treatment.

Ideally, measures of treatment objectives require controlled study to demonstrate that they are indeed connected to the putatively effective treatment. Even in the absence of perfect experimental evidence, however, there is some knowledge of recovery and treatment processes. A credible theoretical basis is an invaluable starting point.

The relationship between the treatment objectives and outcomes valued by patients in the community needs to be understood. Research is needed to establish how much improvement a measure of a functional ability needs to show to be sustained in the community after discharge. The factors that determine whether a functional skill is used or not need to be better understood. Controlled research is needed to clarify the situations and patient attributes that promote long-term growth or at least maintenance of function in the community over the long term.

Treatment objectives may typically be described in terms of what the patient will be able to do upon discharge in rather familiar functional terms (Haffey & Johnston, 1989, 1990; Johnston & Wilkerson, 1992). The following are examples of several systems for measurement of specific disabilities or functional limitations that are promising as measures of treatment objectives:

- To cite an example from brain injury rehabilitation, the Haffey–Johnston Comprehensive Assessment Inventory for Rehabilitation (CAIR) includes both independence in basic adaptive activities of daily living (ADLs) and mobility as well as higher-level household and community skills such as parenting, driving, cooking, shopping, and financial management (Haffey & Johnston, 1989, 1990).

- Treatment objectives in communication also can be expressed relative to functional impairment (e.g., aspects of language) or to achieving success in practical communicative activities (Frattalli, 1992). An example of a real-world performance measure might be a count of the person's frequency of success in purchasing groceries in the market he or she uses or a rating of the quality of the activity (Haffey & Johnston, 1989, 1990). Such treatment objectives are almost certainly responsive to training and experience.
- Some treatment objectives may target a mix of impairments and independent management skills. For instance, bowel and bladder problems involve a mix of continence and independence in self-management. Specification of health self-management objectives would include reduction of the severity of impairment or disease, specific medications or activities, and the objective of achieving reliable self-regulation.
- Musculoskeletal and body movement impairments include general weakness, coordination, balance, endurance, and so forth. Some interventions (e.g., pharmacologic interventions) may directly reduce such impairments. If research shows that a reduction of the impairment of a certain magnitude generally results in sustained increase in the independence of certain patient types, then the reduced impairment may serve as the clinical treatment objective. In other cases, impairment reduction may produce an inconsistent impact on disability. In such cases, a more general measure of the patient's function (e.g., a measure of disability in physical ADLs) may be needed to ascertain whether a useful treatment effect has occurred. Thus, the measure of disability would become the instrument to measure attainment of treatment objectives.
- For many maladaptive social and emotional behaviors, especially behavioral excess syndromes, reduction in counts of frequency and ratings of disruptiveness would be suitable treatment objectives (Haffey & Johnston, 1989, 1990). Measures of psychological syndromes might be outcomes measures for some pharmacologic and psychotherapeutic interventions, provided that their reality and sustained worth in the community have been established.

Developing and validating treatment objectives, as defined here, will require substantial applied research efforts, but the achievement of more cost-effective practice will make the effort worthwhile. Valid long-term treatment objectives may differ from current short-term clinical objectives, because treatment objectives, as defined, require linkage to valued outcomes sustained after discharge. Validation of measures of treatment objectives should also involve improvement relative to a control group rather than improvement per se. Following such research, the worth of the intervention will be known, and long-term follow-up activities can be prioritized. Because of resource constraints, long-term follow-up does not and cannot occur in every case. Research can help practice by specifying when long-term follow-up is most needed and when it is less needed.

There is concern about whether it is possible or desirable to specify concrete treatment objectives in rehabilitation. It is said that rehabilitation is so complex and holistic that specification of processes and their objectives is impossible. An insistence on definite processes and outcomes can lead to a mechanistic inflexibility. Rehabilitation should not lose its holistic sensitivity, flexibility, and care for the individual. Moreover, effects of rehabilitation on the general quality of life and global functional level of patients have been documented. Rehabilitation researchers need to listen to their clinical critics. Rehabilitation in practice is complex—so complex that it can overwhelm research.

At the same time, specification of concrete treatment objectives is hardly inconsistent with quality rehabilitation. Indeed, specification of priority objectives provides focus and organization to the rehabilitation plan for an individual (Haffey & Johnston, 1989; Haffey & Lewis, 1989). Outcomes research that has not specified treatment processes and objectives, although of some value, has frequently had statistically unstable or inconclusive results. Holistic, flexible, and individualized are by themselves pretheoretical and shed little light into the black box. To advance the field, outcomes research needs to clearly specify key aspects of rehabilitative processes and the specifically expected outcomes for common patient problems.

METHODOLOGIES TO INFER EFFECTIVE TREATMENT

Methodologies Needed

Randomized Experiments What medical rehabilitation needs most is rigorous, controlled study of the efficacy and cost-effectiveness of its treatments, with the first priority being RCTs. RCTs are the standard for testing the efficacy of treatment interventions. More than any other research design, the randomized experimental design controls for threats to the validity of inference of treatment effects such as spontaneous recovery or differences in case severity between experimental and control groups. Although there are major difficulties in setting up RCTs in rehabilitation, other fields of health care also experience such difficulties; but they have repeatedly overcome them. Whenever there is no evidence or no clear reason to judge that one rehabilitative intervention is more effective than another, randomized selection is ethical. RCTs also require appropriate measures, clearly defined treatment alternatives, a clear but not necessarily elaborate theoretical basis, and other features discussed later in this chapter. Few RCTs have been done in rehabilitation, but they are not impossible. Past RCTs have provided results that demonstrate the marked effectiveness of certain rehabilitative interventions and the ineffectiveness of others.

Strong Quasi-Experiments Quasi-experimental research designs are potentially very useful alternatives to randomized experiments. However, the technical requirements for truly rigorous quasi-experimental studies are not widely understood. Rigorous quasi-experimental studies are technically more complex than experimental research, and strong quasi-experimental designs are commonly confused with weak ones. Two quasi-experimental designs are especially rigorous and promising: the interrupted time-series design and the regression-discontinuity design (Johnston, Ottenbacher, & Reichardt, 1995).

Both of these research designs are, in practice, two-stage designs. A first-stage study would be needed to test assumptions. In the interrupted time-series design, a prior study is needed to establish the shape of the recovery curve. In the regression-discontinuity design, preliminary work is required to construct a quantitative criterion for choice of treatment. The payoff is that both of these designs can provide rigorous results.

Similar but Nonequivalent Comparison Groups Statistical control studies are commonly employed in outcomes research. Although less rigorous than randomized or strong quasi-experimental research designs, they provide useful information about patient outcomes.

Outcomes research involving a comparison group is potentially much more revealing than research that does not involve any comparison group at all. Nonequivalent comparison group research uses matching or covariance analysis to identify very similar but not equivalent patients. The design hinges on excellent statistical adjustment for case severity and on understanding strong, nontreatment determinants of outcomes and quantifying them. If very similar patients who receive very different treatments can be identified, it may be found that outcomes are highly correlated with variations in treatment but little correlated with residual variations in case severity. In these fortunate circumstances, there may be fairly convincing evidence of a treatment effect (Johnston et al., 1995; Reichardt, 1979). Such correlational techniques are the basic ones used in outcomes research involving large databases.

Pre–Post and Longitudinal Designs Perhaps the most commonly employed research designs in rehabilitation outcomes research have not involved an explicit comparison group at all: Longitudinal research involving measurement of patients is repeated points in time, or simple pre–post, admission–discharge measurement. The rehabilitation literature is replete with such research designs. This research has established much evidence suggesting the effectiveness of rehabilitation. Patients with dismal prognoses have been shown to improve significantly in rehabilitation. With advances in acute medical care, persons with severe injuries, such as severe brain injury or complete tetraplegia, for instance, now survive; with adequate continued care, they can have near-normal life expectancies; and with rehabilitation, they can experience decades of relative independence (DeJong & Sutton, 1995; Stover et al., 1995; Verbrugge, 1984). Pre–post research designs and longitudinal research in rehabilitation have established a formidable fund of knowledge regarding prognosis and predictive factors in rehabilitation.

However, too much research has interpreted correlations (e.g., between rehabilitation admission and patient improvement) as evidence of causation, without searching for plausible alternative causes (e.g., natural recovery processes). It is unusual for correlational research to yield unambiguous evidence of a causal process. The absence of a correlation between treatment and patient outcomes (e.g., between intensity of therapy and functional gain per day in inpatient rehabilitation) may not always imply absence of a treatment effect if variation in treatment is highly limited (e.g., all patients may receive about 3 hours per day of therapy). Without variation in treatment, correlations with outcomes will be zero. Many past studies of rehabilitation outcomes compared only subtle or relatively small variations in treatment strategy or intensity (e.g., Garraway, Akhtar, Prescott, & Hockey, 1980; Heinemann et al., 1995). The effectiveness of rehabilitation may be evident only when substantial variations in treatments are studied across very similar patient groups.

Individual correlational studies typically suffer from major validity threats, but a series of correlational studies can provide convincing evidence of treatment effectiveness, provided that results are congruent and validity threats are heterogeneous across the studies (Cordray, 1990; Johnston, Ottenbacher, & Reichardt, 1995). Reviews of the biomedical literature have repeatedly found that weakly controlled studies commonly report that a treatment is effective; subsequent randomized trials typically have demonstrated that these reports are exaggerated or even mistaken (Freedman, Pisani, Purves, & Adhikari, 1991). Rigorous research is needed to identify the optimal rehabilitative interventions required for different patient groups.

Preparatory Research

Research is needed to prepare for controlled studies of treatment effectiveness. Literature syntheses, descriptive work, measure development, and studies of predictive factors are required.

Literature Syntheses In major outcomes-related research (e.g., studies by the Agency for Health Care Policy and Research), literature syntheses occupy a prominent place. Literature synthesis is prominent in outcomes research because real patient outcomes are determined by more factors than can be investigated in any one study. Furthermore, rehabilitation, like family practice or pediatric medicine, is eclectic. It uses technologies from medicine, pharmacology, nursing, engineering, social work, physical therapy, occupational therapy, speech-language pathology, psychology, and other therapies. *Rehabilitation* itself has even been defined as the orchestration of these technologies. Synthesis of the best available knowledge from the component technologies is fundamental to outcomes research in rehabilitation.

Descriptive Research A first step in any research or science is to describe the phenomena of interest. Description of the frequency and relative severity of problems experienced by patients, interventions applied, and so on is needed to understand rehabilitation and to plan controlled research. Descriptive research identifies areas for future study. Knowledge of the variance of an outcomes measure is needed to estimate the sample size necessary for detecting a given treatment effect. Qualitative research methodologies reveal the complexities of rehabilitation to help avoid oversimplification.

The body of literature describing rehabilitative processes and outcomes, however, is already large. Descriptive studies by definition lack control groups. Many quantitative methodologies lack validated measures or definite methods of discriminating more desirable from less desirable outcomes. Although there may be exceptions, it is hard to see how even more descriptive research can advance the field.

Measure Development Like any scientific endeavor, outcomes research depends on the quality of its measurement tools and the field's understanding of them. Progress has been slow but substantial since the 1960s, with the development of many instruments useful in medical rehabilitation outcomes research. Outcomes researchers now have several hundred fairly well-developed measures or indices of health status to use in their research (Cole, Finch, Gowland, & Mayo, 1994; Lohr, 1992; McDowell & Newell, 1996; Spilker, 1990; Stewart & Ware, 1992; Wade, 1991).

Nagi (1991) and Wood (WHO, 1980) attempted to provide a framework for the profusion of measures and domains relevant to health status assessment. An orderly understanding of these measures can be based on the WHO's (1980) concepts of impairment, disability, and handicap, augmented by concepts such as pathology and the subjective experience of illness or personal well-being.

Rehabilitation has contributed substantially to this larger movement (e.g., Fuhrer, 1987; Granger et al., 1996; Johnston, Keith, & Hinderer, 1992; McDowell & Newell, 1996; Spilker, 1990). The emphasis in rehabilitation has been on largely physical ADLs and mobility. The Functional Independence Measure (FIM) (State University of New York at Buffalo, 1993) has emerged as the most widely used outcomes measure in U.S. rehabilitation facilities (Granger et al., 1995). As a whole, the FIM has been demonstrated to be highly reliable (Hamilton, Laughlin, Fiedler, & Granger, 1994). Substantial progress also has been made in other domains important to rehabilitation (e.g., neuropsychology). Research in the field has seen large numbers of unique, poorly developed measures. The increased recognition that face validity alone is an insufficient basis for assessment in rehabilitation led to publication of *Measurement Standards for Interdisciplinary Medical Rehabilitation* (Johnston, Keith, & Hinderer, 1992).

Long-standing, continuing problems in rehabilitation outcomes measurement include the following:

- Ceiling and floor artifacts. Most existing instruments measure function over a limited range (Velozo, Magalhaus, Pan, & Leiter, 1995). Common measures of independence in ADLs, for instance, do not measure the small changes in functioning important in various minimally responsive states or variations in need of skilled nursing care, nor do they measure high-level improvements in function important for household management, community mobility, or vocational productivity. Outcomes research needs measures that work across settings and over the entire spectrum of recovery, from acute medical instability to community integration.
- The need to expand the domain of measurement beyond physical ADLs and mobility to include cognition, instrumental ADLs, social life, work capacity, emotion, life satisfaction, and individual differences in valuation of outcomes.
- Rater biases.
- Losses to follow-up.
- Measures that do not clearly distinguish capacity from performance, or need from actual care received. The standard for outcomes measurement has been that actual performance, rather than judged ability, be assessed. Although this standard remains justifiable as a priority, it is essential to distinguish ability from performance in many extremely important circumstances (e.g., in disability assessment for Social Security benefits, to decide whether a person needs more supervision or daily attendant care).
- Confusion in the term *handicap,* which has multiple component attributes (Johnston et al., 1996). The term is most closely related to problems in normative social role performance, but roles are complex and heterogeneous and reflect cultural expectancies that can be questioned

(e.g., age and gender stereotypes). Norms are unclear, changing, and multiethnic in the United States. *Handicap* also contains the idea of disadvantage, and perceived disadvantage is individualized.

- A lack of systematic research on methods of optimal patient involvement and empowerment. Little research has been done to develop reliable means of eliciting differences in individual patients' preferences or the value of alternative feasible outcomes and how these optimally change over time. Patient involvement is more than a theoretical problem in rehabilitation; therapy optimally begins by asking the patient what he or she wants.

Glueckauf (1993) noted that the primary problem with current assessment methods in rehabilitation is the "failure to meet fundamental scientific standards for utility in practice"; assessment techniques in rehabilitation should not only measure a target domain but also suggest factors that influence the behavior or domain and "lead to a specific plan of treatment" (pp. 135–136). Although these problems are long-standing, substantial progress can be made in the near future:

- Rasch analysis should help in the development of additive-conjoint measures of function that are more nearly equal interval, more unidimensional, and span a greater range of function (Fisher, Harvey, Taylor, Kilgore, & Kelly, 1995; Velozo et al., 1995). Rasch analysis might be described as the next step beyond factor analysis. The technique clearly reveals ceiling and floor problems. Scales developed by Rasch analysis can be briefer than those developed by traditional true score models. More brevity, if possible without reducing reliability, can greatly enhance the practical utility of functional measurement. At the same time, there are circumstances where traditional methods, such as factor analysis, remain useful (Smith, 1996).

- With sufficient concurrent validity data, it may be possible to develop true "gold standards" for measures (Fisher et al., 1995). Measures of a functional domain can become so well understood that it may be possible to reliably and quantitatively translate between one measurement tool and another, leading to communication in terms of levels of domains of human function, such as physical ADLs, rather than in terms of the particular tool used.

- Certain measures from general health outcomes research should be applicable to rehabilitation populations. The applicability of these instruments and their limitations when applied to patient groups served in rehabilitation will be understood with further research.

- Several studies are underway to develop improved measures of disability and handicap, of cognitive and communicative disability, of family support, and of other outcomes domains important to rehabilitation. Continuation of these efforts is necessary to advance the field of rehabilitation.

The development of improved measures of general impairments, certain kinds of disabilities, and aspects of handicap (i.e., determinants of social disadvantage) deserves continued effort. The existing indicators, although they have limitations, should be sufficient to characterize the outcomes of many aspects of medical rehabilitation, particularly of physical disability in ADLs and mobility. The necessity for improved measures need not delay controlled study of the effectiveness of many kinds of rehabilitation interventions.

Prediction of Outcomes   The understanding of predictive relationships, or prognosis, is basic to outcomes research. Information on prognosis is also of substantial importance in clinical case management and forms the basis for severity adjustment in outcomes research. Information on predictive relationships is the basis for blocking to increase the power in experimental outcomes research.

Knowledge of robust, independent predictive relationships yields valuable clues regarding likely causes. Evidence of an unexpected degree of improvement following an intervention may suggest that the intervention was effective, but it does not prove this. Too much past research in rehabilitation (and other fields) has claimed that outcomes *after* an intervention are outcomes *because* of the intervention. Such claims should not be treated as acceptable in rehabilitation research. As a rule, the result of longitudinal and pre–post research designs is not knowledge of causation but knowledge of prognosis.

If the accuracy of prediction is very high and well established, more effective rehabilitation can be inferred in principle if conspicuous deviations from the expected outcomes repeatedly occur. Such accuracy of prediction or such extreme deviations are rare, however, in health care.

A substantial amount of research has already been done on predictors of outcomes for major diagnostic groups seen in rehabilitation such as stroke, spinal cord injury, and acquired brain injury (Dikmen & Machamer, 1995; Evans et al., 1992; Johnston, Kirshblum, et al., 1992; Stover et al., 1995). The following are some typical findings:

- Functional recovery can be nonlinear, and the shape of the recovery curve can differ, depending on initial severity (Carey, Matyas, & Oke, 1993; Collins & Horn, 1991; Dikmen & Machamer, 1995; Evans et al., 1992; Johnston, Kirshblum, et al., 1992).
- It is also essential to have models or quantitative theories about growth or recovery. Without such models, it is not possible to determine the optimal statistical method that should be used to compute or model gain scores (Collins & Horn, 1991; Collins & Johnston, 1995).

- Outcomes prediction is typically substantially more accurate if multiple predictors are used; outcomes are multiply determined (e.g., Evans et al., 1992; Inouye et al., 1993; Johnston, Kirshblum, et al., 1992; Stineman, Maislin, & Williams, 1993).
- Chronicity is an essential consideration in understanding prognosis. For sudden-onset diseases, *chronicity* would be operationally defined in terms of the time between onset and rehabilitation admission. Following moderately severe injury to the central nervous system, and following the period of acute medical instability, there is typically a period of spontaneous recovery lasting for several months. Even after neurologic stability is reached, improvement in some adaptive skills may continue for many more months or even for years (Dikmen & Machamer, 1995; Evans et al., 1992; Johnston, Kirshblum, et al., 1992; Stover et al., 1995).
- Understanding when a group of persons with an impairment becomes functionally asymptomatic as a group is pivotal in outcomes research, because control procedures and inference of effectiveness depend on whether participants are expected, on average, to improve, deteriorate, or remain the same in function in the absence of the experimental treatment.
- There is also evidence that functional recovery is influenced by non-medical factors such as previous life role, prior employment status, prior living arrangement, preinjury function, and other factors in the social and physical environment (e.g., Adler et al., 1993; Haley, Cost-ner, & Binda-Sundberg, 1994; Inouye et al., 1993; Johnston, Kirshblum, et al., 1992; Stineman et al., 1993; Verbrugge & Jette, 1994).
- Functional recovery also has features that can be best understood in terms of stages or qualitative developments. Stage theories need quantitative, empirical testing. Special methods need to be used if recovery is to be treated qualitatively (i.e., categorically) or as a series of stage-sequential or ordinal developments (Collins & Johnston, 1995).

Although outcomes may appear to be predictable when computing statistical averages from data on the experience of groups of persons with disabilities, when confronted with an individual patient in the present, future outcomes often appear to be unpredictable. Clinical professionals in rehabilitation have emphasized that effective rehabilitation is tailored to the individual and is a complex interaction of innumerable factors in the person and the environment. At the same time, research properly attempts to discern patterns of person–treatment interaction that are reliably associated with better outcomes. There is a great deal yet to be learned about determinants of rehabilitation outcomes, that is, strong predictors that are relatively independent of other confounding predictive factors.

Prediction research is important and central to most outcomes research; however, the authors believe that prediction research should be a somewhat lower priority than research comparing the effectiveness or efficacy of different rehabilitative interventions. If research comparing different interventions reveals no treatment effects, there still may be information on predictive relationships; but longitudinal research on persons undergoing similar or poorly defined treatments will not reveal what works best in helping persons with disabilities.

Case Severity Adjustment Scrupulous measurement or modeling of case severity is unequivocally essential in rehabilitation outcomes research. The quality of the input measures is as essential as the outcomes measures in rehabilitation outcomes research. Quantification of case severity is critical: Patients are selected for rehabilitation because they are disabled, yet they have some potential for improvement. Comparison of outcomes to unselected patients of the same diagnosis can be utterly misleading. Even among those selected for rehabilitation, there can be variation in severity of disability, comorbidities, and psychosocial factors that affect outcomes.

Measurement of severity in terms of disease stage, general pathology, or general impairment has logical advantages in medical rehabilitation research: It connects the research to the established biologic models of disease. Such measures can be (but are not always in practice) highly objective, and they give insight into potentially critical underlying processes.

From an outcomes research perspective, however, there are difficulties with most indicators of impairment and pathology. Even within one disease group, hundreds to thousands of specifically important biologic indicators, from the molecular level to the organ-system level, could be measured. As indicators become more specific, it typically becomes more difficult to understand the organism or the person as a whole. Many specific impairments or pathology indicators have only a small correlation with overall function or quality-of-life outcomes, or they apply well to only a small fraction of cases.

Measures of disability have advantages as indicators of case severity. Disability measures have been shown to have robust, cross-diagnostic prognostic power. As performance measures, they tap patients' strengths as well as their weaknesses. Disability measures are in widespread use, and most have a simple basis in answering questions such as the following:

1. Can the person walk?
2. Can the person dress independently?
3. Can the person take care of his or her own bathroom needs?

Such questions have a clear relationship to valued, practical, real-world needs and outcomes. However, disability measures typically do not provide the insight into key biologic processes that measures of impairment and pathology provide.

Indicators of both impairment and disability need to overcome problems of reliability and validity of measurement (Johnston, Keith, & Hinderer, 1992). The relative importance and interplay of impairment and biologic, disability, and social measures should be a continuing topic of empirical research. The connection between disabilities and their biologic substrates is a central topic in rehabilitation. At the biologic level, what is needed for rehabilitation outcomes research is the identification of the biologic factors that are most central or powerful in different situations. To be useful in outcomes research, measures of impairment or pathology that have robust correlations with humanly significant outcomes for large patient groups need to be identified. An example of such an impairment measure is the Fugl-Meyer measure of motor dysfunction (Fugl-Meyer, Jääskö, Leyman, Olsson, & Steglind, 1975) following stroke. It has what is probably the strongest well-documented correlation with ADL and mobility outcomes, as measured by the Barthel Index (Mahoney & Barthel, 1965), of any known measure (Duncan et al., 1992); it can predict FIM scores at discharge even more highly than FIM scores at admission (Chae, Johnston, Kim, & Zorowitz, 1995). Similarly, neurologic level of injury is the key severity indicator in research on outcomes following spinal cord injury (Stover et al., 1995).

However, researchers must not overdraw the impact of even robust pathology and impairment measures. Although pathology and impairment are central to medical science, it does not mean that personally or socially valuable outcomes are strongly coupled with any particular pathology or impairment. Subjective well-being, for instance, has been related to health, income, social activities, and perceived control, although the relationships are not always strong or consistent (Fuhrer, 1994). Physical impairments and even disabilities often have a weak or inconsistent relationship to reported subjective well-being (Fuhrer, 1994).

Moreover, epidemiologic studies have shown that access to medical care in general explains only a portion of the variability in mortality and morbidity status of human populations; income, education, health-related behaviors, attitudes, stress, control over one's life, ethnicity, and other social factors are also essentially connected to health in society as a whole (Adler et al., 1993). Environmental factors are also critical in understanding rehabilitation outcomes. Institutionalization of persons with disabilities has been shown to depend as much on the level of family help available as on patient's disability (Johnston, Zorowitz, & Nash, 1994).

In sum, to understand long-term rehabilitation outcomes, research must measure factors exogenous to medical rehabilitation per se, such as preinjury function, comorbidities, personal motivation, and the physical and especially the social environment, as well as severity of impairment and disability. In addition, laboratory research is needed to understand the basis of recovery and treatment processes and the proximal effects of these for different patient groups. Information from all these sources needs to be synthesized into theories or models that link rehabilitative processes to outcomes.

CONCLUSIONS

The Problem of Complexity

The complex and multidisciplinary nature of medical rehabilitation creates difficulties. Traditional research methods are optimized for a single defined treatment applied to a homogeneous patient group with a single expected outcome. Rehabilitation applies multiple interventions to a diverse group of patients and has multiple expected outcomes. Complex processes are always more difficult to elucidate than simple ones.

Although there are no easy solutions to the methodologic problems facing rehabilitation research, there are research strategies that will help deal with multifaceted (but definable) rehabilitative processes and outcomes (Whyte, 1994). Useful methods include the following:

- Measurement of multiple highly relevant inputs, processes, and outcomes
- Study of more common patient groups, syndromes, and treatment patterns, so that sufficiently large sample sizes are feasible
- Multivariate techniques such as path analysis, multiple regression, recursive partitioning, factor analysis, and others
- Prioritization of hypotheses to permit formal hierarchical analysis (e.g., Cohen & Cohen, 1983) (With a limited sample size and numerous variables, only a few a priori hypotheses can be tested definitively. Many relationships can be examined post hoc to provide a more complete understanding of processes involved, to suggest promising possibilities for future research, and to retain a sense of the complexity of the whole.)
- Synthesis of findings of controlled research from other fields so that some treatment effects can be assumed and need not be reinvestigated
- Study of treatments that are sufficiently well defined to be used in a clinical practice guideline that explicates variations in approach as a function of patient characteristics

Finally, there are rehabilitative interventions that are too complex and ill defined to support clear research results. Study of defined treatment–outcome issues can be a priority, provided that the issues are not too narrow.

Simplifying Factors

Although the complexity of rehabilitative systems is often daunting, there are several important factors that simplify rehabilitation research. First, diagnosis has already been established in most cases. Because the illness or injury is already known at admission to rehabilitation, it is possible to test the effectiveness of treatment by departure from baseline projections. Admittedly, obtaining stable pretreatment baseline data involves a change in ordinary clinical procedures and overcoming political barriers to collaborate with referring physicians who see patients before they enter rehabilitation. A major barrier is simply that the necessary strong time-series designs are not widely understood or used (Johnston et al., 1995).

Second, physical disability, the focus of most rehabilitation interventions, is clearly observable, and there are many useful albeit imperfect instruments for measuring it, such as the FIM (State University of New York at Buffalo, 1993) and the Barthel (Mahoney & Barthel, 1965; see also, e.g., Cole et al., 1994; Lohr, 1992; Spilker, 1990). Likewise, there are many useful measures for assessing neurologic disability (McDowell & Newell, 1996; Wade, 1991) and neuropsychologic impairment (Lezak, 1983).

Third, although the multiplicity of diagnoses and impairments seen in medical rehabilitation is a barrier to some types of purely medical or physiologic research, it is not an insuperable barrier to studies of classic rehabilitation interventions, which concentrate on improvement of function using techniques that theoretically should work across a range of impairments.

Rehabilitation has a humanistic tradition of treating the person with a disability as a person, honored as an equal participant in the process. Although this realization is of little advantage to purely physiologic research, it *is* an advantage to outcomes research. Patients' viewpoints and honest expressions, provided that there is rapport between the researchers and the patients and the researchers do not bias patient responses, offer a sound beginning for outcomes research, particularly in selecting dimensions of greatest value. The authors are not saying that patients understand themselves after a new injury, that patients' statements should be taken at face value, or that self-report measures do not have many reliability and validity issues. Instead, we are saying that the patients' evaluation of the care received, their experience, and their evaluation of the quality of their own lives should be treated as having fundamental validity, at least until proved to be mistaken, and even then it is incumbent on the researcher to distinguish sources of misunderstanding from areas of true understanding.

Finally, the eclectic nature of rehabilitation makes it possible to borrow a great deal from other fields. Medical rehabilitation outcomes research can test the effectiveness of interventions, based on established theories and findings from other fields, when applied to patient groups with severe disability or multiple problems.

All biomedical research faces complexity, but this does not prevent progress. Well-specified rehabilitative treatment processes are grounded in learning theory, physiology, or other established biomedical processes. Putative causal mechanisms need to be established by highly controlled experiments. Given the multiplicity of diagnoses and problems treated in medical rehabilitation, it is advantageous for rehabilitation outcomes research to encompass some breadth and flexibility in approach. The generalizability and cost-effectiveness of rehabilitative interventions need to be tested in real-world studies using both randomized and strong quasi-experimental research designs. Rehabilitation needs to develop validated measures of treatment objectives, embedded in treatment protocols with a sensible theoretical basis. Researchers especially need to understand when rehabilitative treatment effects are transient and when they are enduring.

There is a substantial literature on treatment approaches in rehabilitation. There are hundreds of small-sample studies, using weak if any control procedures, that report intriguing but unreplicated findings (Ottenbacher, 1995). This literature, properly studied and understood, can provide invaluable background and pilot data for larger-sample outcomes research involving a higher degree of experimental control, such as randomization or a strong quasi-experimental research design. The search for new and more efficacious interventions needs to be thoroughly grounded in existing knowledge.

Controversies abound in rehabilitation, and questions of its worth are recurrently heard. Highly controlled, comparative outcomes studies, however, have rarely been attempted in medical rehabilitation. The power of randomized experiments, not to mention strong quasi-experimental research designs, has largely been unexploited. The time is ripe for study of many interventions thought to be effective in medical rehabilitation. The preeminent need is for well-controlled studies of the efficacy and effectiveness of defined rehabilitative interventions compared with practical alternatives. Medical rehabilitation should prove to be a fertile but challenging field for the application of controlled research methods.

REFERENCES

Adler, N.E., Boyce, T., Chesney, M.A., Folkman, S., & Syme, L. (1993). Socioeconomic inequalities in health. *Journal of the American Medical Association, 269*(24), 3140–3145.

Arokiasamy, C.V. (1993). A theory for rehabilitation? *Rehabilitation Education, 7*(2), 77–98.

Bach-y-Rita, P. (1990). Brain plasticity as a basis for recovery of function in humans. *Neuropsychologia, 28*(6), 547–554.

Barry, M.J., Fowler, F.J., Jr., Mulley, A.G., Jr., Henderson, J.V., Jr., & Wennberg, J.E. (1995). Patient reactions to a program designed to facilitate patient participation in treatment decisions for benign prostatic hyperplasia. *Medical Care, 33*(8), 771–782.

Beckerman, H., Bouter, L.M., van der Heijden, G.J., de Bie, R.A., & Koes, B.W. (1993). Efficacy of physiotherapy for musculoskeletal disorders: What can we learn from research? *British Journal of General Practice, 43*(367), 73–77.

Ben-Yishay, Y., & Diller, L. (1993). Cognitive remediation in traumatic brain injury: Update and issues. *Archives of Physical Medicine and Rehabilitation, 74,* 204–213.

Bender, G.A. (1961). *Great moments in medicine.* Detroit, MI: Parke-Davis.

Carey, L.M., Matyas, T.A., & Oke, L.E. (1993). Sensory loss in stroke patients: Effective training of tactile and proprioceptive discrimination. *Archives of Physical Medicine and Rehabilitation, 74,* 602–611.

Chae, J., Johnston, M., Kim, H., & Zorowitz, R. (1995). Admission motor impairment as a predictor of physical disability after stroke rehabilitation. *American Journal of Physical Medicine and Rehabilitation, 74,* 218–223.

Cohen, J., & Cohen, P. (1983). *Applied multiple regression/correlation analysis for the behavioral sciences* (2nd ed.). Hillsdale, NJ: Lawrence Erlbaum Associates.

Cole, B., Finch, E., Gowland, C., & Mayo, N. (1994). *Physical rehabilitation outcome measures.* Toronto, Ontario: Canadian Physiotherapy Association.

Collins, L.M., & Horn, J.L. (1991). *Best methods for the analysis of change.* Washington, DC: American Psychological Association.

Collins, L.M., & Johnston, M.V. (1995). Analysis of stage-sequential change in rehabilitation research. *American Journal of Physical Medicine and Rehabilitation, 74*(2), 163–170.

Cordray, D.S. (1990). Strengthening causal interpretations of nonexperimental data: The role of meta-analysis. In L. Sechrest, E. Perrin, & J. Bunker (Eds.), *Conference proceedings: Research methodology: Strengthening causal interpretations of non-experimental data* (pp. 151–172) (DHHS Pub. No. [PHS] 90-3454). Rockville, MD: U.S. Department of Health and Human Services, Public Health Service, Agency for Health Care Policy and Research.

Dahmer, E.R., Shilling, M.A., Hamilton, B.B., Bontke, C.F., Englander, J., Kreutzer, J.S., Ragnarsson, K.T., & Rosenthal, M. (1993). A model systems database for traumatic brain injury. *Journal of Head Trauma Rehabilitation, 8*(2), 12–25.

DeJong, G., & Sutton, J.P. (1995). Rehab 2000: The evolution of medical rehabilitation in American health care. In P. Kitchell Landrum, N.D. Schmidt, & A. McLean, Jr. (Eds.), *Outcome-oriented rehabilitation: Principles, strategies, and tools for effective program management* (pp. 3–42). Gaithersburg, MD: Aspen Publishers, Inc.

DeLisa, J.A., Martin, G.M., & Currie, D.M. (1993). Rehabilitation medicine: Past, present, and future. In J.A. DeLisa et al. (Eds.), *Rehabilitation medicine: Principles and practice* (pp. 3–27). Philadelphia: J.B. Lippincott.

Dikmen, S., & Machamer, J.E. (1995). Neurobehavioral outcomes and their determinants. *Journal of Head Trauma Rehabilitation, 10*(1), 74–86.

Dobkin, B.H. (1993). Neuroplasticity: Key to recovery after central nervous system injury. *Western Journal of Medicine, 159*(1), 56–60.

Duncan, P.W., et al. (1992). Measurement of motor recovery after stroke: Outcome assessment and sample size requirements. *Stroke, 23,* 1084–1089.

Evans, R.W., Baskin, D.S., & Yatsu, F.M. (Eds.). (1992). *Prognosis of neurological disorders.* New York: Oxford University Press.

Falconer, J.A., Roth, E.J., Sutin, J.A., Strasser, D.C., & Chang, R.W. (1994). The critical path method in stroke rehabilitation: Lessons from an experiment in cost containment and outcome improvement. *Quality Review Bulletin, 19*(1), 8–16.

Field, M.J., & Lohr, K.N. (Eds.). (1990). *Clinical practice guidelines.* Washington, DC: National Academy Press, Institute of Medicine.

Fisher, W.P., Jr., Harvey, R.F., Taylor, P., Kilgore, K.M., & Kelly, C.K. (1995). Rehabits: A common language of functional assessment. *Archives of Physical Medicine and Rehabilitation, 76,* 113–122.

Frattali, C.M. (1992). Functional assessment of communication: Merging public policy with clinical views. *Aphasiology, 6*(1), 63–83.

Freedman, D., Pisani, R., Purves, R., & Adhikari, A. (1991). *Statistics* (2nd ed.). New York: Norton.

Fugl-Meyer, A.R., Jääskö, L., Leyman, I., Olsson, S., & Steglind, S. (1975). The post-stroke hemiplegic patient: I. A method for evaluation of physical performance. *Scandinavian Journal of Rehabilitation Medicine, 7,* 13–31.

Fuhrer, M.J. (1987). Overview of outcome analysis in rehabilitation. In M.J. Fuhrer (Ed.), *Rehabilitation outcomes: Analysis and measurement* (pp. 1–15). Baltimore: Paul H. Brookes Publishing Co.

Fuhrer, M.J. (1994). Subjective well-being: Implications for medical rehabilitation outcomes and models of disablement. *American Journal of Physical Medicine and Rehabilitation, 73*(5), 358–364.

Fuhrer, M.J. (1995). Conference report: An agenda for medical rehabilitation outcomes research. *American Journal of Physical Medicine and Rehabilitation, 74,* 243–248.

Garraway, W.M., Akhtar, A.J., Hockey, L., & Prescott, R.J. (1980). Management of acute stroke in the elderly: Follow-up of a controlled trial. *British Medical Journal, 281,* 827–829.

Garraway, W.M., Akhtar, A.J., Prescott, R.J., & Hockey, L. (1980). Management of acute stroke in the elderly: Preliminary results of a controlled trial. *British Medical Journal, 280,* 1040–1043.

Glueckauf, R.L. (1990). Program evaluation guidelines for the rehabilitation professional. In M.G. Eisenberg & R.C. Grzesiak (Eds.), *Advances in clinical rehabilitation* (Vol. 3, pp. 250–264). New York: Springer.

Glueckauf, R.L. (1993). Use and misuse of assessment in rehabilitation: Getting back to the basics. In R.L. Glueckauf, L.B. Sechrest, G.R. Bond, & E.C. McDonel (Eds.), *Improving assessment in rehabilitation and health* (pp. 135–155). Newbury Park, CA: Sage Publications.

Granger, C.V., Hayes, K.M., Johnston, M.V., Deutsch, A., Braun, S., & Fiedler, R.C. (1996). Quality and outcome measures. In R.L. Braddom & R. Buschbacher (Eds.), *Physical medicine and rehabilitation* (pp. 239–254). Philadelphia: W.B. Saunders.

Granger, C.V., Ottenbacher, K.J., & Fiedler, R.C. (1995). The Uniform Data System for Medical Rehabilitation: Report of first admissions for 1993. *American Journal of Physical Medicine and Rehabilitation, 74*(1), 62–66.

Haffey, W.J., & Johnston, M.V. (1989). An information system to assess the effectiveness of brain injury rehabilitation. In R. Wood & P. Eames (Eds.), *Models of brain injury rehabilitation* (pp. 205–233). London: Chapman & Hall.

Haffey, W.J., & Johnston, M.V. (1990). A functional assessment system for real world rehabilitation outcomes. In D. Tupper & K. Cicerone (Eds.), *The neuro-*

psychology of everyday life: Assessment and basic competencies (pp. 99–124). Boston: Kluwer Academic.

Haffey, W.J., & Lewis, F.D. (1989). Programming for occupational outcomes following traumatic brain injury. *Rehabilitation Psychology, 34,* 147–158.

Haley, S.M., Costner, W.J., & Binda-Sundberg, K. (1994). Measuring physical disablement: The contextual challenge. *Physical Therapy, 74*(5), 443–451.

Hamilton, B.B., Laughlin, J.A., Fiedler, R.C., & Granger, C.V. (1994). Interrater reliability of the 7-level Functional Independence Measure (FIM). *Scandinavian Journal of Rehabilitation Medicine, 26,* 115–119.

Heerkens, Y.F., Brandsma, J.W., Lakerveld-Hyl, K., & van Ravensberg, C.D. (1994). Impairments and disabilities—the difference: Proposal for adjustment of the International Classification of Impairments, Disabilities, and Handicaps. *Physical Therapy, 74*(4), 430–442.

Heinemann, A.W., Hamilton, B., Linacre, J.M., Wright, B.D., & Granger, C. (1995). Functional status and therapeutic intensity during inpatient rehabilitation. *American Journal of Physical Medicine and Rehabilitation, 74*(4), 315–326.

Indredavik, B., Bakke, F., Solberg, R., Rokseth, R., Haaheim, L.L., & Holme, I. (1991). Benefit of a stroke unit: A randomized controlled trial. *Stroke, 22*(8), 1026–1031.

Inouye, S.K., Wagner, D.R., Acampora, D., Horwitz, R.I., Cooney, L.M., Jr., Hurst, L.D., & Tinetti, M.E. (1993). A predictive index for functional decline in hospitalized elderly medical patients. *Journal of General Internal Medicine, 8*(12), 645–652.

Jellinek, M.S., & Nurcombe, B. (1993). Two wrongs don't make a right: Managed care, mental health, and the marketplace. *Journal of the American Medical Association, 270,* 1737–1790.

Johnston, M.V., & Granger, C.V. (1994). Outcomes research in medical rehabilitation: A primer and introduction to a series. *American Journal of Physical Medicine and Rehabilitation, 73*(4), 296–303.

Johnston, M.V., Hall, K., Carnevale, G., & Boake, C. (1996). Functional assessment and outcome evaluation. In L.J. Horn & N.D. Zasler (Eds.), *Medical rehabilitation of traumatic brain injury* (pp. 197–226). Philadelphia: Hanley & Belfus.

Johnston, M.V., Keith, R.A., & Hinderer, S. (1992). Measurement standards for interdisciplinary medical rehabilitation. *Archives of Physical Medicine and Rehabilitation, 73*(Whole Suppl. No. 12-S), S6–S23.

Johnston, M.V., Kirshblum, S., Zorowitz, R., & Shiflett, S.C. (1992). Prediction of outcomes following rehabilitation of stroke patients. *NeuroRehabilitation, 2*(4), 71–96.

Johnston, M.V., Ottenbacher, K., & Reichardt, K. (1995). Strong quasi-experimental designs for research on the effectiveness of rehabilitation. *American Journal of Physical Medicine and Rehabilitation, 74*(5), 383–392.

Johnston, M.V., & Wilkerson, D.L. (1992). Program evaluation and quality improvement systems in brain injury rehabilitation. *Journal of Head Trauma Rehabilitation, 7*(4), 68–82.

Johnston, M.V., Zorowitz, R., & Nash, B. (1994). Family help available. *Topics in Geriatric Rehabilitation, 9*(3), 38–53.

Joynt, R.L., Findley, T.W., Boda, W., & Daum, M.C. (1993). Therapeutic exercise. In J.A. DeLisa et al. (Eds.), *Rehabilitation medicine: Principles and practice* (pp. 526–554). Philadelphia: J.B. Lippincott.

Kalra, L., Dale, P., & Crome, P. (1993). Improving stroke rehabilitation. *Stroke, 24,* 1462–1467.

Keith, R.A. (1995). Conceptual basis of outcome measures. *American Journal of Physical Medicine and Rehabilitation, 74,* 73–80.

Keith, R.A., & Lipsey, M.W. (1993). The role of theory in rehabilitation assessment, treatment, and outcomes. In R.L. Glueckauf, L.B. Sechrest, G.R. Bond, & E. McDonel (Eds.), *Improving assessment in rehabilitation and health* (pp. 33–58). Newbury Park, CA: Sage Publications.

Landefeld, C.S., Palmer, R.M., Kresevic, D.M., Fortinsky, R.H., & Kowal, J. (1995). A randomized trial of care in a hospital medical unit especially designed to improve the functional outcomes of acutely ill older patients. *New England Journal of Medicine, 332*(20), 1338–1344.

Lezak, M.D. (1983). *Neuropsychological assessment* (2nd ed.). New York: Oxford University Press.

Lipsey, M.W. (1990). Theory as method: Small theories of treatments. In L. Sechrest, E. Perrin, & J. Bunker (Eds.), *Conference proceedings: Research methodology: Strengthening causal interpretations of non-experimental data* (pp. 33–52). (DHHS Pub. No. [PHS] 90-3454). Rockville, MD: U.S. Department of Health and Human Services, Public Health Service, Agency for Health Care Policy and Research.

Lohr, K.N. (Ed.). (1992). Advances in health status assessment. *Medical Care, 30*(Suppl.), MS1–MS293.

Mahoney, F.I., & Barthel, D.W. (1965). Functional evaluation: The Barthel Index. *Maryland State Medical Journal, 14,* 61–65.

McDowell, I., & Newell, I. (1996). *Measuring health: A guide to rating scales and questionnaires* (2nd ed.). New York: Oxford University Press.

Nagi, S. (1991). Disability concepts revisited: Implications for prevention. In A. Pope & A. Tarlov (Eds.), *Disability in America: Toward a national agenda for prevention* (pp. 309–337). Washington, DC: National Academy Press.

National Center for Medical Rehabilitation Research. (1993). *Research plan for the National Center for Medical Rehabilitation Research.* (NIH Pub. No. 93-3509). Bethesda, MD: U.S. Department of Health and Human Services, Public Health Service, National Institute of Child Health and Human Development.

Office of Technology Assessment, U.S. Congress. (1978). *Assessing the efficacy and safety of medical technologies.* Washington, DC: U.S. Government Printing Office.

Ottenbacher, K.J. (1995). Why rehabilitation research does not work (as well as we think it should). *Archives of Physical Medicine and Rehabilitation, 76,* 123–129.

Post-Stroke Rehabilitation Guideline Panel. (1995). *Clinical practice guideline number 16: Post-stroke rehabilitation.* (AHCPR Publication No. 950662). Rockville, MD: U.S. Department of Health and Human Services, Public Health Service, Agency for Health Care Policy and Research.

Province, M.A., Hadley, E.C., Hornbrook, M.C., Lipsitz, L.A., Miller, J.P., Mulrow, C.D., Ory, M.G., Sattin, R.W., Tinetti, M.E., & Wolf, S.L. (1995). The effects of exercise on falls in elderly patients: A preplanned meta-analysis of the FICIT trials. *Journal of the American Medical Association, 273*(17), 1341–1347.

Reichardt, C.S. (1979). The statistical analysis of data from non-equivalent group designs. In T.D. Cook & D.T. Campbell (Eds.), *Quasi-experimentation: Design and analysis issues for field settings* (pp. 147–206). Boston: Houghton Mifflin.

Reuben, D.B., Borok, G.M., Wolde-Tsadik, G., Ershoff, D.H., Fishman, L.K., Ambrosini, V.L., Liu, Y., Rubenstein, L.Z., & Beck, J.C. (1995). A randomized trial of comprehensive geriatric assessment in the care of hospitalized patients. *New England Journal of Medicine, 332*(20), 1345–1350.

Rubenstein, L.Z., Josephson, K.R., Wieland, G.D., English, P.A., Sayre, J.A., & Kane, R.L. (1984). Effectiveness of a geriatric evaluation unit: A randomized clinical trial. *New England Journal of Medicine, 311,* 1664–1670.

Sachs, O. (1995). *An anthropologist on Mars.* New York: Knopf.

Smith, R.M. (1996). A comparison of methods for determining dimensionality in Rasch measurement. *Structural Equation Modeling, 3*(1), 25–40.

Spilker, B. (Ed.). (1990). *Quality of life assessment in clinical trials.* New York: Raven.

State University of New York at Buffalo. (1993). *Guide for the Uniform Data Set for Medical Rehabilitation (Adult FIM), version 4.0.* Buffalo, NY: Author.

Stewart, A.L., & Ware, J.E., Jr. (Eds.). (1992). *Measuring functioning and well-being.* Durham, NC: Duke University Press.

Stineman, M.G., Maislin, G., & Williams, S.V. (1993). Applying quantitative methods to the prediction of full functional recovery of adult rehabilitation patients. *Archives of Physical Medicine and Rehabilitation, 74,* 787–795.

Stover, S.L., DeLisa, J.A., & Whiteneck, G.G. (1995). *Spinal cord injury: Clinical outcomes from the model systems.* Gaithersburg, MD: Aspen Publishers, Inc.

Strasser, D.C., Falconer, J.A., & Martino-Saltzmann, D. (1994). The rehabilitation team: Staff perceptions of the hospital environment, the interdisciplinary team environment, and interprofessional relations. *Archives of Physical Medicine and Rehabilitation, 75,* 177–182.

Tinetti, M.E., Baker, D.I., McAvay, G., Claus, E.B., Garrett, P., Gottschalk, M., Kock, M.L., Trainor, K., & Horwitz, R.I. (1994). A multifactorial intervention to reduce the risk of falling among elderly people living in the community. *New England Journal of Medicine, 331*(13), 821–827.

Ueda, S. (1994, August). *Implications of the concepts of ICIDH and OOL for medical rehabilitation outcomes research.* Paper presented at An Agenda for Medical Rehabilitation Outcomes Research: National Invitational Conference. National Center for Medical Rehabilitation Research, National Institute of Child Health and Human Development, National Institutes of Health, and the Agency for Health Care Policy and Research, Bethesda, MD.

Velozo, C.A., Magalhaus, L., Pan, A., & Leiter, P. (1995). Differences in functional scale discrimination at admission and discharge: Rasch analysis of the Level of Rehabilitation Scale–III (LORS–III). *Archives of Physical Medicine and Rehabilitation, 76*(8), 705–712.

Verbrugge, L.M. (1984). Longer life but worsening health? Trends in health and mortality of middle-aged and older persons. *Milbank Quarterly, 62,* 475–519.

Verbrugge, L.M., & Jette, A.M. (1994). The disablement process. *Social Science and Medicine, 38*(1), 1–14.

Wade, D. (1991). *Measurement in neurological rehabilitation.* Oxford, England: Oxford University Press.

Wennberg, J.E. (1990). Small area analysis and the medical care outcome problem. In L. Sechrest, E. Perrin, & J. Bunker (Eds.), *Conference proceedings: Research methodology: Strengthening causal interpretations of non-experimental data* (pp. 177–206). (DHHS Pub. No. [PHS] 90-3454). Rockville, MD: U.S. Department of Health and Human Services, Public Health Service, Agency for Health Care Policy and Research.

Whiteneck, G.G. (1992). Outcome evaluation and spinal cord injury. *Neuro-Rehabilitation, 2*(4), 31–41.

Whyte, J. (1994). Toward a methodology for rehabilitation research. *American Journal of Physical Medicine and Rehabilitation, 73,* 428–435.

World Health Organization. (1980). *International classification of impairments, disabilities, and handicaps.* Geneva, Switzerland: Author.

CHAPTER 2

Distinctive Methodologic Challenges

John Whyte

Medical rehabilitation outcomes research poses some special methodologic challenges. For the purposes of discussing and clarifying these challenges, *medical rehabilitation outcomes research* is defined broadly to include research on both *focal outcomes* and *global outcomes,* recognizing that these are arbitrary labels along a continuum. *Focal outcomes* means the outcome of a specific treatment intervention intended to improve an impairment or specific disability, for example, the improvement in gait resulting from application of a brace or the improvement in memory from treatment with a drug. *Global outcomes* means outcomes such as hospital discharge destination, independent living status, or employment success, which are generally the product of a health care delivery system rather than any individual treatment intervention.

HISTORICAL OVERVIEW

The quantity and quality of medical rehabilitation outcomes research have been generally regarded as inadequate since at least 1981 (Fowler, 1981; Fuhrer, 1981). A number of reasons have been suggested for this state of affairs, including too few trained researchers, too little funding for rehabilitation research, and too many competing clinical demands for a relatively small population of rehabilitation specialists. Fortunately, a number

This chapter was supported by the National Institute of Neurological Disorders and Stroke under Grant R29 NS27715 and by MossRehab Hospital and Moss Rehabilitation Medicine, Inc. The author wishes to thank Myrna Schwartz, Ph.D., and Mark V. Johnston, Ph.D., for helpful commentary on the issues discussed in this chapter, as well as many of the participants at the NCMRR- and AHCPR-sponsored conference on medical rehabilitation outcomes research for their helpful questions and criticisms. Thanks are also due to Ron Kalstein and Wesley Hilton for preparation of the figures and to Mary K. Lombardi for typing the manuscript.

of developments have occurred that may help alleviate some of these obstacles. The founding of the National Center for Medical Rehabilitation
Research (NCMRR) within the National Institutes of Health symbolizes an
increased federal awareness of the importance of rehabilitation research. A
significant portion of NCMRR's funding as well as funding from the National Institute on Disability and Rehabilitation Research within the Department of Education has been earmarked specifically to train future
rehabilitation researchers. Furthermore, extramurally supported projects
from various agencies have helped advance the state of measurement of
rehabilitation outcomes and the development of consensus tools for outcomes measurement.

Despite these very positive developments, this chapter presents some
basic methodologic issues that represent additional obstacles to progress in
the field. Simply providing increased research training in traditional research disciplines and increased research funding will not completely solve
the problem. This chapter also discusses the conceptual hierarchy that un-
derlies rehabilitation practice and research, how this hierarchy shapes the
types of research strategies that are of interest and feasible to perform, and
what implications this conceptual framework has for research training and
research practice.

THE CONCEPTUAL HIERARCHY

The World Health Organization (WHO) defined a conceptual framework
of human function that extends from disease or pathology at the most
microscopic level to handicap at the most macroscopic level (WHO, 1980).
Somewhat similar conceptual systems have been proposed by Nagi (1991)
and the Advisory Board of NCMRR (Association of Academic Physiatrists,
1991). Although the boundaries and details of the different levels vary from
system to system, each system shares the view that one can look at dysfunction within individuals' organs or body parts, dysfunction of the whole
individual, and dysfunction of the individual as he or she interacts with a
more or less supportive environment.

In brief, *pathology* refers to changes in the structure or function of
the body or of a specific tissue or organ. Pathology need not be manifested
in any symptoms or functional limitations. *Impairment* refers to a loss or
abnormality of a psychologic, physiologic, or anatomic system without
regard to its etiology. Thus, for example, early muscular dystrophy may
result in detectable pathology at the biochemical level without producing
an impairment in muscular strength. Conversely, a person may have impaired strength from a variety of etiologies. A key property of impairments
is that they can be defined objectively and are not related to an individual's
goals, social roles, and so forth. *Disability* refers to the net effects of one

or more impairments on an individual's normal level of skill, activity, or ability. *Handicap,* in contrast, refers to the net effects of a set of disabilities interacting with the physical and social environment on an individual's performance of typical social roles.

These levels are presented as a hierarchy, not to imply either gradations of importance or that higher levels exert control over lower levels. Rather, the term *hierarchy* is applied in a manner similar to the taxonomic hierarchy used in classifying living things. Elements high in the hierarchy are (potentially) influenced by more variables below them than are elements low on the hierarchy. For example, more factors determine whether one can work than whether one can extend one's leg, just as a great many more organisms are members of the animal kingdom than of the species *Homo sapiens.*

It is also important to note that these levels are probably not as discrete as they appear, but rather form more of an ascending continuum. For example, a disability in self-feeding might be affected by whether an individual lives in a culture that uses chopsticks or spoons, even though cultural and environmental factors are generally thought to play a role primarily at the handicap level.

The levels of disability and handicap are often referred to as functional levels because it is only once the whole person is addressed that human function takes on meaning. Quality of life and subjective well-being represent other important global outcomes, which were not explicitly placed in the WHO hierarchy. How quality of life relates to the four previously defined levels remains a subject of some controversy (Fuhrer, Rintala, Hart, Clearman, & Young, 1992; Lawton, 1991).

In rehabilitation practice, it is generally the levels of disability, handicap, and quality of life that are of primary interest. For example, in clinical discussions, a therapist may mention a patient's impairment of an elbow contracture. However, an astute colleague will be quick to ask, "Yes, but does it interfere with her activities of daily living?"

POTENTIAL LEVELS OF TREATMENT
INTERVENTION AND OUTCOMES ASSESSMENT

The conceptual hierarchy has relevance both for defining treatment interventions and for measuring outcomes. In principle, treatments can be directed at any of these four levels (see Figure 1). Treatments of pathology or disease are commonplace in acute care medicine and would include, for example, antibiotics to cure an infection. Treatments of impairments would include exercises to improve the strength of paretic muscles, serial casting to elongate contracted soft tissues, and memory-enhancing drugs to improve a memory impairment. Treatments aimed at the level of disability

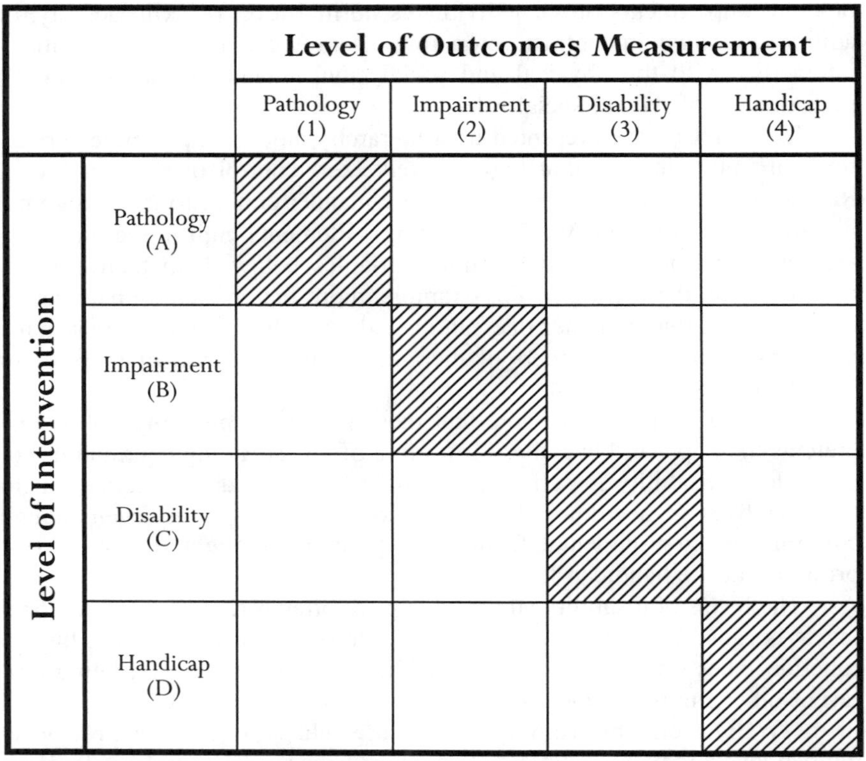

		Level of Outcomes Measurement			
		Pathology (1)	Impairment (2)	Disability (3)	Handicap (4)
Level of Intervention	Pathology (A)	/////			
	Impairment (B)		/////		
	Disability (C)			/////	
	Handicap (D)				/////

Figure 1. Four hierarchical levels of analysis along the vertical axis represent the possible points of treatment intervention, and four hierarchical levels of analysis along the horizontal axis represent the possible points of outcomes assessment. Cells along the main diagonal (striped) represent congruent intervention and assessment. These and the cells above the main diagonal are generally most relevant to treatment research, whereas the cells below the diagonal are most relevant in longitudinal assessment. (Adapted with permission from Whyte, J. [1994]. Toward a methodology for rehabilitation research. *American Journal of Physical Medicine and Rehabilitation, 73,* 431.)

include compensatory strategies such as wrist tenodesis for an individual with quadriplegia and a prescription for a wheelchair for an individual with lower-extremity paralysis. Finally, treatments aimed at the handicap level can be conceptualized as interventions to change the physical or social environment to be more accommodating to individuals with disabilities. For example, the reasonable accommodation clause of the Americans with Disabilities Act (ADA) of 1990 (PL 101-336) could be viewed as a handicap-level treatment.

Some have argued that a variety of training interventions aimed to increase the skills of individuals with disabilities in negotiating the social environment should be viewed as handicap-level interventions (B. Willer, personal communication, August 29, 1994). Perhaps this is no more than a semantic point, but because these interventions involve imparting skills to individual patients rather than systematically seeking to alter the environmental context, for the purposes of this discussion these interventions are placed within the ability or disability level that refers to the skills of individual people.

Special consideration should be given to educational or training interventions that represent a large proportion of the business of the rehabilitation system. Many training interventions need to be conceptualized as operating simultaneously at two levels of the hierarchy (Whyte, 1994). Consider the example of training a person to self-administer insulin for tight glucose control. On the one hand, this treatment is operating at the level of disease because its intended effect is to control blood sugar and the adverse consequences of elevated blood sugar. On the other hand, insulin injection also represents a skill of a whole person. Thus, poor blood sugar control as an outcome might conceivably be due to either an inappropriate dose of insulin or inadequate injection technique or frequency.

In systems of medical rehabilitation service delivery, most treatments are directed at the levels of impairment and disability. However, in the rehabilitation policy arena, treatment extends to the handicap level.

INTERRELATIONSHIPS BETWEEN THE HIERARCHICAL LEVELS

As shown in Figure 2, the variables at these different levels are interrelated. At the onset of disease or trauma, these relationships are predominantly

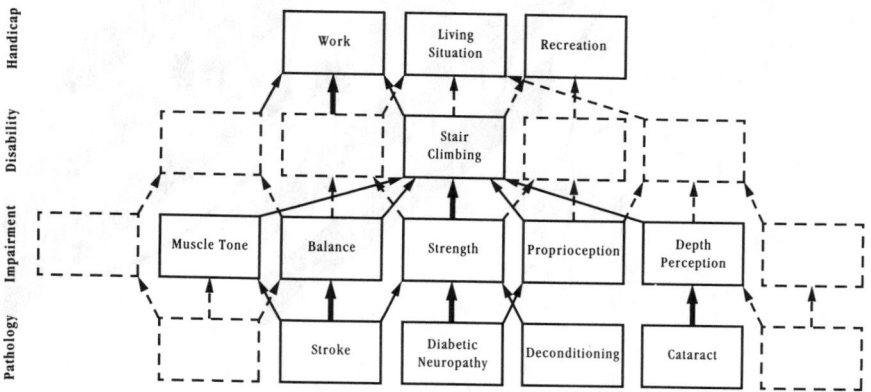

Figure 2. Hypothetical interactions among variables at the four hierarchical levels showing upward causal arrows reflective of immediate relationships. Note that variables at higher levels are potentially influenced by a large number of variables at lower levels. (From Whyte, J. [1994]. Toward a methodology for rehabilitation research. *American Journal of Physical Medicine and Rehabilitation, 73,* 429; reprinted by permission.)

ascending; that is, it is generally assumed that disease or pathology leads to one or more impairments that lead to one or more disabilities that (in combination with the environment) lead to one or more handicaps. As represented in the diagram, there is no direct relationship between pathology and disability or handicap. Rather, any such relationship is mediated by variables at the intervening levels. However, this is really more of an assertion than an empirical finding and needs to be explored through research that simultaneously measures outcomes at a variety of levels. Furthermore, it is likely that quality of life may be influenced directly from any of these levels. For example, the loss of a limb may reduce quality of life by virtue of limiting mobility, interfering with employment, and so forth; but it is also possible that loss of a limb directly lowers quality of life.

Although the immediate effects of disease operate in this ascending fashion, longitudinally there exists the possibility of descending influences. For example, a person with no vocational or social-recreational roles may spend more time in bed and get less exercise, ultimately leading to skin breakdown or weakness. Thus, over time, it is possible for a handicap-level variable to lead to pathology or impairments (see Figure 3).

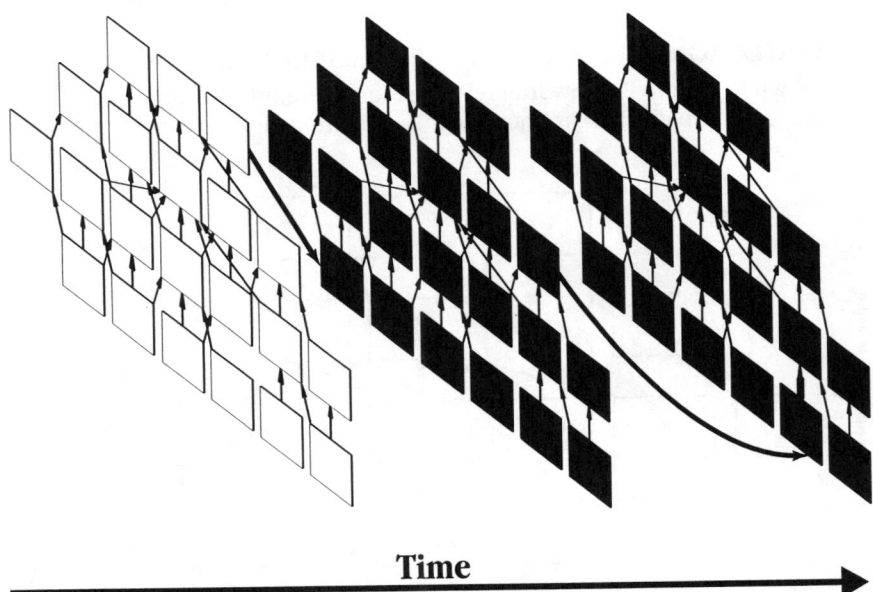

Time

Figure 3.   Hypothetical interactions among variables at the four hierarchical levels with the passage of time, demonstrating that downward causal influences can develop over time. Passage of time is represented horizontally.

THE BIOMEDICAL CAUSAL MODEL

The bulk of biomedical research has not directly addressed questions of function. Yet there has been an underlying assumption that reversal of pathology or disease should translate into restoration of function. In this sense, there is a presumed linear relationship between pathology and function. In biomedical research, both the treatments and the measured outcomes are generally at the pathology level (Cell A1 in Figure 1). Thus, one evaluates the efficacy of antibiotic treatment of pneumonia with reference to chest X ray, blood gasses, and culture, but rarely with reference to return to work.

However, such a simple linear causal model applies only in the most limited situations. Effective cures for many diseases are still lacking. Thus, for many individuals, cure of their disease is not even a feasible route to improved function. In addition, many ongoing diseases and conditions lead to the development of secondary physical and psychological impairments that are not automatically reversed by resolution of the underlying pathology. For example, a kidney transplant, which restores kidney function, does not automatically improve aerobic capacity, mood, or social outlets, all of which may have deteriorated during the course of chronic renal failure (Manninen, Evans, & Dugan, 1991). Some treatments that are effective in controlling disease lead to additional impairments. Antihypertensive drugs, though useful in preventing the complications of hypertension, may lead to depression, cognitive blunting, or sexual dysfunction (Chang et al., 1991; Croog et al., 1986). Thus, overall human function may or may not be improved by such drugs. A more extreme example is treatment that, though lifesaving, produces substantial morbidity. Thus, radiation therapy may prevent recurrence of leukemia but may lead to cognitive deficits in children (Bleyer et al., 1990). Clearly, there are many reasons that treatment of pathology may be either unavailable or unable to produce the desired improvement in function.

Conversely, it is sometimes possible to improve human function without affecting pathology. This is the business of much rehabilitation treatment. Braces or surgical contracture releases may improve gait without affecting the neurologic or orthopedic condition that led to the gait disorder (Little & Merritt, 1988; Ragnarsson, 1988). Anticholinergic drugs or self-catheterization may improve continence without affecting intrinsic bladder control (Opitz, Thorsteinsson, Schutt, Barrett, & Olson, 1988).

Finally, the number of situations is increasing where no single disease or pathologic process accounts for the bulk of an individual's disability. This is particularly common in trauma, where people may sustain multiple independent pathologic insults. It is also common in the aging population as the prevalence of independent disabling conditions, such as cardiovascular disease, arthritis, and diabetes, accumulates. In such instances (as shown in Figure 2), it may be difficult to attribute a particular functional problem to any specific disease.

For all these reasons, the correspondence between disease and resolution of disease on the one hand and dysfunction or improvement in function on the other is exceedingly complex. Many variables are likely to be at work in this relationship in any individual person. A different pattern of variables is likely to account for disability from person to person. Furthermore, in seeking to explain more global levels of function (i.e., disability, handicap, quality of life), the number of explanatory variables that may come into play grows rapidly.

APPROACHES TO THE COMPLEXITY

Given what appears to be a hopelessly complex interrelationship among variables at different levels of analysis, how can outcomes be understood and improved? Most biomedical research seeks to make the problem more manageable by focusing both treatment and outcomes assessment at the same level of analysis. Assessing antibiotic efficacy against elimination of culturable microorganisms successfully eliminates many extraneous variables from study. A similar strategy can be applied at the other levels:

1. The effectiveness of strengthening exercises can be evaluated by measuring torque generated.
2. The effectiveness of the wheelchair in improving mobility can be assessed by measuring mobility speed in the wheelchair.
3. The impact of ADA legislation can be assessed by looking at numbers of people with disabilities employed before and after the passage of the ADA.

Such approaches, represented by cells along the diagonal in Figure 1, maximize explanatory power. Conversely, in accounting for variables that are one, two, or three levels removed from the site of intervention (Cells A2–A4, B3–B4, C4), the amount of variance that can be accounted for inevitably drops.

Although such an approach makes conceptual sense from a measurement standpoint, it fails to encompass much of the real work of rehabilitation professionals. In acute rehabilitation, much effort is devoted to reducing impairments in the hope that this will lead to improvements at the disability or handicap level. Similarly, disability-level interventions are often undertaken in the hope that they will lead to more fulfilling social roles at the handicap level. Assessment of such interventions would be precluded by the strategy previously discussed.

THE IMPLICATIONS FOR MEDICAL
REHABILITATION OUTCOMES RESEARCH DESIGN

The strategy just presented may be referred to as *congruent outcome assessment*. When the treatment is aimed at the disability level (Figure 1, Cell C3), this represents an excellent research strategy. The researcher can be both rigorous and relevant by also measuring the impact of that treatment at the disability level. Similarly, the appropriate level at which to evaluate handicap policy interventions or environmental modifications would be the level of role fulfillment of affected individuals. However, there are many other important outcomes measurement questions in rehabilitation. A number of applicable research strategies are discussed below.

Ascending Assessment of Individuals with Predominant Impairments

To understand the effect of an impairment-level treatment on a disability-level outcome (Figure 1, Cell B3), it makes sense to start studying the intervention using subjects who have a single, or at least a predominant, impairment related to that disability. For example, to study the impact of good pain control on mobility function, participants should be selected who have normal strength, normal aerobic capacity, normal balance and coordination, and so forth. In this way, the relationship between their level of pain and their level of mobility would be more likely to approximate the simple linear relationship that is so rarely found. However, it should be kept in mind that, even in this simple case, *linear* is probably a misnomer; *monotonic* may be more accurate. It might be found that a certain level of pain control is required before any mobility begins to occur and that, once pain is in a mild range, mobility is no longer sensitively related to further improvements in pain control. Nevertheless, it would be important to understand this type of relationship before confounding it with additional impairments that may influence mobility function.

Although studying individuals with single impairments is a starting place for rehabilitation outcomes research, it clearly cannot be the ending place. The bulk of real-world rehabilitation patients have multiple impairments. Thus, treatments found to be effective in the simple case are likely to be ineffective in more complex situations. Further systematic steps are required to generalize the findings from the pure cases to the complex ones.

Ascending Assessment Using Single-Subject Experimental Designs

Single-subject experimental designs begin to address the complexity found in individuals with multiple impairments. For example, to improve ambulation function, an ambulation outcome can be assessed at baseline. It can then be hypothesized which set of impairments is producing that ambulation dysfunction, leading to intervention in succession with each impairment. By measuring the outcome at both the impairment and disability levels, this relationship can be clarified, as illustrated in Figure 4. For example, suppose weakness is believed to be the main cause of stair-climbing deficit. If muscle strength improves and so does stair climbing (upper-right cell), this tends to support a causal relationship. If strength improves but climbing does not (upper-left cell), it is clear that muscle weakness alone cannot account for the disability. If neither strength nor climbing improves, the hypothesis may still be correct; but the treatment chosen is ineffective even at the impairment level (lower-left cell). Finally, if strength does not improve but climbing nevertheless improves (lower-right cell), other causes must be considered (e.g., spontaneous recovery, increased motivation) for the functional improvement.

Single-subject experimental designs allow the investigation of the relationship between multiple impairments and disabilities in an individual subject, even though this precise pattern of impairments and disabilities may be unique to that subject. However, this approach poses some challenges to the development of more general models of such relationships. To return to the previous example, suppose a significant improvement in strength failed to improve climbing; when the next intervention, pain control, was added, however, ambulation improved dramatically (see Figure 5). Does this indicate that pain alone was the limiting factor for ambulation? Or does this indicate that weakness and pain together were limiting

DISABILITY OUTCOME

	No Change	Improvement
IMPAIRMENT OUTCOME — Improvement	Causal connection incomplete or disconfirmed	Causal connection confirmed
IMPAIRMENT OUTCOME — No Change	Ineffective treatment	Improvement by alternate mechanism

Figure 4. Measured changes at both the impairment and disability levels create a 2 × 2 matrix of possible outcomes and resulting interpretations. This allows clearer conclusions than can be drawn by measurement at only one level.

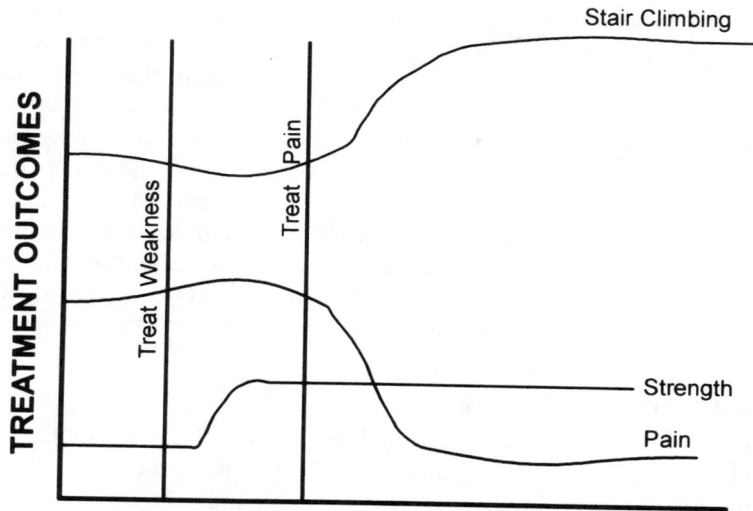

Figure 5. Results of a hypothetical single-subject experiment demonstrate the impact of two different impairment-level treatments (strengthening and pain control) on a disability-level outcome (stair climbing). Stair climbing improves only after the second treatment intervention.

climbing and that both required treatment? Distinguishing between the effects of combined treatments versus the trial-and-error identification of individual effective treatments may be difficult in a single subject. Furthermore, the process of reaching conclusions about "the generic individual with an ambulation dysfunction" is unclear from single-subject methods alone.

Multivariate Research Designs

If many different variables at one level may influence a variable at a higher level, why not study them all? For example, a study might measure muscle strength, balance, endurance, coordination, and so forth and also measure ambulation function. A multivariate model then could be developed that provides different weights to the different impairments in leading to ambulation dysfunction. Presumably, treatment of an impairment that has the greatest weight (assuming an effective treatment exists) should have the highest chance of leading to an improved ambulation outcome. However, if the highest weight is associated with an impairment for which no effective treatment exists, this would suggest a very limited prognosis despite successful intervention with the remaining impairments.

This should be viewed as the ultimate goal of theory building within rehabilitation and studies of integrated human function. However, its achievement is a long way off, except in very limited realms. If the variable to be explained is as global as, for example, return to work, then the number of impairments and disabilities that might contribute to that outcome becomes unmanageable. Additionally, just as the relationship between pairs of variables may not be simple and linear, this is also true in a complex multivariate model. It may be that weakness is relevant to gait dysfunction only if it is greater than a certain degree, or it may be that pain interacts with weakness in ways that differ from those experienced by individuals who have pain or weakness alone, and so on. Thus, such model building represents a late stage following systematic study of simple functional areas, improvements in quantitative measurement in many of the relevant impairments and disabilities, and improvements in statistical procedures for examining nonlinear and interactive relationships among variables.

Clinical Trials of Decision Algorithms

In everyday life, rehabilitation clinicians assign collections of treatments to patients. Although rarely studied explicitly, the process of treatment assignment implicitly involves a mental model similar to the formal model discussed previously. That is, the clinician determines that an individual has a particular disability, determines that he or she has a set of impairments, and develops hypotheses about the causal relationships between those impairments and the disability. An informal estimate can be made of the relative importance of each of the impairments in producing the disability and the likelihood of success in treating each of these impairments. If this implicit process is made explicit, then it can be tested in terms of the outcomes it produces.

Suppose an ambulation dysfunction treatment algorithm were developed. The algorithm would accept all individuals with an ambulation dysfunction and would take their scores on a variety of impairments as input variables (see Figure 6). Depending on those scores, a different collection of treatments might be assigned to different individuals, but the desired outcome would be improved ambulation in all cases. Despite the heterogeneity of the patients, the efficacy of the treatment algorithm, rather than the individual treatments, could be tested. This approach has been employed to reduce the incidence of falls in older adults (Tinetti et al., 1994).

Such an approach requires a great deal of background work in making explicit the implicit knowledge of experienced clinicians. However, this process is beginning through the development of practice parameters and clinical guidelines. It is less critical that such guidelines be correct than that they be systematic and lawful. The outcomes data will help determine in what ways these clinical protocols need to be modified. However, this modification will certainly require supplementation with other research strategies. For example, it is quite likely that some patients treated under such an algorithm will have poor functional outcomes, but the reasons for

ASSESSMENT AND TREATMENT ALGORITHM

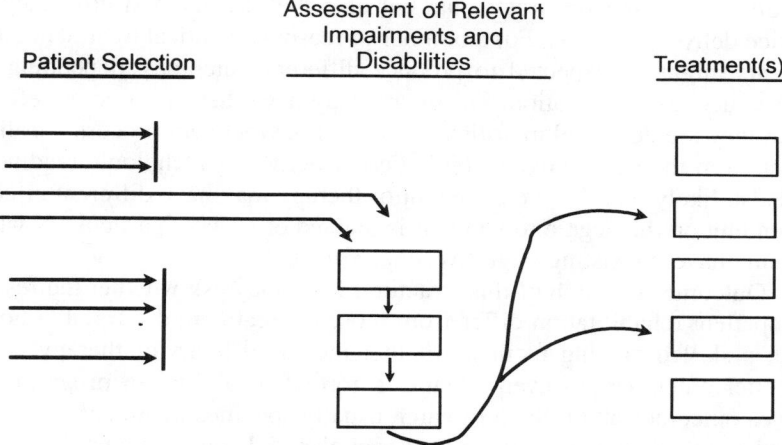

Figure 6.   Screening for a variety of patient selection variables is shown in the left-hand column. Only those patients meeting selection criteria enter the algorithm where the impairments and disabilities relevant to the algorithm are assessed. Assessment results in the application of (in this example) two of many possible treatment interventions.

treatment failure may not be self-evident. Additional formal research will be required to identify the differences between the successes and failures in terms of their impairment and disability patterns at the onset of treatment or in terms of other confounding factors that may not have been included in the treatment algorithm.

Longitudinal Ascending and Descending Designs

Although all of the research designs discussed previously require time to complete, none of them addresses the unfolding of events over time in an explicit manner. However, an additional aspect of research involves this question of longitudinal development. For example, perhaps a certain degree of lower-extremity weakness will not cause any ambulation dysfunction immediately; but if it leads to accelerated joint degeneration, ambulation dysfunction may occur prematurely in the course of the next 10 years. Also, as mentioned previously, problems with vocational and social reintegration may lead to secondary morbidity, rehospitalization, and so forth. Such long-term outcomes questions require supplementation of the basic designs with a longitudinal time frame. Thus, the interrelationships among variables across levels at a given moment in time and how this relationship changes over time need to be investigated.

ASSESSMENT OF SERVICE DELIVERY OUTCOMES

The primary focus of outcomes research in rehabilitation has been not just the efficacy of specific treatments but also the efficacy and efficiency of service delivery systems. For a number of reasons, identical treatment components might be expected to produce different outcomes, depending on their structural organization. Treatments may have their most potent effects when they are delivered in critical periods of the recovery process—critical either from the perspective of biologic plasticity or psychologic readiness. It is also likely that the same amount of therapy may have different effects, depending on the degree to which it is massed or spaced, particularly when patients have coexisting cognitive impairments.

Outcomes research of this structural form may ask whether the results of inpatient rehabilitation differ from those of treatment delivered at home or in a skilled nursing facility, whether increased hours of therapy result in better outcomes, or even whether a formal rehabilitation program improves outcomes at all. Such research usually specifies treatment only very grossly, either categorically (e.g., hospital-based versus home-based) or quantitatively (e.g., number of hours of physical therapy).

Although the results of service delivery system–based outcomes research can potentially lead to more cost-effective achievement of specific outcomes and possibly even to better outcomes, there is a theoretical limit to how far system-based research can lead. Ultimately, all of the slack may be squeezed from existing service delivery systems. At that point, improved outcomes can be achieved only by examining the efficacy of individual components of the black box that constitutes the service delivery system. Thus, researchers need to be concerned not just with the number of hours of physical therapy but also with what actually takes place during that time. In the final analysis, there needs to be an interplay between research focused on individual treatments and that focused on systems of care; the most effective service delivery systems are ultimately those that organize *effective components* into *efficient systems*.

AN INTEGRATED APPROACH

A comprehensive understanding of rehabilitation outcomes is a mammoth undertaking. It requires understanding the outcomes of individual treatments directed at individual impairments and disabilities. It also requires the study of rehabilitation health care delivery systems and how they deploy those treatments within various kinds of infrastructures over various time courses. No single research strategy alone is up to the task, and no one has proceeded far enough along this path to provide authoritative guidelines on the appropriate uses of particular research strategies in particular contexts. Nevertheless, it is appropriate to try to place the different research strategies into some semblance of order.

Some basic methodologic and statistical progress is required to advance outcomes research through any of these methods. Further development and validation of specific measures of the various impairments, disabilities, and handicaps are also critical. Only by developing measures that can be cleanly interpreted as lying at a particular level of analysis can interrelationships among levels be coherently explored. Ideally, this measurement development will result in interval measures suitable for parametric statistical techniques. However, in many instances, it will not be possible to develop interval measures, and even when interval measures are developed, the scores in many rehabilitation populations are likely to deviate so greatly from normality that parametric techniques may not be applied. Thus, it is important to develop sophisticated, multivariate, nonparametric statistical techniques and to speed dissemination of statistical innovations from other disciplines.

Beyond basic tool development is the consideration of the order of application of these various research techniques. Use of relatively pure cases and detailed use of single-subject experimental designs represent good initial phases for outcomes studies intended to understand the effects of specific treatments. As the results of these studies accrue, they can lead to formal testing through multivariate models. Statistical approaches such as structural equations modeling can be used to quantify the causal connections in such complex models (Bentler & Stein, 1992). Further confirmation can occur through intervention trials involving clinical decision algorithms based on those multivariate models. Longitudinal studies represent an additional step because they presume some understanding of the more immediate interrelationships among outcomes at different levels of analysis. Although these strategies are presented in sequence, clearly there needs to be an iterative process whereby failures of the more complex models lead to further detailed studies of specific problem areas through additional single-subject or pure case approaches.

Qualitative research can also be extremely useful in helping to understand atypical cases or deviations from a model. Patients and clinicians can be questioned in an open-ended fashion about their perceptions of why treatments did not work, and these findings can then be tested more formally.

CONCLUSIONS

Medical rehabilitation outcomes research is an ambitious undertaking. It requires consideration of variables at many levels of analysis from tissue to social system, and it is challenged by the fact that suitable definitions, measurements, and statistical and experimental procedures are not fully developed. Although there is a long way to go before the medical rehabilitation outcomes research enterprise can be fully realized, a clear conceptualization of the hierarchy and nature of the obstacles facing medical rehabilitation outcomes research is an essential first step. In addition, this perspective suggests that rehabilitation research training should expose trainees to a broad array of disciplines that cross these levels and should impart to trainees an understanding of where their contributions fit in a much larger picture. Finally, this conceptualization suggests that rehabilitation outcomes research funding must be targeted to help build large, multidisciplinary, collaborative research endeavors, because no individual researcher or research laboratory can adequately address all of the relevant concepts.

REFERENCES

Americans with Disabilities Act (ADA) of 1990, PL 101-336, 42 U.S.C. §§ 12101 *et seq.*

Association of Academic Physiatrists. (1991). National Center for Medical Rehabilitation Research: The disabling process. *Association of Academic Physiatrists Newsletter, 9*(4), 38.

Bentler, P.M., & Stein, J.A. (1992). Structural equation models in medical research. *Statistical Methods of Medical Research, 1,* 159–181.

Bleyer, W.A., Fallavollita, J., Robison, L., Balsom, W., Meadows, A., Heyn, R., Sitarz, A., Ortega, J., Miller, D., Lonstine, L., et al. (1990). Influence of age, sex, and concurrent intrathecal methotrexate therapy on intellectual function after cranial irradiation during childhood: A report from the Children's Cancer Study Group. *Pediatric Hematology and Oncology, 7*(4), 329–338.

Chang, S.W., Fine, R., Siegel, D., Chesney, M., Black, D., & Hulley, S.B. (1991). The impact of diuretic therapy in reported sexual dysfunction. *Archives of Internal Medicine, 151*(12), 2402–2408.

Croog, S.H., Levine, S., Testa, M.A., Brown, B., Bulpitt, C.J., Jenkins, C.D., Klerman, G.L., & Williams, G.H. (1986). The effects of anti-hypertensive therapy on quality of life. *New England Journal of Medicine, 314*(26), 1657–1664.

Fowler, W.M., Jr. (1981). Viability of physical medicine and rehabilitation in the 1980's. *Archives of Physical Medicine and Rehabilitation, 63,* 1–5.

Fuhrer, M.J. (1981). Medical rehabilitation research: Distortions, deflections, and detractions. *Archives of Physical Medicine and Rehabilitation, 63,* 49–54.

Fuhrer, M.J., Rintala, D.H., Hart, K.A., Clearman, R., & Young, M.E. (1992). Relationship of life satisfaction to impairment, disability, and handicap among persons with spinal cord injury living in the community. *Archives of Physical Medicine and Rehabilitation, 73,* 552–557.

Lawton, M.P. (1991). A multidimensional view of quality of life in frail elders. In J.E. Birren, J.E. Lubben, J.C. Rowe, & D.E. Deutchman (Eds.), *The concept and measurement of quality of life in the frail elderly* (pp. 3–27). New York: Academic Press.

Little, J.W., & Merritt, J.L. (1988). Spasticity and associated abnormalities of muscle tone. In J.A. DeLisa (Ed.), *Rehabilitation medicine: Principles and practice* (pp. 430–447). Philadelphia: J.B. Lippincott.

Manninen, D.L., Evans, R.W., & Dugan, M.K. (1991). Work disability, functional limitations, and health status of kidney transplantation recipients posttransplant. *Clinical Transplants,* 193–203.

Nagi, S. (1991). Disability concepts revisited: Implications for prevention. In A.M. Pope & A.R. Tarlov (Eds.), *Disability in America: Toward a national agenda for prevention* (pp. 309–327). Washington, DC: National Academy Press.

Opitz, J.L., Thorsteinsson, G., Schutt, A.H., Barrett, D.M., & Olson, P.K. (1988). Neurogenic bladder and bowel. In J.A. DeLisa (Ed.), *Rehabilitation medicine: Principles and practice* (pp. 492–518). Philadelphia: J.B. Lippincott.

Ragnarsson, K.T. (1988). Orthotics and shoes. In J.A. DeLisa (Ed.), *Rehabilitation medicine: Principles and practice* (pp. 307–329). Philadelphia: J.B. Lippincott.

Tinetti, M.E., Baker, D.I., McAvay, G., Claus, E.B., Garrett, P., Gottschalk, M., Koch, M.L., Trainor, K., & Horwitz, R.I. (1994). A multifactorial intervention to reduce the risk of falling among elderly people living in the community. *New England Journal of Medicine, 331*(13), 821–827.

Whyte, J. (1994). Toward a methodology for rehabilitation research. *American Journal of Physical Medicine and Rehabilitation, 73,* 428–435.

World Health Organization (WHO). (1980). *International classification of impairments, disabilities, and handicaps.* Geneva, Switzerland: Author.

CHAPTER 3

Value Perspectives and the Challenge of Managed Care

Gerben DeJong

Although seldom acknowledged, societal and professional values are central to the outcomes research enterprise. Researchers bring their own values and baggage to the outcomes research process. Many never have to challenge their values, because they work, collaborate, and live with like-minded people who share many, if not most, of the same values. Therein lies both a strength and a weakness. The strength is the ability to proceed with operationalizing key concepts without reopening larger value issues at each turn. The weakness is the possible failure to note the extent to which outcomes measures and the values implicit in them are also a function of the particular community of interest represented.

In short, outcomes measures arise, as do the values implicit in them, from a particular social, professional, and economic context. This context is changing, largely because of the rise of managed care and capitation payment as the dominant methods of health service delivery and financing in the 1990s. The managed care revolution is restructuring the relationships among providers, consumers, and payers and is reshaping the role of health outcomes measures in American health care.

PURPOSE AND SCOPE

The purpose of this chapter is twofold. First, it seeks to underscore how approaches to medical rehabilitation outcomes, and health outcomes in

This chapter was supported in part by the National Rehabilitation Hospital (NRH) Research Center's Research and Training Center on Medical Rehabilitation Services and Health Policy, which is funded by Grant H133B40025 from the National Institute on Disability and Rehabilitation Research. The views expressed are those of the author and do not necessarily reflect the views of the NRH Research Center, the National Rehabilitation Hospital, the Medlantic Research Institute, or any other organization with which the author is affiliated.

general, are a function of values and the represented community of interest (i.e., providers, consumers, payers, researchers) (Banja & Johnston, 1994). Researchers often focus on issues of validity and reliability without asking more fundamental questions about the values implicit in outcomes measures. This chapter argues that people all bring their own baggage to the outcomes research process, but, as a society, Americans share a remarkable consensus about a number of key values that are not always adequately represented in outcomes measures. This chapter makes more explicit the various value assumptions and perspectives that govern approaches to outcomes measurement in medical rehabilitation.

Second, the chapter seeks to determine the likely impact of managed care on the role of medical rehabilitation outcomes in the payer-dominated health care system of the mid-1990s and its probable role in a more consumer-driven health care system that is emerging. This chapter argues that, if it is to be responsive to the anticipated consumer-driven system, the medical rehabilitation community must achieve consensus on outcomes measures that can be used in report cards to rate health plans and provider networks. This chapter also calls for research on the development of meaningful risk adjusters that can be used to compare outcomes across health plans and providers by risk-adjusting outcomes on the basis of facility or program case mix.

This chapter has seven objectives:

1. To identify some of the value perspectives that different provider, consumer, and payer constituencies bring to medical rehabilitation outcomes research
2. To address some of the unacknowledged cross-cultural issues in medical rehabilitation outcomes
3. To identify how some of the different research tools and outcomes measures of various research communities (i.e., trauma care, medical rehabilitation, aging and long-term care, developmental disabilities, mental health, health services) also serve latent professional self-interests, an unacknowledged social value in its own right
4. To address how level of function relates to some of the core societal values shared across various constituencies and to discuss the implications of these core values for the future of outcomes research in medical rehabilitation
5. To describe the impact of managed care on medical rehabilitation service delivery and to note the absence of genuine quality competition
6. To look at the emerging consumer side of the health care market, evaluate its probable impact on the use of medical rehabilitation outcomes measures, and note the need for research on the development of risk-adjustment methods

7. To make more explicit how medical rehabilitation outcomes and their use serve the interests of key stakeholders

DIFFERENT CONSTITUENCIES

Provider Perspectives

The provider perspective has dominated thinking in medical rehabilitation outcomes and has had perhaps the greatest impact on the development of the most commonly used outcomes measures in medical rehabilitation. The provider perspective reflects the manner in which health care, until the rise of managed care, generally has been a provider-driven enterprise where professional autonomy, beneficence, and confidentiality were paramount values.

The medical rehabilitation provider community is not monolithic. It is composed of its own subconstituencies that include administrators, physicians, and allied health professionals (e.g., nursing, physical therapy, occupational therapy, speech-language pathology, psychology, social work, respiratory therapy). Each brings its own perspective. Allied health professionals, for example, place special emphasis on their particular domain of interest. For instance, it has been said somewhat facetiously that occupational therapists are concerned with upper-limb function, physical therapists are concerned with lower-limb function, and nursing is concerned with everything in between.

Nonetheless, medical rehabilitation places a high value on the team approach to patient care. This approach also is reflected in the ability of medical rehabilitation professionals to achieve consensus on a number of outcomes issues and measures. Collectively, the outcomes model that dominates medical rehabilitation is the functional limitations or enhancements model that has its clearest expression in consensus measures such as the Functional Independence Measure (FIM) (State University of New York at Buffalo, 1993). Although the consensus is stable, professional tugs of war continue as different allied health disciplines insist that their domain of interest is not adequately represented and that the FIM is too gross to capture some of the finer increments of functional improvement.

Within medical rehabilitation, especially among administrators, an additional perspective has emerged—namely, a business and marketing perspective that has paralleled the growing commoditization of health care during the 1980s and 1990s, whereby health care is marketed much like other commodities. This perspective emphasizes patient or consumer satisfaction: "Was our consumer pleased with how he or she was treated and with the services received?" The business and marketing perspective of providers converges with many of the issues of immediate concern to the consumer. The marketing perspective is, in a sense, a crossover perspective from the provider side to the consumer side of the market.

Consumer Perspectives

The concept of consumer satisfaction embraces a number of different dimensions that can best be illustrated with a series of questions:

- *Perception of benefit:* Did the consumer believe that he or she benefited from the service obtained?
- *Manner of service delivery:* Was the consumer satisfied with the manner in which the services were rendered in terms of waiting time, level of professional courtesy, and the degree to which the consumer's views were taken into account?
- *Level of accommodation:* Was the consumer satisfied with the accommodations and amenities provided, such as the food service, visiting hours, access to a telephone, noise level, and overall comfort of the room?

To the clinician, some of these issues may seem secondary to the functional outcomes actually achieved. The issue is, Whose perspective should prevail? Increased appreciation for the consumer perspective has made consumer satisfaction an outcomes dimension in its own right, but it is often ascertained apart from other outcomes issues. An increasing number of medical rehabilitation facilities, however, now include consumer satisfaction questions with functional status questions in their follow-up surveys of former patients.

There is another consumer perspective that emerges, not from the consumer of the marketplace but from the adherents of the independent living and disability rights (IL–DR) movement, who emphasize the values of independence, personal autonomy, and self-direction. The values of the IL–DR movement resonate with important American values such as independence, personal responsibility, and control over one's own life. For IL–DR adherents, independence in activities of daily living, which is valued by rehabilitation clinicians, is secondary to independence in making informed choices that lead to control over one's own life. Consider, for example, the definition of *independent living* preferred by the National Council on the Handicapped (1986; now the National Council on Disability), adapted from the definition used by Frieden, Richards, Cole, and Baley (1979):

> Independence is control over one's life based on the choice of acceptable options that minimize reliance on others in making decisions and in performing everyday activities. This includes managing one's day-to-day affairs, participating fully in community life, fulfilling a range of social roles and making decisions that lead to self-determination and the minimization of nonproductive physical and psychological dependence upon others. Independence implies an optimally responsible and productive exercise of the power of choice. It further implies that each

disabled person, regardless of his or her mental or physical ability, should be encouraged and assisted, with due respect for cultural or sub-cultural affiliation, to achieve a high quality of life, and to achieve independence and productivity in the least restrictive environment. Independent living is intended to apply to persons with all types of disabilities. (National Council on the Handicapped, 1986)

Independent living is a fairly straightforward concept that can be captured, in part, by behavioral indicators such as the extent to which a person is living in an unstructured environment or participating in work or other productive activities. The concept of *independence*, in the sense of self-direction, is a more problematic concept that is difficult to operationalize and measure. As a result, it is seldom invoked in social and behavioral science research: "Whereas locus of control, attribution, motivation, perseverance, achievement style, autonomy, learned helplessness, and dependency are well represented in the literature, *the affirmative, composite construct of independence* has not been the subject of extensive analysis" (Nosek, 1987; emphasis added). In other words, the converse of independence—namely, various forms of dependence—is more likely to be evaluated. This state of affairs suggests a preoccupation with social pathology, dysfunction, and what is wrong with the individual rather than what is right. It examines function at or below zero and often misses creative and life-fulfilling function above zero; thus, it fails to capture people with disabilities as people leading full and productive lives.

At the core of the consumer perspective is the notion that the individual consumer is the only and ultimate judge of whether the outcome was good or appropriate. According to this perspective, attempts to evaluate outcomes on the basis of objective criteria, applied across groups of people, are flawed because they do not take into account individual differences and preferences. This is the consumer of the marketplace, where the customer is always right. If taken to its logical conclusion, this perspective would suggest that the concept of consumer satisfaction may ultimately be the only valid measure of outcomes. Self-report, not clinical assessment, then also becomes the only valid way in which to measure outcomes.

It would be easy to dismiss such a perspective because it does not take into account the larger interests of a society that is concerned about how its resources are allocated to help ameliorate the functional losses sustained by people with disabilities. Yet if the objective measures of outcomes do not in some way reflect the central concerns for consumers, then something is missing in the repertoire of outcomes measures.

This is not to suggest that people with disabilities are not concerned with functional enhancement; they are. The goal of functional enhancement may be different for the consumer than for the provider, however. In some instances, functional enhancement may not be important at all. For example, if a certain functional activity—say, dressing—can be done independently but takes 2 hours to achieve, this functional objective may be secondary to other important life goals (e.g., gainful work, supervising minor children) that are not within the immediate province of the medical rehabilitation provider.

The consumer perspective also raises an issue about the direction of accountability. As in many other areas of health and human services, accountability in medical rehabilitation flows in two directions: to the consumer, that is, responsiveness (Accountability 1), and to the funding source (Accountability 2). When an individual pays for services from his or her own pocket, payer and recipient of the service are one and the same, and only Accountability 1 is relevant. When payer and recipient are different, both forms of accountability are relevant.

Accountability 2 requires the development of outcomes criteria that can be applied across groups of people but that do not preclude consumer perspectives. Accountability 2 needs to embrace outcomes concepts that relate to the values of both the target population and the larger society that is paying for the services. Accountability 1 and 2 need not be mutually exclusive; however, it is difficult to embrace fully the values of both within a single measure of outcome.

The term *consumer* is sometimes used to include family members such as parents who advocate for their children and adult children who advocate for an older parent. Although the typical adult consumer is concerned with issues of satisfaction, self-direction, and choice, family members are more concerned with issues such as safety, permanence, stability, and comfort. The onset of a disabling condition in a child invokes the protective instincts of a parent; the onset of a disabling condition in an older parent arouses the concerns of adult children that mom or dad is comfortable and well provided for.

This particular consumer perspective is often at odds with the consumer perspective of the IL–DR movement that values personal autonomy and choice. The initial adherents of the IL portion of the movement were critical, if not hostile, to parents of children with disabilities. The initial adherents were mostly younger and middle-age adults with physical impairments (e.g., spinal cord injury, post-polio, cerebral palsy) who valued their new-found independence from parents and did not want parental values to resurface in their lives through the back door of their own advocacy efforts.

Payer Perspectives

Payer understanding of medical rehabilitation outcomes remains largely underdeveloped. In 1990, the National Rehabilitation Hospital (NRH) Research Center conducted an informal telephone survey of people representing payers who included indemnity insurers, managed care organizations (e.g., HMOs), Medicare, Medicaid (at both the federal and state levels), worker's compensation, reinsurers, and employer-based benefit managers (DeJong, 1990). Each respondent from these organizations had a major responsibility for determining whether his or her organization would pay for medical rehabilitation at either an individual level or a group level.

As a group, respondents demonstrated very little knowledge about what medical rehabilitation is, what it does, and what its outcomes are supposed to be. In discussing *outcomes,* respondents focused primarily on *inputs.* For example, they focused on utilization issues or input issues such as the 3-hour therapy rule and whether length of stay exceeded expected length of stay. A few mentioned postrehabilitation outcomes such as return to work, outdoor mobility (e.g., use of transportation), need for help at home, and impact on family. Issues of functional status (i.e., activities of daily living skills) came up only once.

The level of sophistication varied by type of payer. Representatives of Medicare, the single largest payer of medical rehabilitation, and Medicaid had surprisingly little knowledge of medical rehabilitation. Reinsurers had the best understanding of medical rehabilitation. Because of their long-term liability for the well-being of the patient, reinsurers were especially interested in the ability to avert postrehabilitation medical complications and subsequent use of hospital care.

Much has changed since 1990 in the face of the managed care revolution that has swept American health care. Managed care payers, as noted later in this chapter, still are not as concerned about outcomes as they are about cost and price. As a generalization, it is fair to say that payers are mainly concerned about the financial and cost implications of medical rehabilitation service delivery. As their attention turns more to outcomes issues, they will be particularly concerned about outcomes that have economic consequences such as reduced need for hands-on care and rehospitalization.

CROSS-CULTURAL ISSUES

Medical rehabilitation cannot escape the increasing ethnic and racial diversity of the American population. Immigration, for example, accounted for 30% of the U.S. population growth between 1980 and 1990. Asian and Latino or Hispanic individuals accounted for about 70% of new immigrants during the 1980s. By 2030, the minority population of the United States is expected to be 33%. By 2020, California's Caucasian population, as a proportion of the total population, is projected to fall to 46%, down from 57% in 1990. By 2040, California's Hispanic population is projected to become the largest population group (California Department of Finance,

Demographic Unit, personal communication, November 1993). Across the United States, a disproportionate share of the minority population, in age-adjusted terms, is more likely to have adverse health conditions and is more likely to have participated in violence-prone activities that lead to injury and to a need for medical rehabilitation services.

As indicated earlier, both provider and consumer perspectives reflect many of the values that dominate American culture, such as independence, personal autonomy, choice and informed consent, self-sufficiency, competitiveness, and "making it." These values can be contrasted with some of the values of other cultures that place more emphasis on interdependence, group well-being, parental and family consent, group support, cooperation and reciprocity, and simply "being" as opposed to "making it." (See expanded list of contrasts in Table 1.) The values of other cultures are probably more difficult to operationalize because the benefits often accrue to the group rather than to the individual. Outcomes analysis is usually easier when the unit of observation is the individual rather than a group or family unit.

The values of other cultures are not likely to become a major factor in medical rehabilitation outcomes for two reasons. First, the dominant political themes of the mid-1990s emphasize the primacy of the individual and his or her need to take responsibility for his or her own well-being, despite the rhetoric about family values. If anything, traditional American values are becoming even more pronounced. Second, the cultural values of immigrants are likely to be muted. Many immigrants, especially those

Table 1.   Contrasting values

Dominant Caucasian values	Other cultures' values
Personal control over the environment	Fate
Change	Tradition
Time dominates	Human interaction dominates
Human equality	Hierarchy / rank / status
Central: The individual	Central: Family, group, community
Individualism / privacy	Group welfare
Choice, informed consent	Parental / family consent
Self-help, merit	Birthright, inheritance
Independence	Interdependence
Competition	Cooperation, reciprocity
Future orientation	Past orientation
Action / goal / work orientation, "making it"	"Being" orientation
Informality	Formality
Directness / openness / honesty	Indirectness / ritual / "face"
Practicality / efficiency	Idealism / theory
Materialism	Spiritualism / detachment

Adapted from U.S. Department of Agriculture (1986).

who immigrate for economic reasons rather than for political reasons, are a self-selected group who have values that are congruent with the dominant American culture, such as the willingness to take risks, work hard, become self-reliant, and succeed in the new country.

PERSPECTIVES OF OTHER RESEARCH COMMUNITIES

Medical rehabilitation has developed its own research agenda and its own approach to outcomes measurement. At the same time, medical rehabilitation operates at the intersection of several other research traditions and communities whose approaches to outcomes measurement have influenced medical rehabilitation. These research communities bring both competing and complementary values to the field. Five of these research communities are noted here:

1. Trauma care
2. Aging and long-term care
3. Developmental disabilities
4. Mental health
5. Health services research (see Appendix at end of this chapter)

These communities can be distinguished along seven dimensions:

1. The particular patient or client population served
2. Their linkage to a specific service delivery system
3. Their particular academic base or primary academic disciplines
4. Their respective professional organizations
5. Their respective journals, newsletters, and other publications
6. Their own array of research tools, indices, and outcomes measures
7. Their array of funding sources, that is, federal agencies and private foundations

Each community brings its own history, tradition, research paradigms, values, and particular toolkit to the issue of outcomes.

The juxtaposition of the five research communities along these seven dimensions illustrates how outcomes measures are also a function of the values, perceptions, and outlooks indigenous to a particular research community. To paraphrase Elliot Richardson, former cabinet member in the Nixon administration, "Where I stand is a function of where I sit." Medical rehabilitation is no less exempt from this observation than any other field of inquiry.

More important, the juxtaposition of the five research communities indicates the extent to which outcomes measures may be rooted in the need for professional identity and legitimacy. Thus, outcomes measures directly or indirectly have latent social roles in that they serve to help to legitimize a particular professional endeavor, establish territoriality, and contain a strong element of professional self-interest.

Although seemingly independent at times, each research community is becoming increasingly dependent on the insights and measures of other research communities. For example, as trauma care succeeds in averting preventable deaths, attention inevitably turns to the functional status of survivors as a material outcomes issue for trauma care. Since 1980, as medical rehabilitation has expanded into traumatic brain injury, it has had to look to the cognitive sciences and to the mental health community for measures of function and outcome. Likewise, medical rehabilitation has had to look to the developmental disabilities literature for adapting functional status measures to take into account the developmental stages of a pediatric rehabilitation population.

Four trends in health care are challenging the traditional provincialism, or boundaries, of each research community and its approach to outcomes. First is the health outcomes movement, which seeks, among other things, to define a more generic cross-disciplinary set of outcomes measures that can transcend the perspectives of each research community. The development of the 36-Item Short Form Health Survey (SF-36) is perhaps the clearest example to date of the search for a universal outcomes metric (Stewart & Ware, 1992; Ware & Sherbourne, 1992). The quest for a universal outcomes standard has some inherent limits because no outcomes measure can do justice to all relevant domains of function and still remain short and simple enough to be administered reliably in a variety of settings. Second, as noted earlier, is the growing activism among consumers within each of these communities that is challenging the conventional wisdom of professionals. Third is the drive toward managed care and the development of integrated service networks. Fourth is the emergence of what the author believes will be a consumer-driven health care system, in which consumers will choose health plans on the basis of outcomes and other quality indicators, sometimes in the form of health care report cards. (The notion of an emerging consumer-driven health care system is not to be confused with the consumer activism already present within most communities of interest.)

Medical rehabilitation will have much to offer as the boundaries between research communities become more pervious and as various research communities begin to pool their perspectives with respect to outcomes. Of the various research communities noted here, medical rehabilitation has probably given the most thought to distinctions such as pathology, impairment, functional limitation, and disability. Other research communities often fail to make these conceptual distinctions, which sometimes leads to confusion in outcomes discourse and outcomes measurement.

LEVELS OF FUNCTION AND SOCIETAL PERSPECTIVES

Levels of Function

Wilkerson (1996) made a useful distinction among micro, meso, and macro levels of function—in short, a hierarchy of functions wherein a previous level of function is needed to achieve the next level of function (see Table 2). Although one must be able to do many of the micro-level functions to perform meso-level functions, the relationship between meso- and macro-level functions is not as straightforward. The performance of meso-level functions can aid greatly in the performance of macro-level functions; but the ability to perform macro-level functions is not solely dependent on the ability to perform meso-level functions, because macro-level functions also depend on the level of environmental accommodation. (Wilkerson's [1996] hierarchy or levels of function bear some resemblance to the progression implicit in various disability classification schemes that make distinctions among concepts such as *injury/pathology*, *impairment*, *functional limitation*, *disability*, and *societal limitation*, where each prior state is a risk factor for succeeding states.)

Meso-level functions can also be labeled *skills*, that is, the ability to perform certain activities in socially appropriate ways. Medical rehabilitation is skill enhancement. In other words, medical rehabilitation is

Table 2. Levels of function

Micro
- Range of motion
- Memory
- Cognition
- Strength
- Endurance

Meso
- Activities of daily living
- Walking
- Wheelchair propulsion
- Talking, operating equipment
- Interacting with people

Macro
- Working
- Parenting
- Recreation
- Homemaking
- Social life
- Community participation
- Creating

From Wilkerson, D. (1996). *Level of function as an organizing framework for functional assessment applications.* Manuscript submitted for publication.

largely, though not exclusively, targeted to the acquisition or enhancement of meso-level functions or skills. In one sense, the acquisition of specific skills is a legitimate outcome in its own right. In a larger sense, the acquisition of skills is intended to achieve higher-order outcomes such as those at the macro level (e.g., working, participating in family and community life).

The mere acquisition of skills has little intrinsic meaning if these skills do not enable a person to participate in higher-order (macro-level) activities or roles that have real consequences for the individual and society. An example from education would be knowing whether the skills learned in school translate into jobs, income, and citizen participation in later life. Getting good grades and test scores has little intrinsic value if they do not relate to other life goals. If there is lack of correlation between what is learned in school and success in the workplace, the skills that are being taught are reexamined.

The value that we place on skills (meso-level) versus higher-order (macro-level) activities depends in part on when the assessment is being made. The closer to the actual intervention, the more concern there is about skill enhancement outcomes as opposed to higher-order outcomes such as participation in family and community life. Thus, upon discharge from medical rehabilitation, the outcomes deemed important are those that mainly relate to skill enhancement. At follow-up, the outcomes deemed important begin to shift to a broader array of issues such as where a person lives and whether a person works (Whiteneck, Charlifue, Gerhart, Overholser, & Richardson, 1992; Willer, Rosenthal, Kreutzer, Gordon, & Rempel, 1993).

Some of the more generic outcomes measures that relate to overall health status, such as the Sickness Impact Profile (Bergner, Bobbitt, Carter, & Gelson, 1981) and the SF-36 (Ware & Sherbourne, 1992), represent a blend of functional status (meso-level) and higher-order (macro-level) outcomes. The SF-36, for example, addresses both activities of daily living limitations and work and social activities.

Societal Perspectives

Questions remain with regard to societal perspectives on medical rehabilitation outcomes. Is there a set of outcomes that transcends the various perspectives and values described in this chapter? Does our society subscribe to certain core values that can also be the basis for a consensus set of outcomes measures for medical rehabilitation, especially at the macro level? If searching for such a set of measures, where might one begin to look? A revealing, albeit incomplete, answer can be found in the following scenario.

Imagine being asked to testify before a congressional committee or state legislative committee. Assume also that you believe in the efficacy of medical rehabilitation as a therapeutic intervention. At stake is whether your state government is prepared to include medical rehabilitation services as part of its state Medicaid plan. What common values or outcomes would you invoke to establish medical rehabilitation's claim to resources? What values or outcomes would resonate with consumers, public officials, and society at large? Sooner or later you probably would make reference to one or more of the following three sets of long-term outcomes:

1. The degree to which a person can *live independently*, that is, Can the individual live in a relatively unstructured living arrangement that provides for a maximum degree of self-direction and development and requires a minimum of supervision or hands-on care?
2. The degree to which a person can *live actively and productively*, not only in terms of gainful work but also in terms of contributions to family and community life
3. The degree to which a person can *maintain health* and *avert medical complications* that result in costly medical interventions, especially inpatient care (DeJong, 1987)

These outcomes concepts require operationalization as outcomes measures; some outcomes measures already incorporate one or more of these concepts.

The three outcomes concepts not only resonate with key societal values but also address the economic interests of society. Each outcomes concept contains an inherent economic component: Living in a highly structured environment, remaining inactive or unproductive, and failing to maintain health have enormous economic consequences for both the individual and society. In other words, these outcomes are also surrogates for the economic values and considerations that play a role in resource allocation decisions.

These outcomes are not absolute and may reflect important trade-offs in the lives of people with disabilities. For example, people sometimes need more hands-on assistance to live more actively and productively. Thus, a higher value may be placed on being productive than on being independent in various activities of daily living.

Society's economic interests are likely to become more important in American health care as payers, not providers, come to dominate health care decision making and resource allocation decisions in the future. This has become clear in the rapid rise of managed care as the dominant mode of health care delivery and finance in American health care.

MANAGED CARE

Since the mid-1980s, American health care has been undergoing a major transformation from a provider-driven, fee-for-service system to a payer-driven, managed care system that is significantly altering the financial incentives that shape provider and consumer behaviors. The issue, for purposes of this chapter, is how the transformation to a managed health care system is restructuring the medical rehabilitation industry and how it is likely to redefine the role of medical rehabilitation outcomes.

A central feature of this transformation is the use of capitation financing, in which financial risk is transferred from the payer to the provider, who is at risk for all or part of the costs incurred in delivering patient care. Capitation financing can take many forms. In some instances, an entire network of providers may be at risk for all of the health care needed by a subscriber pool in a given year. In other instances, only selected providers are at risk for an episode of care as in the case of acute care hospitals that participate in the Medicare diagnostic-related groups (DRGs) method of financing, in which hospitals are paid a fixed price for a given diagnosis. Regardless of its exact form, capitation financing creates powerful incentives for providers to restrain or reduce costs and prices.

Impact on Medical Rehabilitation

Until the mid-1990s, medical rehabilitation had been sheltered from the managed care revolution. Because 70% of its revenues come from Medicare, inpatient medical rehabilitation has been largely a Medicare product (DeJong & Sutton, 1995). As of 1995, inpatient medical rehabilitation remained exempt from Medicare's prospective DRG-based method of paying for hospital-based care, and it is still being paid on a cost basis, although several DRG-like methods of payment have been proposed for medical rehabilitation (Harada, Sofaer, & Kominski, 1993; Stineman et al., 1994; Sutton, DeJong, & Wilkerson, 1996; Wilkerson, Batavia, & DeJong, 1992).

Despite its exemption from Medicare's prospective payment system, medical rehabilitation has not been immune from the changes sweeping the United States. In some markets, especially on the West Coast, an increasing number of Medicare subscribers are enrolling in at-risk health maintenance organizations (HMOs). Although only about 10% of Medicare subscribers across the United States are participating in managed care programs, approximately 50% or more are already participating in at-risk HMOs in selected West Coast markets. By 2000, about 80% of all Medicare beneficiaries nationwide are expected to be enrolled in at-risk managed care plans. A similar percentage is expected for the Medicaid program as states rapidly convert their Medicaid programs into managed care programs. Proposals in the 104th Congress during 1995–1996 for reform of the Medicare program and block granting of Medicaid ensure that changes such as these trends are a certainty.

The growth of managed care is already affecting the behavior of medical rehabilitation providers and changing the overall medical rehabilitation landscape. Five trends are briefly mentioned here:

1. Inpatient medical rehabilitation providers are being forced to reduce per diem and total costs to remain as recognized providers within a health plan. Lengths of stay in inpatient medical rehabilitation facilities are declining rapidly from an average of 28 days in 1990 to 23 days in 1993 (Granger, Ottenbacher, & Fiedler, 1995).

2. New settings of care are emerging as alternatives to inpatient medical rehabilitation. Most noteworthy is the growth of subacute medical rehabilitation based in skilled nursing facilities, which provide a somewhat less intensive level of care. Similarly, there has been a dramatic growth of outpatient rehabilitation programs and home-based medical rehabilitation programs.

3. To better position themselves to obtain managed care contracts, medical rehabilitation providers are becoming parts of larger health care provider networks that offer a full continuum of health and medical rehabilitation services within a given market area. This trend is referred to as *vertical integration.*

4. Some medical rehabilitation providers are becoming a part of large regional and national chains of medical rehabilitation providers through mergers and acquisitions. This trend is known as *horizontal integration.*

5. The number and proportion of for-profit medical rehabilitation providers are increasing as medical rehabilitation providers seek to use stockholder equity instead of debt to finance expansion and diversification.

Absence of Quality Competition

Noticeably missing among these trends is a concern about quality or outcomes. Quality and outcomes are examined mainly when deciding whether a particular provider should become part of a provider network or be included in a health plan's list of approved providers. Provider disclosure of outcomes, under these circumstances, tends to be very selective and is limited to those outcomes that give the provider competitive advantage in securing managed care contracts. Outcomes are not being used as the basis for continuous monitoring of provider performance or as the basis for payment.

Managed care organizations do not compete on *price* and *quality* as in most consumer markets, but on *price* and *risk*. In a 1995 study of health plans and medical rehabilitation providers in the three most advanced managed care markets (San Diego, Minneapolis–St. Paul, and Worcester, Massachusetts), the NRH Research Center found little or no effective quality competition (DeJong, Wheatley, & Sutton, 1996; Wheatley, DeJong, & Sutton, 1996). Informants insisted that the three most important criteria in securing managed care contracts were "price, price, and price." "Everything is price-driven," said one respondent.

Risk competition, an enduring feature of American health care, is likely to intensify under managed care. Health plans stand to lose financially when a higher-than-expected number of health plan subscribers are high-need, high-cost cases. This is commonly known as the *adverse-risk selection* problem. Health plans do not want to attract high-cost cases and prefer not to advertise the quality of those services that attract higher-than-average users of health services such as people with disabilities. Under capitation-based managed care arrangements, there are powerful financial incentives not to serve more difficult cases, because primary care gatekeepers are financially disrewarded for using too many downstream services such as medical rehabilitation.

THE EMERGING CONSUMER SIDE OF THE MARKET

If price and risk are the driving forces in managed care markets, what, then, is the role of medical rehabilitation outcomes in managed care? At what stage of managed care market development does quality become important? When does ongoing attention to medical rehabilitation outcomes become an essential element in market competition apart from a provider's attempt to be deemed a quality provider worthy of inclusion in a managed care plan?

Effective quality competition is not likely until the consumer side of the market becomes better organized. There are several keys to effective price-and-quality competition, the most important of which is an *informed consumer* who is able to make informed choices from an array of health plans, each of which represents a network of providers and a subsidiary network of rehabilitation providers. As of 1995, consumers had little or no choice and very little information upon which to make a choice. This is changing, however.

Consumer health plan and health provider information is becoming available in selected markets. A publication providing consumer assessment of health plans and providers, known as *Health Pages*, is available in five markets—Atlanta, Boston, Columbus–Cincinnati, Pittsburgh, and St. Louis—and was expected to become available in four other markets by the end of 1995. In the Washington, D.C., market, a consumer magazine, *Consumer Checkbook*, publishes a less sophisticated plan-by-plan, provider-by-provider review annually. In Cleveland, the Cleveland Health

Quality Choice Program evaluates outcomes and patient satisfaction among people discharged from 29 Cleveland area hospitals. The Cleveland findings are risk-adjusted for patient severity of illness to facilitate hospital-to-hospital comparisons.

One organization deserving mention is the National Committee on Quality Assurance (NCQA). Only a small organization in the early 1990s, NCQA has emerged as an important player in evaluating managed care plans. The principal evaluation tool has been NCQA's Health Plan Employer Data and Information Set (HEDIS), which evaluates health plans on 36 performance measures, including a variety of outcomes and consumer satisfaction measures. The main impetus for the emergence of NCQA has been the large employer that seeks standardized quality information to help it decide which health plans it should make available to its employees. Fortunately, the information needs of large employers overlap with the information needs of small consumers who are also seeking to make informed choices.

The example of large employers using their clout to extract quality as well as price information from health plans and providers illustrates how important it is for consumers to organize themselves into large purchasing blocks that can demand the price-and-quality information needed to make informed choices. Organized consumer-purchasing blocks (e.g., health alliances or health insurance purchasing cooperatives [HIPCs]) were prominent features in several of the health care reform proposals considered in the 103rd Congress (1993–1994). A number of HIPC-like groups are emerging to help organize the consumer side of the market.

As of 1995, the consumer side of the market was still not well organized, but increasing evidence supporting a more consumer-driven health care system is clearly beginning to emerge. DeJong and Sutton (1995) argued that the long-term trend to a more consumer-driven health care system represents the third stage of the contemporary American health care system development: from the provider-driven system that competed on prestige and risk, to the payer-driven system that competes on price and risk, and finally to the consumer-driven system that competes on price and quality.

Reaching the Uninformed Consumer

The challenge for medical rehabilitation in a consumer-driven health care system is how to reach out to and communicate with the consumer who is choosing a health plan. Most consumers, especially younger ones, never envision a need for medical rehabilitation services, and many do not even know what these services are. The need for medical rehabilitation services is often considered by the average consumer to be a remote possibility and, as such, is not carefully scrutinized by the consumer when choosing a health plan. Thus, consumers are not likely to make much of an investment in learning about rehabilitation and the quality of various providers within plans.

DeJong (1995) and DeJong and Sutton (1995) identified four steps that the medical rehabilitation industry must take to effectively reach out to the relatively uninformed consumer of health plans. They argued that the industry needs to do the following:

1. Develop, in collaboration with a more neutral entity, a single standardized rehabilitation score (with possible subscores) by which health plans will be rated based on the capabilities and performance of the plan's entire network of rehabilitation providers. (Such a score would be largely outcomes-based and risk-adjusted. Such a score would also create enormous peer pressure to exclude subpar providers and encourage collaboration to improve the plan's overall rehabilitation score.)

2. Convince various health system governing boards and HIPCs that a rehabilitation rating system is needed to help consumers make their annual side-by-side comparison of competing health plans. Without such a rating, consumers will overlook the rehabilitation component of a health plan, and health plans may not be adequately motivated to include the best possible network of rehabilitation providers.

3. Adopt the single-score concept (with possible subscores) as the basis for rating individual providers. Such ratings would guide consumers, physician gatekeepers, and health plan case managers in selecting a within-plan or out-of-plan provider when a rehabilitation need arises.

4. Undertake an education strategy to inform consumers, physician gatekeepers, and case managers of what rehabilitation scores or ratings mean for the choices they need to make when choosing a plan or selecting a provider.

The types of outcomes measures that will be used in a more consumer-driven health care environment will, in all likelihood, include consumer satisfaction measures and the types of outcomes measures already being used to evaluate short-term outcomes. The system also will need longer-term (macro-level) outcomes measures as outlined earlier in this chapter. The medical rehabilitation industry is already well equipped to address the short-term outcomes but has yet to fully operationalize some of the longer-term measures needed to compete in a more consumer-driven health care system.

The Need for Risk Adjusters

Fair quality or outcomes competition requires the development of risk adjusters that can be used to risk-adjust the populations on which outcomes are being compared (Iezzoni, 1994). Medical rehabilitation lacks a recognized methodology by which outcomes can be adjusted for differences in case mix. In the absence of risk adjusters, providers are prone to resort to a large measure of risk competition to demonstrate good outcomes.

Medical rehabilitation has made important progress toward the development of case-mix indices in the form of function-related groups (FRGs) as a possible basis for a prospective payment system for inpatient medical rehabilitation analogous to the DRGs used in the Medicare prospective payment system for acute care hospitals (Harada et al., 1993; Stineman et al., 1994; Sutton et al., 1996; Wilkerson et al., 1992). FRGs categorize patients into 1 of 50 or more relatively homogeneous groups based on type of impairment, age, functional status, and resource consumption as measured by length of stay. In a sense, FRGs are payment risk adjusters intended to reduce risk competition should inpatient medical rehabilitation providers be paid a fixed price for each qualified admission.

Risk adjusters have yet to be developed for medical rehabilitation outcomes. FRGs used for payment are not adequate risk adjusters for outcomes, because they were normed on resource consumption (as measured by length of stay), not on outcomes. Medical rehabilitation outcomes do not necessarily vary in the same manner as resource consumption. Moreover, outcomes variation within individual FRGs may be greater than the variation between groups.

As a resource-based patient classification methodology, FRGs offer a model of how similar classification schemes might be used as risk adjusters for medical rehabilitation outcomes. One limiting factor with FRGs is that they were designed only for one type of medical rehabilitation setting—namely, inpatient settings. In managed care markets, all but a few impairment groups are being served in inpatient settings, with the remainder going to subacute and other nonhospital settings (DeJong et al., 1996; Wheatley et al., 1996). A risk adjustment methodology for medical rehabilitation outcomes will have to transcend treatment settings if there is to be effective outcomes competition in the more consumer-driven health system.

Risk adjusters are needed to create a more risk-neutral health care system that will help health plans and providers compete on price and quality, not on price and risk. Without risk adjusters or "carve-outs" for high-user populations, health plans will continue to discriminate against people with disabilities, and health care providers such as medical rehabilitation providers will be discouraged from serving people with greater rehabilitation needs. The development of risk adjusters for health plans and health providers is probably the single greatest analytic challenge for the late 1990s and beyond.

HEALTH PLAN REVIEW OF MEDICAL REHABILITATION OUTCOMES

Apart from the types of ongoing outcomes monitoring required in a more consumer-driven health care system, there is another level at which outcomes information is being sought by payers. Health plan managers are constantly reexamining the scope of their benefit packages and want to know whether a particular intervention or therapy has merit and should therefore be included as a benefit in the plan. Health plan managers want to know whether the scientific evidence, based on outcomes, for a particular intervention merits coverage and funding for the intervention in question. A case in point is a study conducted at the NRH Research Center for the Civilian Health and Medical Program of the Uniformed Services (CHAMPUS), the health plan for the 6 million U.S. military dependents and retirees. The study examined all published and unpublished medical rehabilitation research literature that met predetermined standards of methodologic rigor to determine which therapies and interventions based on outcomes merit inclusion in the CHAMPUS health plan.

This type of outcomes review is expected to intensify as health plan managers seek to limit the costs of their plans. They will attempt to weed out therapies and interventions that have little or only marginal benefit. Each year new health care technologies and interventions seek third-party coverage. In the traditional fee-for-service health care system, there is little financial incentive to limit the use of new or marginal interventions. In a system of capitation-based managed care, there are strong incentives to make more discriminating use of both new and long-standing but never before questioned health care interventions.

This type of review presents a special challenge for medical rehabilitation. Although medical rehabilitation has made remarkable advances in standardizing its approach to outcomes measurement, it remains difficult to disaggregate the individual effects of its component therapies and interventions. In a review article on rehabilitation effectiveness for acquired brain injury (ABI), Cope (1995) noted that ABI rehabilitation cannot always be reduced to a single "silver bullet" and that ABI rehabilitation is "multifactorial with many poorly defined elements delivered with variable intensity and expertise over differing time spans." In addressing questions about the overall effectiveness of medical rehabilitation, it often becomes necessary "to consider the rehabilitation process to essentially comprise a 'black box' consisting of various permutations of all these treatments" (Cope, 1995).

In a consumer-driven system, where managed care plans and providers compete on outcomes, the components of the black box become less important because payers will be more concerned about outcomes and results and less concerned about how providers achieved their outcomes. It will be left to the provider to optimize resources in achieving predetermined outcomes. Effective outcomes competition reduces the need for the kinds of managed care micromanagement that providers in the 1990s find so distasteful.

CONCLUSIONS

An understated theme in this chapter is the question of whose interests are being served by 1) what outcomes are being measured, 2) how they are disseminated, and 3) how they are being used. The matter of whose interests is central in understanding the value perspectives and the role of medical rehabilitation outcomes in American health care and provides a way of summarizing some of the chapter's main arguments.

In the provider-driven health care system of the past, the chief role of medical rehabilitation outcomes has been professional legitimacy. In Western society, science is an important tool of social and professional legitimation. Medical rehabilitation physicians have sought that legitimation in part vis-à-vis their physician colleagues in other medical disciplines, especially those in body-system- or organ-specific areas of specialization (e.g., neurology, cardiology, nephrology) who work with more defined end points such as the elimination of pathology and patient survival. Medical rehabilitation's focus has been not on pathology, but on function, a domain that includes social and environmental components that, at times, seem removed from the concerns of medical science. Medical rehabilitation has attempted to develop a science, but a science requires known end points or outcomes.

Within medical rehabilitation, each allied health discipline has sought to ensure that its domain of interest is adequately represented in consensus outcomes measures. The absence of representation brings into question the very existence and legitimacy of an allied health discipline. Some allied health disciplines question the adequacy of consensus measures and propose their own measures to supplement consensus measures.

Medical rehabilitation's stature has increased among the health professions, partly because it has defined and articulated its therapeutic end points. More important, however, other medical specialties have come to realize that the removal of pathology and survival are no longer adequate end points and have had to look to broader outcomes that reflect the inherent chronic nature of the conditions they address. Here is where medical rehabilitation stands to be a leader in the health sciences community.

The interests of providers become more transparent when the perspectives of medical rehabilitation are compared with the perspectives of other research communities, and each research community is juxtaposed in terms of the seven dimensions outlined in the Appendix: client population, service delivery system, academic base, professional organization, journals, research/tools/indices, and funding sources.

The IL–DR movement brings its own interests to the outcomes debate. First, it seeks to broaden the domain beyond the activities of daily living level to include the various social and environmental issues that affect the daily lives of people with disabilities. Moreover, the focus of independent living centers, the chief institutional expression of the IL movement, is on the social and environmental dimensions of human existence. Second, the movement seeks to wrest from the provider the right to determine who should be the ultimate judge of what works and what does not.

At the stage of managed care development in 1995, payers are largely uninterested in medical rehabilitation outcomes, except in a global way, in determining whether medical rehabilitation should be included as a benefit in their health plans. Their interests are mainly economic: Subscribers are needed who are willing to pay premiums, and costs need to be curtailed for payers to remain viable and profitable. Their interests are more transparently economic than those of either providers or consumers.

This chapter noted several trends that are challenging the interests and perspectives of individual provider and consumer communities. Noted were the increased integration of health care provider networks because of managed care, the development of more global health status and medical outcomes measures, the increasing stake of society as a payer of health services for people with chronic health conditions, and the eventual development of a more consumer-driven health care system in which outcomes will have to be expressed and reported to the general consumer.

As society's interests become stronger and as American health care becomes more consumer-driven, there will be more complete disclosure of medical rehabilitation outcomes. In the provider-dominated system, medical rehabilitation facilities considered their outcomes data to be confidential. Large databases in medical rehabilitation, such as the Uniform Data System for Medical Rehabilitation and the National Spinal Cord Injury Data Base, still reflect these provider-centered values and contain strict safeguards against disclosure of facility-specific data. In the payer-driven system, there is selective disclosure of outcomes by individual facilities that are seeking to demonstrate their capabilities to prospective payers. In the consumer-driven system, where an informed consumer is the hallmark of a truly competitive market-based system, eventually there will be complete disclosure of medical rehabilitation outcomes data.

Medical rehabilitation providers would be remiss if they were to see this type of disclosure as a loss of power. They have already lost power in the payer-driven marketplace of the 1990s. A consumer-driven system that includes full outcomes disclosure (risk-adjusted) is very much in the interest of providers who seek a more level playing field in a more consumer-driven, risk-neutral, market-based health care system. Medical rehabilitation outcomes are essential to creating a more balanced and efficient health care system.

REFERENCES

Banja, J., & Johnson, M. (1994). Ethical perspectives and social policy. *Archives of Physical Medicine and Rehabilitation, 75,* SC19–SC26.

Bergner, M., Bobbitt, R., Carter, W., & Gelson, B. (1981). The Sickness Impact Profile: Development and final revision of a health status measure. *Medical Care, 19,* 955–962.

Cope, D.N. (1995). The effectiveness of traumatic brain injury rehabilitation: A review. *Brain Injury, 9*(7), 649–670.

DeJong, G. (1987). Medical rehabilitation outcome measurement in a changing health care market. In M.J. Fuhrer (Ed.), *Rehabilitation outcomes: Analysis and measurement* (pp. 261–271). Baltimore: Paul H. Brookes Publishing Co.

DeJong, G. (1990, October). *Outcome measurement from a third party payor perspective.* Paper presented at the annual meeting of the American Congress of Rehabilitation Medicine, Phoenix, AZ.

DeJong, G. (1995, June). *Empowering the consumer and enabling the provider in an era of managed care.* The 5th Annual John W. Goldschmidt lecture presented at the National Rehabilitation Hospital, Washington, DC.

DeJong, G., & Sutton, J. (1995). Rehab 2000: The evolution of medical rehabilitation in American health care. In P. Kitchell Landrum, N.D. Schmidt, & A. McLean, Jr. (Eds.), *Outcome-oriented rehabilitation: Principles, strategies, and tools for effective program management* (pp. 3–42). Gaithersburg, MD: Aspen.

DeJong, G., Wheatley, B., & Sutton, J. (1996). Medical rehabilitation undergoing major shakeup in advanced managed-care markets. *BNA Managed Care Reporter, 2,* 138–141.

Frieden, L., Richards, L., Cole, J., & Baley, D. (1979). *ILRU source-book: A technical assistance manual on independent living.* Houston, TX: Institute for Rehabilitation and Research.

Granger, C., Ottenbacher, K., & Fiedler, R. (1995). Uniform Data System for Medical Rehabilitation: Report of first admissions for 1993. *American Journal of Physical Medicine and Rehabilitation, 74,* 62–66.

Harada, N., Sofaer, S., & Kominski, G. (1993). Functional status outcomes in rehabilitation: Implications for prospective payment. *Medical Care, 31*(4), 345–357.

Iezzoni, L. (1994). *Risk adjustment for measuring health care outcomes.* Ann Arbor, MI: Health Administration Press.

National Council on the Handicapped. (1986). *Toward independence: An assessment of federal laws and programs affecting people with disabilities, with legislative recommendations. A report to the President and the Congress of the United States* [Appendix]. Washington, DC: U.S. Government Printing Office.

Nosek, M. (1987). Outcome analysis in independent living. In M.J. Fuhrer (Ed.), *Rehabilitation outcomes: Analysis and measurement* (pp. 71–83). Baltimore: Paul H. Brookes Publishing Co.

Stewart, A., & Ware, J. (1992). *Measuring functioning and well-being: The medical outcomes study approach.* Durham, NC: Duke University Press.

State University of New York at Buffalo. (1993). *Guide for the Uniform Data Set for Medical Rehabilitation (Adult FIM), version 4.0.* Buffalo, NY: Author.

Stineman, M., Escarce, J., Goin, J., Hamilton, B., Granger, C., & Williams, S. (1994). A case-mix classification system for medical rehabilitation. *Medical Care, 32,* 366–379.

Sutton, J.P., DeJong, G., & Wilkerson, D. (1996). Function-based payment for inpatient medical rehabilitation: An evaluation. *Archives of Physical Medicine and Rehabilitation, 77,* 693–701.

U.S. Department of Agriculture. (1986). Untitled document.

Ware, J., & Sherbourne, C. (1992). The MOS 36-Item Short Form Health Survey (SF-36). I: Conceptual framework and item selection. *Medical Care, 30,* 473–483.

Wheatley, B., DeJong, G., & Sutton, S. (1996, Spring). How managed care is transforming American health care: A survey of rehabilitation providers in leading markets. *Georgetown Public Policy Review,* 1–15.

Whiteneck, G., Charlifue, S., Gerhart, K., Overholser, J., & Richardson, G. (1992). Quantifying handicap: A measure of long-term rehabilitation outcomes. *Archives of Physical Medicine and Rehabilitation, 73,* 519–526.

Wilkerson, D. (1996). *Level of function as an organizing framework for functional assessment applications.* Manuscript submitted for publication.

Wilkerson, D., Batavia, A., & DeJong, G. (1992). The use of functional measures for payment of medical rehabilitation services. *Archives of Physical Medicine and Rehabilitation, 73,* 111–120.

Willer, B., Rosenthal, M., Kreutzer, J., Gordon, W., & Rempel, R. (1993). Assessment of community integration following rehabilitation for traumatic brain injury. *Journal of Head Trauma and Rehabilitation, 8,* 75–87.

Appendix

Six Different Research Communities

Note: This is not an exhaustive listing.

1. **Trauma/Emergency Medical Services**
   Client population: TBI, SCI, Hfx, MI
   Service delivery systems: Trauma centers, emergency medicine
   Academic base: Emergency medicine, public health, epidemiology, biostatistics, biomechanics
   Professional organization: APHA, American College of Surgeons, AAAM
   Journals: Journal of Trauma, Annals of Emergency Medicine, Critical Care Medicine, Journal of Safety Research, Accident Prevention and Analysis
   Research/tools/indices: ISS, AIS, GCS, RTS
   Funding sources: CDC, NHTSA, NIOSH

2. **Medical Rehabilitation**
   Client population: TBI, SCI, Hfx, CVA, Amp, Ortho
   Service delivery systems: CIR, SAR, CORF, day rehabilitation, home-based rehabilitation
   Academic base: Physiatry, psychology, OT, PT, SLP, P&O rehabilitation, rehabilitation engineering
   Professional organization: AAPM&R, ACRM, IRMA, AAP_1, AAP_2, AOTA, APTA, ASHA, ASIA
   Journals: Archives of Physical Medicine and Rehabilitation, Journal of Neurological Rehabilitation, Journal of Head Trauma Rehabilitation, American Journal of Physical Medicine and Rehabilitation, Rehabilitation Management, and PT, OT, SLP journals
   Research/tools/indices: FIM, PECs, LADs/LORs, Barthel, GCS, CIQ, CHART
   Funding sources: NIDRR, NCMRR, NINDS, CDC

3. **Aging/Long-Term Care**
   Client population: Hfx, CVA, UI, Alzheimer's disease, dementia, osteoporosis

Service delivery systems: H&CBS, AAA, CCRCs, assisted living, nursing facilities

Academic base: Gerontology, aging studies, geriatrics, human development

Professional organization: GSA, ASA, AGS

Journals: Journal of American Geriatrics Society, Age and Aging, Generations, Gerontologist, Caring, Journal of Gerontology, Journal of Aging and Health

Research/tools/indices: Katz Scale, Kronofsky, MDS–RAI, Zarit-Burden, Mini-Mental, DSM-III

Funding sources: NIA, ASPE, HCRA, CDC, RWJF, Pew, Hartford Research Retirement Fund

4. Developmental Disabilities

Client population: MR, CP, MD, SB, JA, autism, learning disabilities, epilepsy

Service delivery systems: Special education, ICF, DD councils, adult services

Academic base: Pediatrics, special education, psychology, social work, PT, OT, SLP, pediatric rehabilitation

Professional organization: AAUAP, AAMR, ACN, Academy of CP, AAP_2, NAPAS, ASMRPDs, CEC, TASH, NDSC

Journals: Journal of Special Education, American Journal on Mental Retardation, Successful Children

Research/tools/indices: Pediatric FIM, IQ (Binet, Wechsler), Adaptive behavior intervention

Funding sources: U.S. Department of Education, ADD, NIDRR, NICHD, NINDS

5. Mental Health

Client population: Depression, bipolar, schizophrenia

Service delivery systems: Private practice, CMHCs, group homes, psychiatric hospitals, day centers, rehabilitation centers

Academic base: Psychiatry, psychology, psychiatric nursing, psychiatric social worker

Professional organization: APA_1, APA_2, NMHA, MHLP, NAPAS, NAMI

Journals: Hospital and Community Psychiatry, Administration and Policy in Mental Health, American Journal of Psychiatry, American Psychologist, Psychiatric Hospital, Journal of Mental Health Administration, Journal of Psychiatric Research, Mental Health Report, Policy and Perspective Focus, New Directions

Research/tools/indices: Beck's Depression, DSM-III, Mini-Mental

Funding sources: NIMH, CMHS, HCFA, HSRA, MacArthur Foundation, RWJF, Pew

6. **Health Services Research**
   Client population: All conditions
   Service delivery systems: All settings
   Academic base: Public health, health policy, health economics, bioethics, community medicine
   Professional organization: APHA, AHSR, ISTAHC
   Journals: HSR, JHPPL, *Health Affairs, Health Care Financing Review, Hospitals, Journal of the American Medical Association, Journal of Health Economics, Inquiry, Medical Care, Milbank Quarterly, New England Journal of Medicine*
   Research/tools/indices: SIP, HSQ, SF-36, MedisGroups, quality-of-life measures
   Funding sources: AHCPR, HCFA, ASPE, RWJF, Pew

List of Acronyms and Abbreviations

AAA	Area Agency on Aging
AAAM	American Association for Automotive Medicine
AAMR	American Association on Mental Retardation
AAP_1	Association of Academic Physiatrists
AAP_2	American Academy of Pediatrics
AAPM&R	American Academy of Physical Medicine and Rehabilitation
AAUAP	American Association of University Affiliated Programs
ACN	American College of Nursing
ACRM	American Congress of Rehabilitation Medicine
ADD	Administration on Developmental Disabilities
AGS	American Gerontological Society
AHCPR	Agency for Health Care Policy and Research
AHSR	Association for Health Services Research
AIS	Abbreviated Injury Scale
Amp	amputation
AOTA	American Occupational Therapy Association
APA_1	American Psychiatric Association
APA_2	American Psychological Association
APHA	American Public Health Association
APTA	American Physical Therapy Association
ASA	American Society on Aging

ASHA	American Speech-Language-Hearing Association
ASIA	American Spinal Injury Association
ASMRPDs	American Society of Mental Retardation Program Directors
ASPE	Assistant Secretary for Planning and Evaluation
CCRC	Community Care Residential Centers
CDC	Centers for Disease Control
CHART	Craig Handicap Assessment Reporting Technique
CIQ	Community Integration Questionnaire
CIR	comprehensive inpatient rehabilitation
CMHCs	community mental health centers
CMHS	community mental health services
CORF	comprehensive outpatient rehabilitation facility
CP	cerebral palsy
CVA	cerebral vascular accident
DD	developmental disabilities
DSM-III	*Diagnostic and Statistical Manual of Mental Disorders–3rd Edition*
FIM	Functional Independence Measure
GCS	Glasgow Coma Scale
GSA	Gerontological Society of America
H&CBS	home- and community-based services
HCFA	Health Care Financing Administration
Hfx	hip fracture
HSQ	Health Status Questionnaire
HSR	Health Services Research
HSRA	Health Services Resource Administration
ICF	intermediate care facility
IQ	intelligence quotient
IRMA	International Rehabilitation Medicine Association
ISS	Injury Severity Scale
ISTAHC	International Society for Technology Assessment in Health Care
JA	juvenile arthritis
LORs	Level of Rehabilitation Scale
MD	muscular dystrophy
MDS–RAI	Minimum Data Set–Resident Assessment Instrument
MH	mental health
MHLP	Mental Health Law Project
MI	myocardial infarction
MR	mental retardation
NAMI	National Alliance for the Mentally Ill

NAPAS	National Association of Protection and Advocacy Systems
NCMRR	National Center for Medical Rehabilitation Research
NDSC	National Down Syndrome Congress
NHTSA	National Highway Traffic Safety Administration
NIA	National Institute on Aging
NICHD	National Institute of Child Health and Human Development
NIDRR	National Institute on Disability and Rehabilitation Research
NIMH	National Institute of Mental Health
NINDS	National Institute of Neurological Diseases and Stroke
NIOSH	National Institute of Occupational Safety and Health
NMHA	National Mental Health Association
Ortho	orthopedic
OT	occupational therapy
P&O	prosthetics and orthotics
PECs	Patient Evaluation and Conference System
Pew	Pew Family Trust
PT	physical therapy
RTS	Revised Trauma Score
RWJF	Robert Wood Johnson Foundation
SAR	subacute rehabilitation
SB	spina bifida
SCI	spinal cord injury
SF-36	Short Form 36
SIP	Sickness Impact Profile
SLP	speech-language pathology
TASH	The Association for Persons with Severe Handicaps
TBI	traumatic brain injury
UI	urinary incontinence

CHAPTER 4

Elaborating the Model of Disablement

Gale G. Whiteneck,
Patrick Fougeyrollas, and Kenneth A. Gerhart

The dominant theoretical model for describing the consequences of the disablement process is the World Health Organization's (WHO) International Classification of Impairments, Disabilities, and Handicaps (ICIDH) (WHO, 1993). It is the thesis of this chapter—the result of a developing conceptualization (Whiteneck, 1994)—that the WHO model of disablement can serve as an appropriate conceptual basis for evaluating rehabilitation outcomes if it is elaborated by emphasizing handicap as a key outcome, considering the lifetime nature of disablement, including the subjective perceptions of people with disabilities, and recognizing the importance of environmental factors in determining the consequences of disablement.

THE WHO MODEL OF DISABLEMENT

In General

The major contribution of the WHO model of disablement has been the conceptual distinctions between three levels of disablement outcomes:

1. Impairments at the organ level
2. Disabilities at the person level
3. Handicaps at the societal level

Differentiating the performance of organ systems from the performance of activities of daily living (ADL) from performance as members of society

This chapter was supported in part by the U.S. Department of Education's National Institute on Disability and Rehabilitation Research via the Model Spinal Injury System program. In addition, the authors are grateful to Kathy Quick for her assistance.

greatly clarifies the distinct but interrelated effects that the disablement process can have on individuals.

In the WHO model, the most basic consequence of a disease, injury, or congenital abnormality is an *impairment* at the individual organ or organ-system level, which has been defined as "any loss or abnormality of psychological, physiological or anatomical structure or function" (WHO, 1993, p. 27). The ICIDH provides an elaborate classification scheme for a range of impairments, including paralysis, amputation, loss of vision, and others. The severity of impairment is typically assessed by using instruments designed for the specific disease, injury, or condition. For example, the American Spinal Injury Association Motor Score describes the extent of paralysis for spinal cord injury (American Spinal Injury Association, 1990), the Glasgow Coma Scale (Teasdale & Jennett, 1974) quantifies the severity of acquired brain injury, and various visual screening tools are used to define degrees of visual impairment.

Impairments may lead to *disability* at the person level, which is defined as "any restriction or lack (resulting from an impairment) of ability to perform an activity in the manner or within the range considered normal for a human being" (WHO, 1980, p. 28). Disability is typically measured in terms of degree of independence with which an individual can perform ADL. Many different impairments can cause similar disabilities, whereas similar impairments can result in different disabilities. Many disability measures have been developed to apply across a range of impairments, including the early Barthel Index (Mahoney & Barthel, 1965) and the Functional Independence Measure (FIM) (State University of New York at Buffalo, 1993). Other examples include the Pulses (Moskowitz & McCann, 1957), Patient Education Conference System (Harvey & Jellinek, 1981), and the Level of Rehabilitation Scale (Carey & Posavac, 1978).

Impairment or disability may lead to *handicap*. This term is not meant pejoratively as used in ordinary conversation, but rather as a concept that emphasizes the roles of an individual in society. *Handicap* is defined as "a disadvantage for a given individual that limits or prevents the fulfillment of a role that is normal (depending upon age, sex, social and cultural factors) for that individual" (WHO, 1993, p. 29). Handicap includes such expected social roles as friend, student, worker, and family and community member. It also includes such dimensions as orientation, physical independence, mobility, occupation, social integration, and economic self-sufficiency. Instruments such as Whiteneck, Charlifue, Gerhart, Overholsen, and Richardson's (1992) Craig Handicap Assessment and Reporting Technique and Willer, Rosenthal, Kreutzer, Gorden, and Rempel's (1993) Community Integration Questionnaire (Willer, Linn, & Allen, 1993) have been developed to provide a quantitative measure of handicap.

Variants of the WHO Model

Considerable conceptual confusion has emerged as various U.S. government agencies have adopted conceptual frameworks similar to the WHO model but have used quite different terminology (National Institutes of Health [NIH], 1993). For example, the Institute of Medicine and the National Center for Medical Rehabilitation Research have adopted the terminology first suggested by Saad Nagi (Pope & Tarlov, 1991), which replaces the WHO term of *disability* with the term *functional limitations.* Furthermore, in this scheme, the term *disability* is used to describe what the WHO model of disablement refers to as *handicap.* Similarly, the Public Health Service Task Force describes *impairment* as simply the "organ level," *disability* as the "person level," and *handicap* as the "interaction of environment on person" (NIH, 1993, p. 33). Although subtle differences exist among these models (Pope & Tarlov, 1991), all share commonality with the WHO model in that they differentiate three broad arenas: 1) organ system performance, 2) performance of ADL at the person level, and 3) role performance as a member of society.

Multiple, competing sets of terminology have proliferated and at times have led to confusion. Although the WHO can be faulted for its sometimes provocative and often less-than-descriptive use of the term *handicap,* its model of disablement is internationally recognized and widely used. Moreover, it is a dynamic and responsive model, with an international team already working to revise the ICIDH by 2000. Consequently, the WHO terminology of *impairment, disability,* and *handicap* is used in this chapter to signify the three domains of disablement.

REHABILITATION OUTCOMES: MINIMIZING DISABLEMENT

In the WHO model (1980), disablement is viewed as a process that starts with a disease, injury, or abnormality. It becomes recognized as an impairment at the organ level, manifests as disability in the performance of ADL, and ultimately may lead to a handicap or inability to fulfill social roles. The WHO model and its variants provide a useful conceptualization of the potentially cascading series of events that make up the disablement process. In contrast, the process of rehabilitation may be viewed as a series of interventions intended to minimize disablement by breaking this chain of events. Minimizing impairment for given levels of pathology through effective medical management is an appropriate goal of acute rehabilitation. Maximizing functional independence and minimizing disability for a given level of impairment have been the typical foci of medical rehabilitation. A few of the interventions used to accomplish this goal include rehabilitation therapies, ADL training, and adaptive equipment. Minimizing handicap for given levels of impairment and disability by reintegrating people with disabilities into their communities as active, independent, productive members of society also is a frequently cited goal of rehabilitation (Carey & Posavac, 1978; Frey, 1984; Kemp & Vash, 1971; Pflueger, 1977; Wagner, 1987).

Because many rehabilitation interventions are possible at several different points in time, can be delivered in numerous different formats, and are targeted at people with various disabilities, outcomes research is needed to identify the most effective and efficient interventions. Therefore, the concepts of impairment, disability, and handicap can be viewed as outcomes measures for rehabilitation, and the WHO model itself can serve as the conceptual basis. However, a few shifts of emphasis, clarification, and elaboration are needed to enhance the model.

Emphasizing Handicap

Although their goal is reducing handicap, rehabilitation facilities often focus on measuring impairments and disabilities to the neglect of handicap assessment. This may be explained partly by a perception that handicap is a more nebulous, global concept than is function and hence is more difficult to measure objectively than is impairment or disability. Furthermore, the view of rehabilitationists is that they have more direct control over disability than handicap; thus, they are more willing to judge their effectiveness on the basis of reducing disability than on the basis of reducing handicap.

Nonetheless, in contrast to the focus in rehabilitation on *disability* assessment, the national goal, as called for by the Americans with Disabilities Act (ADA) of 1990 (PL 101-336), is the reduction of handicap through the full participation in society of people with disabilities. Community integration is the true goal of rehabilitation and the ultimate goal of consumers of rehabilitation services. Therefore, all three dimensions of the disablement process (impairment, disability, and handicap) are appropriate outcomes measures for rehabilitation and need to be included in both the conceptual emphasis and the practical measurement of rehabilitation outcomes. There needs to be an emphasis on handicap as an equally important and appropriate outcomes measure for rehabilitation.

Emphasizing the Lifetime Perspective: Secondary Conditions

The lifetime nature of many disabling conditions needs to be emphasized in the WHO model of disablement. Although often viewed as stable, disabling conditions are anything but static (Marge, 1988). The Centers for Disease Control has focused attention on secondary conditions that occur throughout the lifetime of an individual living with a primary disabling condition. These secondary impairments, secondary disabilities, and secondary handicaps are associated with, and are the outcomes of, the disabling condition. They may occur either because the primary disabling condition is a risk factor for the secondary conditions or because the primary disability itself necessitates alterations in how the secondary condition is treated (State University of New York at Syracuse, 1994).

After the onset of a primary impairment, secondary impairments represent merely those additional, related impairments that may occur throughout the individual's life. Examples include loss of muscle strength decades after the initial onset of polio and shoulder pain and joint disease associated with years of using a wheelchair as a result of spinal cord injury. Likewise, secondary disabilities further reduce the independence with which individuals perform ADL. The need for additional help as an individual with a physical disability ages is one example. Secondary handicaps represent further limitations in role fulfillment that occur over the individual's lifetime. These may include the need for early retirement or the increased social isolation that often occurs as people with a disability grow older. Therefore, an emphasis on secondary conditions is needed if the WHO model is to serve as a comprehensive model of rehabilitation outcomes. Indeed, any model of disablement must acknowledge its dynamic nature and that, at any point in time, an individual's level of disability and handicap is the sum of all primary and secondary impairments, disabilities, and handicaps that have affected him or her over the course of a lifetime.

Incorporating Subjective Perceptions and Quality of Life

Elaboration of the WHO model of disablement to include the subjective perceptions of individuals with disabilities is also necessary if the model is to serve as a basis for conceptualizing rehabilitation outcomes. Although rehabilitationists can objectively quantify the degree of impairment, disability, and handicap by measuring organ system performance, ADL performance, and social role performance in comparison to people without disabilities, such objective assessments tell only half of the story. The subjective perceptions of people regarding their own impairments, disabilities, and handicaps are equally valid and merit equal attention. From the subjective perspective of the individual, the sum of all primary and secondary impairments might be viewed as *perceived health*. From the subjective perspective of the individual, the sum of all primary and secondary disabilities might be viewed as *perceived activity limitations*. Similarly, from the subjective perspective of the individual, the sum of all primary and secondary handicaps might be viewed as *perceived role limitations*. These internal perceptions of reality would be related to, but distinct from, the more objective assessments of impairment, disability, and handicap.

Perceived health, activity limitations, and role limitations are closely related to quality of life. As such, there is growing consensus for conceptualizing quality of life as a global subjective assessment of well-being, hierarchically composed of subjective perceptions in broad domains (Spilker, 1990). Quality of life might therefore be considered (but not limited to) the subjective perceptions of health, activity limitations, and role limitations. Figure 1 summarizes elaborations of the WHO model of disablement in the areas of secondary conditions and subjective perceptions, including quality of life.

Incorporating Environmental Factors

A final area needing elaboration is that of environmental factors. The foreword to the ICIDH states that "an important task in the revision of the ICIDH will be to improve the presentation and illustration of the way in which external factors affect the ICIDH components" (WHO, 1993, p. 5).

A major criticism of the WHO model of disablement has been its implied causality. Indeed, the WHO model described disablement as originating with pathology, leading to impairment, which in turn produces disability and, finally, handicap. Although this conceptualization is well grounded in the medical model, it fails to acknowledge the importance of the environment as a major contributor to the disablement process, a contributor that can either restrict or enhance the performance of an individual.

Disability activists and organizations of people with disabilities have been quick to point out that, in the WHO model, the causes of disablement are limited to disease and trauma and that the interventions to address disablement are also limited to medical care and rehabilitation of the individual. They argue that equally important causes of disablement lie in the environment. As such, interventions directed at changing the physical,

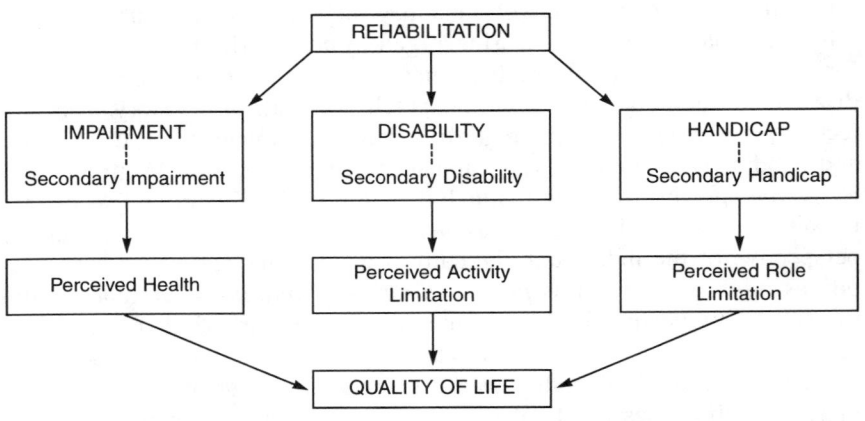

Figure 1. Secondary conditions and subjective perceptions in the WHO model of disablement. (From Whiteneck, G.G. [1994]. Measuring what matters: Key rehabilitation outcomes. 44th annual John Stanley Coulter lecture. *Archives of Physical Medicine and Rehabilitation, 75,* 1075; reprinted by permission.)

social, and policy environments in which people with disabilities find themselves are just as important. For example, architectural barriers and inaccessible transportation isolate people in wheelchairs. Negative attitudes of employers and financial disincentives may keep qualified people with disabilities from working. All of these affect their ability to fulfill roles and their level of handicap. Thus, in addition to medical research and effective rehabilitation, social changes, environmental adaptations, and program access also can lessen, mitigate, or "cure" disabilities and handicaps.

Thus, the final needed elaboration of the WHO's model of disablement is to explicitly add the concept of environmental factors to the disablement process, listing the elements and the characteristics of the environment that should be considered and that determine its impact. This retains the strengths of the original model while correcting its weaknesses by adding an emphasis on external influences.

Environmental factors are theoretically important in all aspects of the disablement process. However, the most relevant nature of the environment differs, depending on what aspect of disablement is being considered. For pathology that occurs at the cellular level, the cellular environment is most relevant. The traditional interventions of medicine take these environmental factors into consideration. Steroid treatments, for example, may decrease local cord swelling and damage immediately following spinal cord injury, whereas antibiotics may enhance the ability of white cells to fight infection. For impairment at the organ level, the environment expands to related organ systems. Again, medical treatments constitute the most appropriate interventions, such as the use of alternative urologic management methods to treat neurogenic bladders. For disability at the person level, the environment would include the techniques and technologies of rehabilitation that assist in the performance of ADL tasks. The extensive use of adaptive equipment is a prime example. Finally, for handicap, environmental factors include such things as accessibility, discrimination, and availability of resources. Often the interventions are not so much medical as societal.

These examples illustrate that environmental factors are present at all levels of disablement. They also demonstrate that they are implicitly included in and addressed by both the medical and WHO models for pathology, impairment, and disability. However, it is at the level of handicap where environmental factors and appropriate interventions go well beyond the boundaries of both the medical model and the WHO model of disablement. It is these social, cultural, and physical dimensions—dimensions that constitute the very organization and context of human society—that seem to have been neglected or overlooked. Therefore, it appears most critical that environmental factors be incorporated in the ICIDH revision at the level of handicap.

Environmental Factors as External Determinants of Handicap To understand the role of environmental factors in influencing handicap, a distinction must first be made between the internal and external determinants of handicap. *Internal factors* are the array of individual characteristics that can be further subdivided into those characteristics directly related to the disablement process and those that existed before or outside of the disablement process. Within the disablement category, impairment and disabilities are the traditional focus. However, compensatory abilities also must be considered. The term *personal identity* has been proposed to encompass the many demographic and life experience characteristics that are distinct from the disablement process (Fougeyrollas, 1995).

In contrast to these internal individual characteristics, environmental factors represent the external determinants of handicap. It is only through the examination of the unique impairments and abilities and disabilities of a given individual, interacting with his or her unique personal identity and environmental factors that the particular handicaps that result can be understood (see Figure 2).

In general terms, *environmental factors* can be defined as all social, cultural, and physical dimensions that constitute the organization and context of a human society. Relating more specifically to handicap, *environmental factors* can be defined as all characteristics external to an individual with an impairment or disability that influence that individual's performance as a member of society. Environmental factors are the external influences on handicap.

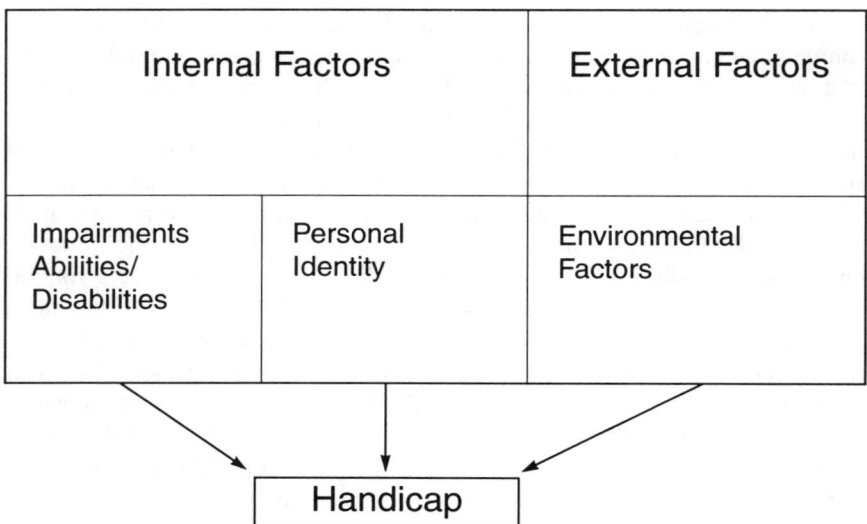

Figure 2. Determinants of handicap.

Characteristics of the Environment To improve the understanding and categorization of environmental factors, three approaches are proposed. First, the general elements of the environment common to all people (whether or not they have a disability) are presented. Second, three levels from which to analyze the environment are suggested, ranging from the immediate personal environment to the broad societal environment. Finally, five general characteristics of environments that influence how poorly or how well an individual becomes an active, productive member of society are listed.

Elements of the environment common to all individuals include both natural and constructed physical environments as well as the cultural, political, economic, social, and legal environments. The three levels of analysis from which to view the environment are micro, meso, and macro. The micro level consists of the immediate personal environment of the individual, with the focus being on physical and functional characteristics such as access and accommodations. The meso level consists of the somewhat broader community environment and focuses on the attitudes and beliefs held by people whom the individual encounters. The macro level consists of the broadest societal environment, focusing on the policy issues of resource allocation and equality (Fougeyrollas, 1995). Examining the many elements of the environment from these levels has led to the identification of five characteristics of the environment that have significant influence on handicap:

1. Accessibility
2. Accommodation
3. Resource availability
4. Social support
5. Equality

Accessibility answers the question, "Can you get where you want to go?" It is defined in terms of physical access and includes architectural barriers such as steps and inaccessible bathrooms as well as the accessibility of transportation. These aspects of the environment either restrict or facilitate an individual's ability to move about freely in his or her community.

Accommodation addresses the question, "Can you do what you want to do?" It is defined in terms of the equipment, services, or modifications to tasks that facilitate full participation and independent living. Areas of accommodation include home, workplace, school, other businesses and organizations, and other community settings. This aspect of the environment either restricts or facilitates an individual's ability to participate in an activity once he or she is at the location of that activity.

Resource availability addresses the question, "Are your special needs met?" It is defined in terms of the availability and provision of services and resources made necessary by the particular disability. These may include medical care, personal assistant services, and income security. This category assesses the degree to which the extra resources needed by a person with a disability are available.

Social support addresses the question, "Are you accepted by those around you?" It is defined in terms of the attitudes and prejudices of others that either discourage community integration or provide a supportive environment that allows community integration to flourish. Social support may be provided by family and friends, employers and teachers, neighbors and peers, and other community members. This category focuses on the social barriers that can be remedied only by attitude change in others. Extra funding is not likely to solve these particular problems.

Equality addresses the question, "Are you treated equally with others?" It is defined in terms of the degree to which the policies and regulations of governments and institutions ensure equality of opportunity for people with disabilities. Included in this category are discrimination, financial disincentives, health care management and rationing, and legislative mandates.

These five environmental characteristics form useful criteria for evaluating environments. However, they must be applied to each individual's situation, because the same environment may restrict one person but not another. In each case, these five environmental characteristics can be assessed on a continuum ranging from restrictive barriers to inclusive facilitators.

CONCLUSIONS

The elaborations of the WHO model of disablement suggested in this chapter represent four major shifts in emphasis that are needed to effectively pursue medical rehabilitation outcomes research. First, greater emphasis must be placed on understanding and measuring handicap. Handicap has been a long-neglected but important outcome of rehabilitation. At the national level, the ADA expresses the goal of minimizing handicap by ensuring a quality of opportunity, full participation, independent living, and economic self-sufficiency. Brown (1993) suggested that these four stated goals of the ADA closely parallel the dimensions of handicap identified by the WHO. Thus, with the concept of handicap at the heart of both rehabilitation programs and national policy, the need to emphasize handicap is clear.

The second major shift is the greater recognition of the lifelong, dynamic nature of disablement. Secondary impairments, secondary disabilities, and secondary handicaps deserve as much attention as the primary disabling condition. Successfully controlling lifelong secondary conditions is the mark of quality rehabilitation and is just as important as controlling medical complications and maximizing independence during initial hospitalization.

A third major shift in emphasis is the commitment to measure quality of life and the recognition of subjective perceptions as legitimate outcomes. Subjective perceptions are needed to fill the gaps left by traditional objective assessments. Perceived health, perceived activity limitations, perceived role limitations, and perceived quality of life must be incorporated into outcomes measures.

Finally, the role of environmental factors in determining handicap must be acknowledged and emphasized. The medical model is not adequate in and of itself to completely explain the consequences of disablement. For some conditions, the impact of environmental barriers on handicap may even outweigh the impairments and disabilities themselves. The inclusion of environmental factors in both conceptual modeling and outcomes research designs is necessary to develop an understanding of the relative importance of internal versus external factors in the disablement process.

REFERENCES

American Spinal Injury Association. (1990). *American Spinal Injury Association standards for neurological classification of spinal injury patients*. Chicago: Author.

Americans with Disabilities Act (ADA) of 1990, PL 101-336, 42 U.S.C. §§ 12101 *et seq.*

Brown, S.C. (1993). Revitalizing handicap for disability research: Developing tools to assess progress in quality of life for persons with disabilities. *Journal of Disability Policy Studies, 4*(2), 57–76.

Carey, R.G., & Posavac, E.J. (1978). Program evaluation of a physical medicine and rehabilitation unit: A new approach. *Archives of Physical Medicine and Rehabilitation, 59,* 330–337.

Fougeyrollas, P. (1995). Documenting environmental factors for preventing the handicap creation process: Québec contributions relating to ICIDH and social participation of people with functional differences. *Disability and Rehabilitation, 17*(3/4), 145–153.

Frey, W.D. (1984). Functional assessment in the '80s. In A.S. Halpern & M.J. Fuhrer (Eds.), *Functional assessment in rehabilitation* (pp. 11–43). Baltimore: Paul H. Brookes Publishing Co.

Harvey, R.F., & Jellinek, H.M. (1981). Functional performance assessment: A program approach. *Archives of Physical Medicine and Rehabilitation, 62,* 456–461.

Kemp, B.J., & Vash, C.L. (1971). Productivity after injury in a sample of spinal cord injured persons: A pilot study. *Journal of Chronic Disease, 24,* 259–275.

Mahoney, F.I., & Barthel, D.W. (1965). Functional evaluation: The Barthel Index. *Maryland State Medical Journal, 14,* 61–65.

Marge, M. (1988). Health promotion for persons with disabilities: Moving beyond rehabilitation. *American Journal of Health Promotion, 2,* 29–35.

Moskowitz, E., & McCann, C.B. (1957). Classification of disability in the chronically ill and aging. *Journal of Chronic Disease, 5,* 342–346.

National Institutes of Health (NIH). (1993). *Research plan for the National Center for Medical Rehabilitation Research* (NIH Publication No. 93-3509). Washington, DC: U.S. Department of Health and Human Services.

Pflueger, S.S. (1977). *Independent living: Emerging issues in rehabilitation.* Washington, DC: Institute for Research Utilization.

Pope, A.M., & Tarlov, A.R. (Eds.). (1991). *Disability in America: Toward a national agenda for prevention.* Washington, DC: National Academy Press.

Spilker, B. (1990). *Quality of life assessments in clinical trials.* New York: Raven Press.

State University of New York at Buffalo. (1993). *Guide for the Uniform Data Set for Medical Rehabilitation (Adult FIM), version 4.0.* Buffalo, NY: Author.

State University of New York at Syracuse, Health Sciences Center. (1994). *Conversation on disability issues: Secondary conditions and aging with a disability.* Syracuse, NY: Author.

Teasdale, G., & Jennett, B. (1974). Assessment of coma and impaired consciousness: A practical scale. *Lancet, 2,* 81–84.

Wagner, K.A. (1987). Outcome analysis in comprehensive medical rehabilitation. In M.J. Fuhrer (Ed.), *Rehabilitation outcomes: Analysis and measurement* (pp. 19–28). Baltimore: Paul H. Brookes Publishing Co.

Whiteneck, G.G. (1994). Measuring what matters: Key rehabilitation outcomes. 44th annual John Stanley Coulter lecture. *Archives of Physical Medicine and Rehabilitation, 75,* 1073–1076.

Whiteneck, G.G., Charlifue, S.W., Gerhart, K.A., Overholser, D., & Richardson, G.N. (1992). Quantifying handicap: A new measure of long-term rehabilitation outcomes. *Archives of Physical Medicine and Rehabilitation, 73,* 519–526.

Willer, B.S., Linn, R.T., & Allen, K.M. (1993). Community integration and barriers to integration for individuals with brain injury. In M.A.J. Finlayson & S. Garner (Eds.), *Brain injury rehabilitation: Clinical considerations* (pp. 355–375). Baltimore: Williams & Wilkins.

Willer, B., Rosenthal, M., Kreutzer, J.S., Gorden, W.A., & Rempel, R. (1993). Assessment of community integration following rehabilitation for traumatic brain injury. *Journal of Head Trauma Rehabilitation, 8*(2), 75–87.

World Health Organization (WHO). (1980). *International classification of impairments, disabilities, and handicaps: A manual of classification relating to the consequences of disease.* Geneva, Switzerland: Author.

World Health Organization (WHO). (1993). Foreword. In *International classification of impairments, disabilities, and handicaps: A manual of classification relating to the consequences of disease.* Geneva, Switzerland: Author.

CHAPTER *5*

The Measurement
of Disability

Carl V. Granger and Roger C. Fiedler

The Americans with Disabilities Act of 1990 (PL 101-336) mandates integration of people with disabilities into society. Because approximately 35 million Americans have a disability, it has become clear that "disability is an issue that affects every individual, community, neighborhood, and family in the United States. It is more than a medical issue; it is a costly social, public health, and moral issue" (Pope & Tarlov, 1991, p. 1). It is further estimated that the annual national costs of disabilities exceed $170 billion, including an estimated $85 billion in federally supported programs for benefits and services to people with disabilities (Pope & Tarlov, 1991).

As these figures indicate, rehabilitation has become a national priority. The increasing survival of infants with major developmental delays, the enhanced capacity to stabilize people following major disabling trauma, the disproportionate effects of disablement on minorities and lower socio-economic groups (Centers for Disease Control, 1992), and the growing proportion of the older adult segment of the population have highlighted the need to develop and assess effective and efficient rehabilitation services.

These factors have increased attention on medical rehabilitation and have raised questions about what medical rehabilitation is, what it does, how it is done, why it is done, and what its costs are. Questions about why medical rehabilitation is done have resulted in an emphasis on research on the goals, costs, and outcomes of medical rehabilitation.

Medical rehabilitation outcomes research has been limited by the absence of a uniform language and terminology to provide a conceptual basis for understanding the roles of medical rehabilitation and the outcomes of disabilities. It also has been hampered by inadequate funding, the lack of high-quality measurement tools, scant epidemiologic data, and a scarcity of well-trained and productive rehabilitation scientists (National Center for

Medical Rehabilitation Research, 1992). This absence of uniformity and conceptual models for understanding and communicating about medical rehabilitation outcomes and the scarcity of well-designed measurement tools to translate conceptual models into observable and measurable outcomes to compare alternative interventions have been the primary barriers preventing major advances in medical rehabilitation. The translation of conceptual models into measurement of functional status and disability has become key to monitoring, tracking, and accounting for recovery from disability. It is the measurement of disability built on a foundation of a uniform conceptual model that allows for assessing patient progress and predicting positive and negative outcomes following rehabilitation, both across disciplines and across the life span.

This chapter discusses three primary concerns for medical rehabilitation outcomes research: 1) the conceptual basis for measuring rehabilitation outcomes, 2) the measurement of disability in outcomes research across disciplines and across the life span, and 3) the need for future research efforts to advance the field. The chapter begins by describing a new conceptual model for studying medical rehabilitation outcomes and then establishes a link between the concepts in the model and their translation into clinical practice using a uniform measurement system for tracking patients and their outcomes. It is argued here and elsewhere (Johnson & Wolinsky, 1994; Wilson & Cleary, 1995) that understanding research on medical rehabilitation outcomes begins by defining the conceptual basis for outcomes within a comprehensive theoretical framework and then operationally defining these concepts through measurement. Once these steps are accomplished, the process of medical rehabilitation becomes more universally understood, and research using measures of outcomes may proceed in light of this understanding.

A CONCEPTUAL FRAMEWORK
FOR DEFINING OUTCOMES MEASURES

Measuring outcomes in medical rehabilitation must begin with an understanding of what is to be measured, and this understanding must be grounded in theory and connected to a comprehensive model for meeting the needs of the patient. One of the critical problems that has hampered the development of good measurement tools in medical rehabilitation has been the inability of health care professionals to speak a common language. Several conceptual and theoretical models have been developed that have provided differing definitions of patient impairment, disability, and handicap (Nagi, 1965; World Health Organization, 1980).

Although some progress has been made on these issues and some consensus has been reached, more detailed conceptual models are needed to cover the broad expanse of medical rehabilitation. In the mid-1990s, some authors attempted to provide detailed and comprehensive conceptual models for understanding the role of medical rehabilitation (Johnson & Wolinsky, 1994; Verbrugge & Jette, 1994; Wilson & Cleary, 1995; Ziebland, Fitzpatrick, & Jenkinson, 1993). As Wilson and Cleary (1995) pointed out, "The relationships between traditional clinical variables and health status measures have not been adequately conceptualized in much of the research to date" (p. 63). These authors argued that the conceptualization and measurement of these relationships will provide key insights into the link between diagnosis and therapy. Current measures of disability alone may not be easily interpreted without concomitant measures of patient health perceptions and measures of environmental factors. They also argued, as did Johnson and Wolinsky (1994), that causal relationships need to be established and tested if outcomes research is to move forward. These authors argued that the conceptualization and measurement of disability should not be limited to functional status alone, but that patient perceptions and environments must be considered as well within an overall context of general life satisfaction and quality of life. It is these latter concepts that have helped to form the basis of a new model for studying disability.

These examples of conceptual models make it clear that medical rehabilitation is quite comprehensive in its goals, including treating patient problems along a continuum from the molecular and cellular level to the complex overall quality-of-life level. This suggests that medical rehabilitation outcomes can be measured at a variety of levels or stages, including the physical, cognitive, and emotional levels, but that they should be measured within the context of the choices, demands, and expectations that are held by the patient, family, and environment. Thus, any comprehensive model of medical rehabilitation outcomes must consider the physical, cognitive, and emotional capacities of the individual while recognizing the match between those capacities and the demands of the environment within which that individual is expected to function. This must all be balanced by considering the differing expectations of individuals for functioning within their own capacities within their own environmental demands.

To begin the process of comprehensively defining and measuring medical rehabilitation outcomes, the following new operational definition of *quality of daily living* is offered: Quality of daily living is the ever-changing balance between one's choices, options, and expectations versus the physical, cognitive, and emotional demands of daily living. This definition focuses attention on the functional outcomes of medical rehabilitation and moves the focus of attention away from other concepts of quality of life. Thus, the concept and its definition provide the context within which medical rehabilitation outcomes may be more easily understood. This definition also leads directly to a new and comprehensive conceptual model for understanding disability outcomes in medical rehabilitation. This new conceptual model is represented in the diagram shown in Figure 1. This figure represents a dynamic model for challenges to the quality of daily living in anticipation of an integrated science of medical rehabilitation based on a firm foundation of theory and scientific measurement principles.

The model proposed in Figure 1 allows for the development, measurement, and testing of an entirely new organizing and unifying model for studying disablement and subsequent medical rehabilitation outcomes. This model focuses on a new conceptual framework of challenges to the quality of daily living and covers a range of concerns being debated by the field of medical rehabilitation in the mid-1990s. The model presented in Figure 1 views fulfillment as a result of achieving a dynamic balance in life between the functional opportunities available to the individual and the functional requirements or demands placed on the individual. It is clear from Figure 1 that the dynamic balance between functional opportunities and functional demands that influences a patient's overall sense of fulfillment is a constant challenge to maintain and that the measurement of disability is complicated by this ever-changing balance.

The challenges to the quality of daily living model developed from the work of the noted American psychologist Abraham Maslow (1954). Maslow advanced a new theory of human motivation that challenged some of the orthodox principles of Freudian and Skinnerian psychology. Before

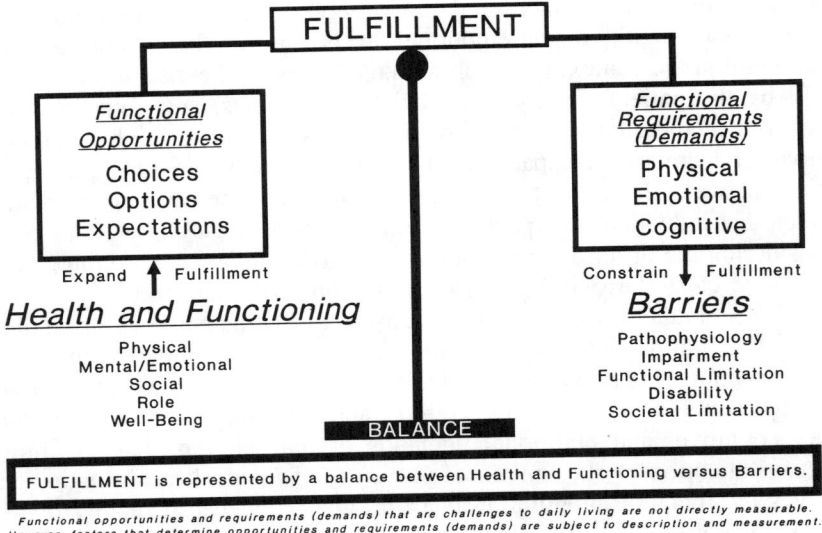

Figure 1. Model for challenges to the quality of daily living. (From Granger, C.V., Kelly-Hayes, M., Johnston, M., Deutsch, A., Braun, S., & Fiedler, R.C. (1996). Quality and outcome measures for medical rehabilitation. In R.L. Braddom (Ed.), *Physical medicine and rehabilitation* (p. 240). Philadelphia: W.B. Saunders; reprinted by permission.)

Maslow, it had been considered appropriate to control and manipulate employees in the workplace. In the 1960s, Maslow developed the Eupsychian Management way of thinking to encourage a more humanistic relationship between management and employees. From this, Maslow evolved a hierarchy of needs that would support self-actualization. At the base of his conceptual pyramid lay the physical needs for survival. At progressively higher levels were satisfaction of needs for security, social interaction, and self-esteem. As lower-level needs were satisfied, successively higher levels of need became relatively more important as motivators of behavior. Ultimately, the fully evolved individual would achieve self-actualization, a term that describes the full use of human capacities to perceive, feel, learn, acquire skill, exercise intellectual capabilities, create, and love—in short, based on self-esteem and respect for others, to grow in competence and ability to live a fulfilling life (Maslow, 1954).

Maslow's concepts form the conceptual framework for the study of medical rehabilitation outcomes. Medical rehabilitation is a system of interdisciplinary interventions designed to facilitate fulfillment and the quality of daily living for individuals with disabilities. Medical rehabilitation needs measurement that can reflect effectiveness and efficiency of the process. Yet, to a large extent, fulfillment and quality of daily living are not directly measurable. However, to account for the challenges to fulfillment and the quality of daily living, the factors that determine the opportunities and requirements (demands) must be identified. Figure 1 proposes that an individual's fulfillment and quality of daily living are a result of achieving a balance between functional opportunities (left column) and functional requirements or demands (right column). Functional opportunities are expressed as the individual's choices, options, and expectations; and functional requirements are expressed in physical, cognitive, and emotional terms. To achieve fulfillment and to maximize the quality of daily living, there must be a balance between improved opportunities through an individual's health and functioning (left column) and the reduction or removal of life's barriers causing constraints (right column). This model reflects Maslow's (1954) industrial psychological beliefs that health and functioning result from the individual being presented with life's work in the form of barriers and systematically overcoming them. The model further reflects Maslow's hierarchical beliefs in that it views the individual with disabilities as meeting progressively higher needs of function through the work of medical rehabilitation. The field of medical rehabilitation recognizes the need for balance between functional demands and functional opportunities and progressively presents to the patient both the demands and the ways to achieve the opportunities in the form of challenges to the quality of daily living while moving up the hierarchy from the basic physical needs to the satisfaction of the need for security, social interaction, and self-esteem. The ultimate goal of medical rehabilitation then becomes, in Maslow's terms, self-actualization, the full use of the human capacities to perceive, feel, create, and love, in the form of fulfillment through the everyday efforts to challenge barriers and overcome them.

Figure 1 includes several measurable factors that serve as domains of health and functioning (left column) such as physical, mental and emotional, social, role performance, and subjective well-being, and measurable barriers (right column), including pathophysiology, impairment, functional limitation, disability, and societal limitation. This unifying model for medical rehabilitation fits well with existing theoretical frameworks (e.g., the open systems theory models of von Bertalanffy [1968]; and Kielhofner & Burke [1980]) across the many disciplines involved in medical rehabilitation of hierarchical structures and of expanding and constraining relationships between levels of the hierarchy, and it provides an organizing conceptual framework for measuring disability across disciplines in medical rehabilitation. The model also includes many of the concepts described by the models of other medical rehabilitation researchers (Johnson & Wolinsky, 1994; Wilson & Cleary, 1995; Ziebland et al., 1993). Under the heading of health and functioning, the model considers the patient's choices, options, and expectations that expand fulfillment. These include the concepts of patient perceptions of disability such as perceived health (Johnson & Wolinsky, 1994) and general health perceptions (Wilson & Cleary, 1995), which are viewed as ways that patients can increase health and functioning, as well as perceptions that may decrease health and functioning, as indicated by the concept of subjective distress (Ziebland et al., 1993). On the other side of the model are considered the barriers to fulfillment, including the concepts of disease and pathology, impairment, disability, functional limitations, and societal limitations (handicap). These fit well with the Johnson and Wolinsky (1994) model of disease, disability, functional limitation, and perceived health. Also on this side of the balance are the concepts of environmental and family factors (Wilson & Cleary, 1995), which can either present barriers or remove barriers to fulfillment and push toward the improvement of the quality of daily living.

As previously described, the model recognizes that functional opportunities and requirements that serve as the challenges to the quality of daily living are not directly measurable, but that the factors that determine the opportunities and requirements are subject to description and measurement. The next critical step in developing a comprehensive model for conceptualizing and measuring medical rehabilitation outcomes is to translate the functional opportunities and requirements or demands into measurable constructs that may then be used in models to establish causal relationships.

THE MEASUREMENT OF DISABILITY IN MEDICAL REHABILITATION

To operationally define the concepts in the model, the field of medical rehabilitation has already moved forward in developing measures of the quality of daily living. Of considerable importance has been the development and widespread international acceptance of the Functional Independence Measure (FIM^{SM}) (State University of New York at Buffalo, 1993a) as one of the primary tools for assessing disability in medical rehabilitation patients (Hamilton, 1991). However, this uniform measure has been available only since 1987. Before the FIM, the multiplicity of functional status outcomes scales used in different rehabilitation hospitals contributed to confusion regarding outcomes of medical rehabilitation. Many of these scales, which are used in studying a variety of outcomes in medical rehabilitation, may be found together in several texts (Basmajian, 1994; Granger & Gresham, 1984; Wade, 1992). However, these scales reflect the differences in conceptualization of disability in the field and have contributed to confusion by providing scores that were not comparable across disciplines or impairments. Thus, the FIM was developed to offer the field a uniform method for describing the severity of disability and the functional outcomes of medical rehabilitation.

The construction of the FIM was unique in that it evolved through a process of national consensus followed by a systematic procedure of evaluation. After reviewing 36 published and unpublished functional assessment instruments, the challenge was to select the most common and useful functional assessment items and to decide on an appropriate rating scale that would permit most rehabilitation clinicians to assess severity of disability in a uniform and reliable manner. Sponsoring, cooperating, and endorsing organizations that participated in the development of the FIM included the following: American Congress of Rehabilitation Medicine, American Academy of Physical Medicine and Rehabilitation, American Physical Therapy Association, American Occupational Therapy Association, American Speech-Language-Hearing Association, Association of Rehabilitation Nurses, National Association of Rehabilitation Facilities (now the American Rehabilitation Association), Commission on Accreditation of Rehabilitation Facilities (now CARF . . . The Rehabilitation Accreditation Commission), American Hospital Association—Section for Rehabilitation Hospitals and Programs, National Association of Research and Training Centers, American Spinal Injury Association, National Head Injury Foundation, and National Easter Seal Society. These organizations helped to provide the initial consensus for the FIM from a variety of clinical standpoints.

The FIM was thus developed through a broad consensus of clinicians and researchers in the field and included 18 items measuring six subscales in two domains of key importance to the field. The initial FIM was thought to be comprehensive yet easy to administer, but it required the usual steps of testing for its measurement properties, including its reliability, validity, and feasibility in clinical practice. To more clearly identify and standardize the process of examining new tools developed for studying clinical outcomes in medical rehabilitation, a set of measurement standards was developed by Johnston, Keith, and Hinderer (1992). According to these authors, the key questions to address when designing or evaluating a scale involve identifying its purpose, whether the scale is practical for clinical use, whether its items and scoring systems are acceptable and useful, and whether it has standardized procedures for administration and scoring, as well as testing whether the scale is reliable and valid. Scales failing to meet these standards may be judged to be suspect in their benefits to patients (Merbitz, Morris, & Grip, 1989) because they may not be useful indicators of medical rehabilitation outcomes. All scales in medical rehabilitation should be evaluated under this set of standards to judge the scales' value to the profession and its patients.

The initial investigations of the FIM were carried out in three phases: pilot, trial, and implementation. These investigations focused on determining the measurement properties of the FIM and also studied its clinical applicability and ease of administration. As with any comprehensive model for assessment of medical rehabilitation outcomes, the translation of concepts into measurement and the application of good measurement principles to test the translation process become key to evaluating the promise of the model.

The pilot study of the FIM (Hamilton, Granger, Sherwin, Zielezny, & Tashman, 1987) was completed in 1985, using 11 facilities and 110 patients to determine FIM face validity and ease of administration. The intent of the trial, completed in 1986, was to assess interrater reliability, validity, precision, and time to administer the data set. Data for the trial were obtained at admission, discharge, and, when feasible, follow-up after discharge in 25 facilities across the United States. A sample of 250 patients was assessed, and 891 clinician assessments were performed (Hamilton et al., 1987). The implementation phase evaluation of the FIM in 18 facilities with 303 patients in 1987 finalized the seven-level scale, revised it from the original four-level scale, and confirmed the face validity and precision findings of the trial. The results also showed improvement in the interrater reliability (FIM total score intraclass correlation of .95) (Hamilton, Laughlin, Fiedler, & Granger, 1994) and demonstrated an average FIM learning time of 41 minutes and FIM administration time by clinicians of 32 minutes (Hamilton et al., 1987).

The FIM measures a patient's performance of basic activities of daily living using 18 items within the six subscales of self-care (eating, grooming, bathing, dressing upper and lower body, and toileting), sphincter control (bladder and bowel management), mobility (transfers to bed/chair/wheelchair, toilet, and tub/shower), locomotion (walking/wheeling and stair climbing), communication (comprehension and expression), and social cognition (social interaction, memory, and problem solving). The seven levels of performance reflect the extent to which the activities are performed independently or require the help of another person. A higher score means that the person is more independent. A score on the FIM is a way of representing the burden of care or cost of disability in terms of the amount of effort needed from another person and the costs in terms of consumption of social and economic resources.

The Measurement Properties of the FIM

Precision The ability of the FIM to detect meaningful change in level of function has been observed to be high. For a sample of 309 patients with acquired brain injury (ABI) admitted to five ABI model systems hospitals in the United States, the admission FIM average score was 59, with a 95% confidence range of ± 3.2. Discharge FIM average score was 100, with a 95% confidence range of ± 2.8 (Dahmer et al., 1993).

Feasibility of Use Feasibility of use of the FIM has been observed to be acceptable. Feasibility may be estimated by documenting the learning time and administration time for a clinician using the instrument. During the implementation phase, the average time required to learn to use the FIM was reported to be almost 40 minutes and the average time required to evaluate a patient was about 30 minutes. Telephone interviews have been used to assess function on the FIM and take approximately 20–30 minutes (Hamilton et al., 1987).

Interrater Reliability The most recent test of interrater agreement was performed by having two or more pairs of clinicians assess each of 1,018 patients undergoing inpatient medical rehabilitation at 89 Uniform Data System for Medical Rehabilitation (UDSmr^SM) subscribing hospitals. The results were as follows: total FIM intraclass correlation coefficient (ANOVA), .99; self-care, .98; sphincter control, .97; mobility, .98; locomotion, .97; communication, .97; and social cognition, .98. FIM item kappas ranged from .69 to .84 (Hamilton et al., 1994). It was concluded that the seven-level FIM demonstrated good interrater agreement among clinicians. Efforts to improve and refine testing of interrater reliability and internal consistency reliability are ongoing. Research in functional assessment is addressing use of the FIM to predict clinical outcomes and resource need.

Validity In general, validity is the extent to which an instrument measures what it is intended to measure or the extent to which there is agreement between the measure and a criterion. No instrument is inherently valid; rather, an instrument is valid with regard to a specific purpose, range, and sample (Granger, Cotter, Hamilton, & Fiedler, 1993; Granger, Cotter, Hamilton, Fiedler, & Hens, 1990; Granger, Divan, & Fiedler, 1995; Heinemann, Hamilton, Granger, Linacre, & Wright, 1992; Heinemann, Hamilton, Granger, Wright, & Linacre, 1991; Heinemann, Linacre, Wright, Hamilton,

& Granger, 1993). Validity of the FIM has been assessed in several ways. Acceptable content and face validity were achieved by clinicians' responses to three questions: 97% said there were no unnecessary items, 83% said there was no need for more items, and an average response of 3.5 on a Likert scale (poor = 1 to excellent = 5) was achieved regarding adequacy of the FIM as a measure of disability. Construct validity of the FIM has been assessed with home visits by clinicians who documented minutes of help per day using a journal and stopwatch procedure. For participants with multiple sclerosis, the amount of variance explained in predicting minutes of help per day by FIM scores was .77 (Granger et al., 1990); for subjects after stroke, .65 (Granger, Cotter, Hamilton, & Fiedler, 1993); for spinal cord injury, .76 (Hamilton, 1991); and for ABI, .94 (Granger, Divan, & Fiedler, 1995).

These studies also compared the FIM with other existing measures of disability in predicting burden of care, operationally defined as minutes of help per day. The FIM was a better predictor than were the Environmental Status Scale (International Federation of Multiple Sclerosis Societies, 1985; Mellerup et al., 1981), the Brief Symptom Inventory (Derogatis & Melisaratos, 1983), the Sickness Impact Profile (Bergner, Bobbitt, Carter, & Gelson, 1981), the Dartmouth COOP Functional Health Assessment Scales (Beaufait et al., 1992), the Community Integration Questionnaire (Willer, Linn, & Allen, 1993), and the Fatigue Severity Scale (Krupp, LaRocca, Muir-Nash, & Steinberg, 1989). However, for each of these studies, the FIM was not as good a predictor of overall life satisfaction as it was for minutes of help per day. Thus, the conceptual model described previously and echoed by other theorists in the field shows that disability measured by functional status and disability measured by life satisfaction are not perfectly correlated. To achieve a balance of functional opportunities and demands as shown in Figure 1, the individual must not only improve health and functioning but also overcome environmental barriers to overall life satisfaction. These areas have been clearly identified as distinctively different by the research on a variety of patient samples using a variety of medical rehabilitation measures.

In summary, the FIM has been shown to be a comprehensive, easy-to-administer, minimal data set that is both highly reliable and valid across a variety of impairment groups. However, researchers have focused on another key aspect in the measurement process of disability. Merbitz et al. (1989) suggested that ordinal rating scales cannot be used as objective, interval-level measures in studying patients with disabilities. This psychometric concern has generated considerable research focused on understanding and evaluating the process of measurement in medical rehabilitation.

DEFINING MEASUREMENT IN MEDICAL REHABILITATION

The process of measurement always begins with the concept of what is to be measured. Measurement may be as simple as deciding whether an event is present or absent, such as in determining a disease or diagnosis, or measurement may occur along a scale or dimension, such as rating disability or using hard science physical measures to determine heart rate, blood pressure, or nerve conductivity. One of the most immediate issues for measurement in medical rehabilitation has been to determine whether that which is to be measured is observable, which is often the case for functional measures, or whether it must be inferred from subjective evaluations of how the patient feels, which is more common with measures of pain or well-being.

It is useful to compare the measures designed for medical rehabilitation with traditional biologic or physiologic measurements taken in other medical fields. The field of medical rehabilitation is unique in its emphasis on both the pathophysiologic and psychosocial measurement of disablement. The emphasis in the 1990s on developing measures that cut across diagnostic categories and that focus on disablement and measure impairment, disability, and handicap has resulted in measures that are quite broad-based and multidisciplinary. These tools move beyond the physical domain into areas of how patients feel and function. Thus, the functional scales in medical rehabilitation have been viewed by many as designed by physicians and care providers to subjectively assess patients using a broad spectrum of rating scales. Physical functioning, mental and social role functioning, subjective well-being (e.g., patient satisfaction), impairment, disability, and handicap are all measured with more refined scales that have more accuracy, sensitivity, and predictive value. The use of these various scales across patients, sites, and disciplines suggests problems in making fair comparisons at any single point in time. The problem is further compounded when studying changes over time and across the life span for the varieties of patients experiencing medical rehabilitation.

Although traditional examinations and assessments identify and quantify deficits, they "do not show how the individual's deficits might interact with task and environmental demands and, thus, impact on the individual's ability to function" (Special Projects, 1992, p. 52,683). Thus, "functional assessment differs from more traditional assessments by focusing on how individual limitations and strengths interact with the demands of living, working, and learning environments" (Special Projects, 1992, p. 52,684).

These concerns raise two critical points. The first is that measures in medical rehabilitation that are to adequately reflect the aspects of the challenges to the quality of daily living model must reflect the subjective experiences of the patient and the objective amount of time and care in terms of physical assistance needed for the patient. This distinction was made when considering the differences in medical rehabilitation outcomes between minutes of help per day and overall life satisfaction (Granger et al., 1990, 1993, 1995). The second concern is whether subjective measures, which are typically scored on rating scales, have sufficient psychometric properties to be analyzed with parametric statistical procedures in prediction models for determining patient outcomes, and whether they can serve as adequate outcomes measures in themselves. The latter issue is tied closely to whether ordinal scales can adequately reflect changes over time.

A considerable amount of controversy and subsequent attention to the issue of ordinality have developed as a result of the study of the FIM. The FIM has been extensively studied for its psychometric properties. These studies have included the examination of reliability and validity as previously described. However, one of the primary concerns for ordinal scales has been whether these scales can be used as interval measures of patient function and progress. This concern has brought a new methodology to the study of the FIM. Rasch analysis (Harvey et al., 1992; Heinemann et al., 1991, 1992, 1993; Wright & Linacre, 1991) has been extensively employed to study in detail the ordinality of the FIM. Rasch analysis provides a way to transform ordinal scale scores into interval-level measures by determining the difficulties of rating scale items on a single interval-level dimension known as a logit line. Rasch analysis requires that the items on a scale placed along the logit item difficulty line must measure only the one dimension reflected by the logit line. Thus, Rasch analysis allows for both a test of a scale's unidimensionality and its transformation from ordinal scores to interval measures.

Rasch (latent trait) analysis of FIM data from 14,799 hospitalized patients has indicated that the 13 motor items and the 5 cognitive items of the FIM can be successfully converted into two unidimensional interval measures (Heinemann et al., 1991). FIM motor and cognitive logit-transformed (Rasch) measures in a sample of 256 patients with ABI admitted to rehabilitation at five ABI model systems hospitals correlated significantly with duration of posttraumatic amnesia, thus indicating its construct validity, and with the Rancho Los Amigos Levels of Cognitive Functioning Scale (Hagen & Malkmus, 1979) and the Disability Rating Scale (Rappaport, Hall, Hopkins, Belleza, & Cope, 1982), thus indicating its concurrent validity (Heinemann et al., 1993). In addition, the 13 FIM motor items on admission were found to be the best predictors of rehabilitation length of stay for nearly all impairment groups studied (Heinemann et al., 1991, 1993).

Cautions About the FIM as an Outcomes Measure

As with all outcomes measures in use in medical rehabilitation, the FIM has its limitations. It is limited in its ability to fully describe the characteristics of disability in patients recovering from head injury and those with high quadriplegia from spinal cord injury. There is a need for some technical refinements with respect to assessment criteria for bladder, bowel, locomotion, comprehension, expression, and stair climbing.

Research using Rasch models has shown that the raw scores are not linear and may not be useful in parametric statistical analyses (Heinemann et al., 1991, 1992). There is controversy involving the appropriate mathematical treatment of such scales when they are used to establish parameters for practice, quality assurance, and program evaluation. Merbitz et al. (1989) argued that data obtained from an ordinal scale would not allow mathematical operations that could directly relate to the real world, and they contended that results of mathematical manipulations performed on ordinal data were not logically valid and could be misinterpreted. Wright and Linacre (1991) proposed a Rasch transformation of ordinal ranked functional status scores into a linear ratio scale so that mathematical operations could be conducted. Harvey et al. (1992) stressed that interval measurement would improve functional status scales by providing unidimensionality and additivity. *Additivity* means that adding one more unit always increases the pool by the same amount.

Using a Rasch-transformed measure permits statistical validity in comparing individuals based on results of using an aggregate score of a scale and permits valid comparison of change in aggregate scores over time. Rasch analysis of the FIM has shown it to have motor and cognitive components, each of which has unidimensional characteristics, additivity, and good reliability. Rasch-converted measures are available. However, it remains to be empirically tested how importantly and to what degree these affect and are useful to the results of research studies.

In summarizing the results of research on the measurement properties of the FIM, it has been found to have utility features of comprehensiveness, effectiveness, efficiency, comparability, and predictability. Comprehensiveness of the FIM is demonstrated by its use as a principal gauge of the major functional and behavioral activities that represent burden of care, meaning that there is need for daily assistance from another person. Effectiveness is demonstrated through changes in the FIM scores that track the status of a person's disability in the direction sought by the program. Efficiency is demonstrated by an analysis of the relationships between the cost and duration of a program and the person's pre- and postrehabilitation levels of functional status. Comparability is facilitated because outcomes of programs are described uniformly. Predictability allows facility administrators and clinicians to use the compiled database to predict which people are best served by the program, the kinds and amounts of services needed, and the likelihood of obtaining the desired results. The major benefit is facilitation of effectiveness and efficiency of rehabilitation services.

This is useful to rehabilitation providers, policy makers, and planners, with the ultimate benefit going to the patients, families, and the community.

The types of questions that the scale may be expected to help answer depend on how the scale is classified: 1) as discriminative, 2) as predictive, or 3) as evaluative. For example, the FIM helps to quantify disability. It is used to discriminate between classes of subjects with respect to severity of disability; it helps to predict discharge to living in the community rather than in a nursing facility or to predict the cost of maintaining a patient with disability if there is no further improvement; and it is evaluative, permitting detection of clinically important change when it occurs.

However, there remain cautions about the use of ordinal scales in medical rehabilitation. The impact of these cautions on the study of outcomes remains unclear. One of the primary directions for research in the field is to continue the investigations started on the measurement properties of the FIM, as well as to examine other scales in use in medical rehabilitation for their metric properties. This would include measures of impairment as well as measures of disability and of handicap. These measurement studies also need to focus on designing new measures for studying health and functioning and the barriers to fulfillment that serve in balancing the challenges to the quality of daily living.

Such a process has already begun with the assessment of physical functioning in terms of body movement and control through the Functional Assessment Screening Questionnaire (FASQ) (Granger & Wright, 1993). A new tool, the Medical Rehabilitation Follow-Along (MRFA), expanded from 5 to 10 items, characterizes upper-body motions (e.g., lifting, reaching, personal care), motions (e.g., kneeling/bending, walking, stair climbing, getting up from a low seat), and static activities (e.g., standing for 30 minutes, sitting for 30 minutes, traveling in an automobile) (Granger, Ottenbacher, Baker, & Sehgal, 1995).

The advantage in using a measure such as this is the ability to register the functioning of individuals comparatively and over time. Furthermore, there are implications for diagnostic analysis based on Rasch analysis of person response and item response. The patterns of response in terms of ease versus difficulty in performance of the items were different for patients with low back pain, neck pain, or upper-limb dysfunction and for patients with other forms of musculoskeletal disorders. Thus, it is possible not only to track change in physical functioning but also to determine whether a particular patient's pattern of response is consistent with the expected pattern for a given disorder. An example of the differential response to three selected items of the FASQ based on the type of disorder is illustrated in Figure 2. Lifting (an upper-body motion) is relatively more difficult for people with neck pain or arm dysfunction; standing for 30 minutes (a

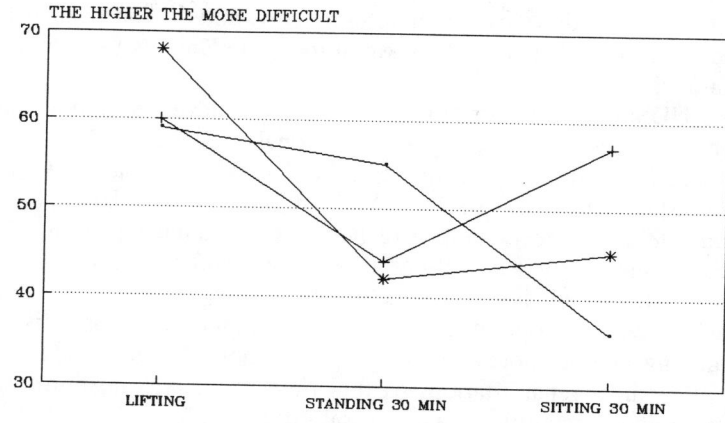

	Musculoskeletal	Low back pain	Neck pain / arm dysfunction
Lifting	59.00	60.00	68.00
Standing 30 minutes	55.00	44.00	42.00
Sitting 30 minutes	36.00	57.00	45.00

Figure 2.   Differential response to three FASQ items: Ease versus difficulty by logits (0–100). (◇ = musculoskeletal, Δ = low back pain, ✕ = neck pain / arm dysfunction.)

lower-body motion) is easier than lifting for all disorders, although it is more difficult for those with general musculoskeletal disorders; and sitting for 30 minutes (a static function) is difficult for people with low back pain and easy for those with general musculoskeletal disorders.

In summary, the results of the many studies of the measurement properties of the FIM indicate that it has met the measurement standards set by Johnston et al. (1992). Because the FIM has been shown to be a reliable and valid measure of disability, it may be combined with other data elements to investigate and understand how to improve the effectiveness and efficiency of medical rehabilitation.

THE UNIFORM DATA SYSTEM FOR MEDICAL REHABILITATION (UDSMR)

To determine how well a conceptual model fits the field of medical rehabilitation, the model must be judged for its comprehensiveness, its ability to be subject to the principles of good measurement, and its practicality in implementation. It also must be rigorously tested by patients, clinicians, and administrators, as well as by researchers in the literature.

The model proposed in Figure 1 is quite comprehensive. It allows for the inclusion of a multidisciplinary approach to the field of medical rehabilitation. The process of translating the model into measurement and the working out of the logistics of implementing it into the clinical arena, where it may be judged by patients, clinicians, and so forth, have begun with the use of the FIM at the UDSMR at the State University of New York at Buffalo.

The UDSMR is a not-for-profit organization developed and managed under the auspices of the Center for Functional Assessment Research, Department of Rehabilitation Medicine, School of Medicine and Biomedical Sciences, State University of New York at Buffalo. The UDSMR, established in 1987, was developed in response to the annual meetings of the American Congress of Rehabilitation Medicine and the American Academy of Physical Medicine and Rehabilitation in November 1983, where a joint task force was appointed to develop a methodology for satisfying a long-standing need to document severity of patient disability and the outcomes of medical rehabilitation. At that time, there was no uniform way to describe and communicate about disability.

The mission of the UDSMR includes the following:

- To establish and maintain a uniform language and definitions for communicating about disability and rehabilitation outcomes (The elements are the data set [descriptors], the database [aggregate of data on patients], data management [quality control and reporting], and other elements of a comprehensive data system.)
- To collect data, provide information, and foster research that uniformly characterizes disability and change in severity through use of uniform language, definitions, and measurements
- To establish and maintain a common data collection and reporting process that the majority of rehabilitation facilities can use and will find beneficial for comparing and evaluating service outcomes

This mission statement reflects the aim of the UDSMR to combine measures of disability (the FIM) with measures of the other patient outcomes proposed by the challenges to the quality of daily living model (see Figure 1). The data for UDSMR are based on a minimum data aggregate made up of demographic, diagnostic, functional, and charge information. The UDSMR provides streamlined data collection forms, software, and standardized directions allowing facilities to uniformly document, monitor, and compare outcomes of rehabilitated patients. Data are forwarded quarterly to the UDSMR for analysis and reporting to participating facilities, providing confidential facility, regional, and national data. The *Guide for the Uniform Data Set for Medical Rehabilitation* (State University of New York at Buffalo, 1993a) is the main form of standardization, and this is periodically updated. An instrument for measurement of disability in children, the WeeFIM (State University of New York at Buffalo, 1993b), has been developed and tested. A reporting system for WeeFIM is being developed that will allow the facility to accumulate and compare repeated patient assessments over time. A UDSMR newsletter is distributed to about 4,500 addresses worldwide, national and international training sessions are conducted, and publications are produced to promote uniformity in use of the data set and to help improve effectiveness and efficiency of the medical rehabilitation process.

The application of the FIM to several other often-studied outcomes, including length of stay, charges, functional change, functional status at discharge, and discharge to community, has been one of the driving forces behind the development of the UDSMR. Each of these outcomes measures serves as an indicator of the quality of daily living model proposed in Figure 1. Measures of length of stay, charges, and discharge destination reflect the efficiency of medical rehabilitation in achieving its goals of returning the patient to a balance of functional opportunities and barriers. Future research needs to focus on how each of these efficiency factors affects the patient's opportunities to achieve health and functioning as well as to overcome the barriers of impairment, disability, and handicap.

The following section focuses on the directions for these future research studies, which need to consider the balance between the efficiency of medical rehabilitation in terms of reducing costs and length of stay and the value of patient functional status as measured by FIM change scores from admission to discharge, functional status at discharge, and family and environmental factors present at the discharge destination. Patient and family perceptions or expectations become key factors in understanding the benefits of medical rehabilitation efficiency and effectiveness. The UDSMR offers a number of uniform descriptors and calculations to subscribers for comparative purposes (Fiedler, Granger, & Ottenbacher, 1996; Granger & Hamilton, 1992, 1993; Granger, Hamilton, & Fiedler, 1992; Granger, Ottenbacher, & Fiedler, 1995).

Measurement of Efficiency

Length of Stay Average change in FIM per day of rehabilitation hospital stay is reported. This is calculated by subtracting admission FIM from discharge FIM and then dividing by length of stay in days. This is a crude but useful measure of care efficiency, with a higher number representing greater efficiency. The advantage of using length of stay (LOS) efficiency is that variation in charges between regions is avoided. LOS efficiency by impairment group is probably the most reliable and useful means of assessing and comparing care efficiency.

Charges Average change in FIM per $1,000 charge is reported. This is calculated by subtracting admission FIM from discharge FIM and then dividing the gain by charges (in dollars), multiplied by 1,000. Multiplying by 1,000 makes the numbers close to 1, which is more easily understood. This is a more conventional expression of cost-efficiency; the higher the number, the higher the efficiency. That is, the higher the benefit (gain) and the lower the cost (charge), the more efficient the care process. However, the same considerations for interpretation must be applied to efficiency as are applied to charges. Region, case mix, and other variables influence charge efficiency. Charge efficiency by impairment group is reported.

Discharge Destination Community discharge is to home, board and care, or transitional living. Long-term care discharge is to intermediate care, skilled nursing facility, or chronic care hospital. Preparing patients for independent living in the community is a major rehabilitation objective. There is generally a correlation between achieving higher levels of function during rehabilitation (e.g., higher FIM) and a greater percentage of patients living independently in the community. Roughly, a FIM score of 80 or better is required for patients returning successfully to the care of a household member, and a FIM score of 100 or better is required if the patient lives alone. Some communities and families are more capable of providing independent living conditions than others, however. These factors influence the percentage of patients going to the community.

Program Evaluation and Performance Index

The program evaluation model provides an example of how a facility may compare its performance in five program objective areas with expected performance using a format similar to that suggested by CARF . . . The Rehabilitation Accreditation Commission. The five program objectives in the model are

1. Achieving a high percentage of patients discharged to independent living in the community
2. Achieving a high effectiveness (FIM gain from admission to discharge)
3. Serving and benefiting individuals with severe disabilities
4. Minimizing rehabilitation length of stay
5. Minimizing the total charges for the rehabilitation length of stay

The performance index is a weighted score of these measures comparing a given facility with the regional and national averages. A score greater than 100 means that a facility has a higher performance index compared with the region or national group, and a score lower than 100 means a lower performance index. The rank ordering of facilities by performance index, developed for each impairment group, gives an indication of where a given facility stands when compared with all others.

The cumulative admission–discharge patient records (plus about 30% follow-up) in the UDSMR database had grown to more than 1 million as of June 1995. Subscribing facilities receive quarterly standard reports showing all patients for the preceding 12 months, first admissions only for the preceding 12 months, and all admissions for the preceding 3 months.

Multifacility corporate reports and other special reports are provided. There are more than 500 U.S. facility subscribers (more than 50% of all U.S. rehabilitation facilities) plus subscribing facilities in Canada, Australia, and Japan. The guide for adults has been translated into Japanese, French, Portuguese, Italian, Spanish, Swedish, Finnish, and German. The WeeFIM has been translated into French and Spanish. The UDSMR continues to establish and maintain fundamental, uniform definitions and measures of disability and care outcomes for the field of medical rehabilitation for use with adults and children in hospital, outpatient, and alternative care settings. Functional assessment research initiatives will continue to advance the care processes and to improve rehabilitation outcomes for people with disability.

This introduction to the UDSMR provides an understanding of how the concepts in the quality of daily living model may be jointly assessed and used in the practice of studying outcomes in medical rehabilitation. With the FIM as its foundation, the UDSMR provides a variety of measures of outcomes, including the presence of a family for overcoming environmental barriers, LOS and charges that reflect economic barriers and options, and discharge location. Each of these measures may be considered within each impairment category as indicated by the UDSMR data. Thus, the UDSMR provides a uniform way of examining outcomes within the conceptual model by including aspects of impairment, disability, and, through follow-up, subsequent handicap, while considering aspects of family and economic barriers within the medical rehabilitation context.

Although this systematic approach to medical rehabilitation outcomes has proved valuable to the field, research on outcomes needs to move forward into additional measurable aspects of the model described in Figure 1. For example, it has become clear that the outcomes of impairment cannot be easily understood without the concomitant study of disability and subsequent health and functioning as well as functional barriers. Patients with stroke are not all the same. They have differing levels of disability, differing lengths of stay and charges, and differing outcomes in terms of functional status at discharge and discharge destination. Future research needs to address these concerns by studying which variables affect these outcomes and how to provide a more standardized way of comparing patient outcomes. Research has developed models for studying such outcomes in the form of the Penn Ability System Function-Related Groups (LOS FIM-FRGs) developed by Stineman et al. (1994).

CONCLUSIONS

With periodic reassessment, changes in patient performance over time can be measured and rehabilitation outcomes can be determined. There are many uses for this type of information. With the advent of cost containment and the need for more efficient and effective programs, managers and administrators are looking to patient improvement as an indicator of institutional productivity. Use of the FIM and the UDSMR will provide medical rehabilitation with critical, timely information that has multiple purposes, including common language and definitions by which the industry can communicate and normative data that will permit assessment of effectiveness and cost-efficiency of care. These have important implications for improving patient outcomes and management of care resources. In addition, clinical and administrative feedback information is provided that can facilitate planning, evaluation, and policy decisions and satisfy requirements of accrediting bodies for quality assurance and program evaluation. Furthermore, the research and education implications of uniform clinical data are substantial. Concurrently, there is a practical, strong economic incentive because of the change in Medicare reimbursement from a cost basis to a prospective system, which means preprice packaging. Facilities presumably will be rewarded for precise goal setting and efficiency in achieving rehabilitation goals. It is possible that the UDSMR or some component will be a potent determinant of how a prospective payment system for medical rehabilitation may be shaped. This avenue of research is being explored by Stineman and co-workers, who developed the FIM-FRG technology (1994). FIM-FRGs form a system for classifying patients to predict LOS and may be used to help in clinical and facility management as well as to form a basis for prospective payment. The FIM-FRGs may also serve as a basis for negotiation of contracts between providers of rehabilitation and managed care companies.

A second avenue of research needs to focus on balancing outcomes in a systematic way to better understand their relationships to each other and the patient. For example, length of stay in medical rehabilitation may be longer or shorter, depending on the goal of the rehabilitation process. If the goal becomes the least costly form of patient care, then it will become of critical value to study how LOS may be reduced to decrease costs while maintaining functional gain. Once again, comparisons of these outcomes have been hampered by confusion over case mix and patient severity at admission. These factors have come under careful study by Stineman et al. (1994). The FIM-FRG models provide a way to standardize patients at admission and compare differing outcomes within relatively homogeneous groups.

A methodology for jointly studying outcomes has been proposed by Fiedler (1995). By comparing like patients at admission with differing outcomes at discharge, it may be hypothesized that differing outcomes would be due to factors other than patient characteristics in studies controlling for FIM-FRG effects because patients would be homogeneous at admission. This would allow for comparisons of factors other than patient case mix.

Another important implication for this avenue of research is to consider the joint impact of outcomes using multivariate approaches and causal models. The models proposed by Johnson and Wolinsky (1994) and Wilson and Cleary (1995) may be tested using path analytic or causal modeling approaches such as Linear Structural Modeling (LISREL) (Joreskog & Sorbom, 1993).

One example of using multivariate approaches is to balance outcomes using efficiency outcomes and functional outcomes on a single standardized metric. For example, if FIM change scores and FIM discharge scores were converted to standard normal scores (z-scores) and LOS and costs were also standardized to the same z-score metric, then the relationships between these outcomes could be compared with one another and could be combined by a simple weighting scheme to form a single composite outcome. It would be interesting to see how these standardized outcomes would appear within FIM-FRG categories to control for the admission impairments and disabilities of the patients.

A second area for future research involves the study of disablement across the life span of individuals. This research has already begun at the UDSMR with the arrival of the WeeFIM. By studying impairment, disability, and handicap at young ages, where developmental measures have been used to indicate a child's progress instead of functional measures, research can begin the process of secondary prevention. By identifying health and functional opportunities as well as the barriers to fulfillment in early childhood, the full continuum of care and the course of disablement and its subsequent outcomes can be better understood.

The final direction for research in measuring outcomes in medical rehabilitation is to broaden the study of the quality of daily living model to include patients not experiencing the traditional inpatient paradigm but who instead are experiencing outpatient treatment for a variety of problems that fit the model in Figure 1. Studying fulfillment in patients out in the community requires new measures of health and functioning that are more sensitive to outpatient problems than are the 1990s version of the FIM. Research at the UDSMR includes measures of outpatient functioning at the levels of physical functioning (including pain assessment), mental and emotional functioning, social functioning, role functioning, and feeling of well-being. There is a growing need for brief and useful measures of daily functioning for rehabilitation outpatients. Nonetheless, the heterogeneous nature of outpatient rehabilitation problems and the importance of factors such as psychosocial functioning and the quality of daily living in the community present unique assessment challenges for this setting. Unfortunately, qualitative information derived from interviewing patients during office transactions does not lend itself easily to the analysis of outcomes. When this information is quantified, clinical decision making can be facilitated.

REFERENCES

Americans with Disabilities Act (ADA) of 1990, PL 101-336, 42 U.S.C. §§ 12101 et seq.

Basmajian, J.V. (Ed.). (1994). Physical rehabilitation outcome measures. Toronto, Ontario: Canadian Physiotherapy Association.

Beaufait, D.W., Nelson, E.C., Landgraf, J.M., Kirk, J.W., Wasson, J.H., & Keller, A. (1992). COOP Measures of Functional Status. In M. Stewart (Ed.), Tools for primary care research. Newbury Park, CA: Sage Publications.

Bergner, M., Bobbitt, R., Carter, W., & Gelson, B. (1981). The Sickness Impact Profile: Development and final revision of a health status questionnaire. Medical Care, 19, 955–962.

Centers for Disease Control. (1992, October). Programs with significant rehabilitation interest. Presentation to the National Advisory Board on Medical Rehabilitation Research, Gaithersburg, MD.

Dahmer, E.R., Shilling, M.A., Hamilton, B.B., Bontke, C.F., Englander, J., Kreutzer, J.S., Ragnarsson, K.T., & Rosenthal, M. (1993). A model systems database for traumatic brain injury. Journal of Head Trauma Rehabilitation, 8, 12–25.

Derogatis, L.R., & Melisaratos, N. (1983). The brief symptom inventory: An introductory report. Psychological Medicine, 13, 595–605.

Fiedler, R.C. (1995, October). Comparing patient outcomes using FIM-FRGs. Paper presented at the Rehab Alliance Conference, Phoenix, AZ.

Fiedler, R.C., Granger, C.V., & Ottenbacher, K.J. (1996). The Uniform Data System for Medical Rehabilitation report of first admissions for 1994. American Journal of Physical Medicine and Rehabilitation, 75, 125–129.

Granger, C.V., Cotter, A.C., Hamilton, B.B., Fiedler, R.C., & Hens, M.M. (1990). Functional assessment scales: A study of persons with multiple sclerosis. Archives of Physical Medicine and Rehabilitation, 71, 870–875.

Granger, C.V., Cotter, A.C., Hamilton, B.B., & Fiedler, R.C. (1993). Functional assessment scales: A study of persons after stroke. Archives of Physical Medicine and Rehabilitation, 74, 133–138.

Granger, C.V., Divan, N., & Fiedler, R.C. (1995). Functional assessment scales: A study of persons after traumatic brain injury. American Journal of Physical Medicine and Rehabilitation, 74, 107–113.

Granger, C.V., & Gresham, G.E. (Eds.). (1984). Functional assessment in rehabilitation medicine. Baltimore: Williams & Wilkins.

Granger, C.V., & Hamilton, B.B. (1992). UDSMR report: The Uniform Data System for Medical Rehabilitation report of first admissions for 1990. American Journal of Physical Medicine and Rehabilitation, 71, 108–113.

Granger, C.V., & Hamilton, B. (1993). The Uniform Data System for Medical Rehabilitation report of first admissions for 1991. American Journal of Physical Medicine and Rehabilitation, 72, 33–38.

Granger, C.V., Hamilton, B.B., & Fiedler, R.C. (1992). Discharge outcome after stroke rehabilitation. Stroke, 23, 978–982.

Granger, C.V., Kelly-Hayes, M., Johnston, M., Deutsch, A., Braun, S., & Fiedler, R.C. (1996). Quality and outcome measures for medical rehabilitation. In R.L.

Braddom (Ed.), *Physical medicine and rehabilitation* (pp. 239–253). Philadelphia: W.B. Saunders.

Granger, C.V., Ottenbacher, K.J., Baker, J.G., & Sehgal, A. (1995). Reliability of a brief functional outcome assessment measure. *American Journal of Physical Medicine and Rehabilitation, 74,* 469–475.

Granger, C.V., Ottenbacher, K.J., & Fiedler, R.C. (1995). The Uniform Data System for Medical Rehabilitation report of first admissions for 1993. *American Journal of Physical Medicine and Rehabilitation, 74,* 62–66.

Granger, C.V., & Wright, B.D. (1993). Looking ahead to the use of functional assessment in ambulatory physiatric and primary care. In C.V. Granger & G.E. Gresham (Eds.), *New developments in functional assessment: Physical medicine and rehabilitation clinics of North America* (pp. 595–605). Philadelphia: W.B. Saunders.

Hagen, C., & Malkmus, D. (1979). *Intervention strategies for language disorders secondary to head trauma.* American Speech-Language-Hearing Association Convention Short Course, Atlanta.

Hamilton, B.B. (1991). *Final report: The cost of disability as measured by the Functional Independence Measure (FIM): Spinal cord injury.* Project H133G90150-90, U.S. Department of Education, State University of New York at Buffalo.

Hamilton, B.B., Granger, C.V., Sherwin, F.S., Zielezny, M., & Tashman, J.S. (1987). A uniform national data system for medical rehabilitation. In M.J. Fuhrer (Ed.), *Rehabilitation outcomes: Analysis and measurement* (pp. 137–147). Baltimore: Paul H. Brookes Publishing Co.

Hamilton, B.B., Laughlin, J.A., Fiedler, R.C., & Granger, C.V. (1994). Interrater reliability of the 7-level Functional Independence Measure (FIM). *Scandinavian Journal of Rehabilitation Medicine, 26,* 115–119.

Harvey, R.F., Silverstein, B., Venzon, M., Kilgore, K.M., Fisher, W.P., Steiner, M., & Harley, J.P. (1992). Applying psychometric criteria to functional assessment in medical rehabilitation: III. Construct validity and predicting level of care. *Archives of Physical Medicine and Rehabilitation, 73,* 887–892.

Heinemann, A.W., Hamilton, B.B., Granger, C.V., Linacre, J.M., & Wright, B.D. (1992). *Rehabilitation efficacy for brain and spinal cord injury: Final report.* Chicago: Rehabilitation Institute of Chicago.

Heinemann, A.W., Hamilton, B.B., Granger, C.V., Wright, B.D., & Linacre, J.M. (1991). *Final report: Rating scale analysis of functional assessment measures.* Chicago: Rehabilitation Institute of Chicago.

Heinemann, A.W., Linacre, J.M., Wright, B.D., Hamilton, B.B., & Granger, C.V. (1993). Relationships between impairment and physical disability as measured by the Functional Independence Measure. *Archives of Physical Medicine and Rehabilitation, 74,* 566–573.

International Federation of Multiple Sclerosis Societies. (1985). *M.R.D. minimal record of disability for multiple sclerosis.* New York: National Multiple Sclerosis Society.

Johnson, R.J., & Wolinsky, F.D. (1994). Gender, race, and health: The structure of health status among older adults. *Gerontologist, 34,* 24–35.

Johnston, M.V., Keith, R.A., & Hinderer, S. (1992). Measurement standards in medical rehabilitation. *Archives of Physical Medicine and Rehabilitation, 73,* S3–S23.

Joreskog, K., & Sorbom, D. (1993). *LISREL eight: Structural equation modeling with the SIMPLIS command language.* Hillsdale, NJ: Lawrence Erlbaum Associates.

Kielhofner, G., & Burke, J. (1980). A model of human occupation: I. Conceptual framework and content. *American Journal of Occupational Therapy, 34,* 572–581.

Krupp, L.B., LaRocca, N.G., Muir-Nash, J., & Steinberg, A.D. (1989). Fatigue Severity Scale. *Archives of Neurology, 46,* 1121–1123.

Maslow, A. (1954). *Motivation and personality.* New York: Harper & Row.

Mellerup, E., et al. (1981). The socio-economic scale. *Acta Neurologica Scandinavica, 64(Suppl. 87),* 130–138.

Merbitz, C.T., Morris, J., & Grip, J.C. (1989). Ordinal scales and foundations of misinference. *Archives of Physical Medicine and Rehabilitation, 70,* 308–312.

Nagi, S.Z. (1965). Some conceptual issues in disability and rehabilitation. In M.B. Sussman (Ed.), *Sociology and rehabilitation* (pp. 100–113). Washington, DC: U.S. Department of Health, Education, and Welfare.

National Center for Medical Rehabilitation Research. (1992). *Report and plan for medical rehabilitation research.* Washington, DC: National Institute of Child Health and Human Development, National Institutes of Health.

Pope, A., & Tarlov, A. (Eds.). (1991). *Disability in America: Toward a national agenda for prevention.* Washington, DC: National Academy Press.

Rappaport, M., Hall, K.M., Hopkins, K., Belleza, T., & Cope, D.N. (1982). Disability rating scale for severe head trauma: Coma to community. *Archives of Physical Medicine and Rehabilitation, 63,* 118–123.

Special Projects and Demonstrations for Providing Vocational Rehabilitation Services to Individuals with Severe Handicaps, 57 Fed. Reg. 52,682 (November 4, 1992).

State University of New York at Buffalo. (1993a). *Guide for the Uniform Data Set for Medical Rehabilitation (Adult FIM), version 4.0.* Buffalo, NY: Author.

State University of New York at Buffalo. (1993b). *Guide for the Uniform Data Set for Medical Rehabilitation for Children (WeeFIM), version 4.0.* Buffalo, NY: Author.

Stineman, M.G., Escarce, J.J., Goin, J.E., Hamilton, B.B., Granger, C.V., & Williams, S.V. (1994). A case-mix classification system for medical rehabilitation. *Medical Care, 32,* 366–379.

Verbrugge, L.M., & Jette, A.M. (1994). The disablement process. *Social Science and Medicine, 38,* 1–14.

Von Bertalanffy, L. (1968). *General system theory: Foundations, development and applications.* New York: Braziller.

Wade, D.T. (1992). *Measurement in neurological rehabilitation.* Oxford, England: Oxford University Press.

Willer, B.S., Linn, R.T., & Allen, K.M. (1993). Community integration and barriers to integration for individuals with brain injury. In M.A.J. Finlayson & S. Garner (Eds.), *Brain injury rehabilitation: Clinical considerations* (pp. 355–375). Baltimore: Williams & Wilkins.

Wilson, I.B., & Cleary, P.D. (1995). Linking clinical variables with health-related quality of life. *Journal of the American Medical Association, 273,* 59–65.

World Health Organization. (1980). *International classification of impairments, disabilities, and handicaps.* Geneva, Switzerland: Author.

Wright, B.D., & Linacre J.M. (1991). *BIGSTEPS: A Rasch-model computer program.* Chicago: MESA.

Ziebland, S., Fitzpatrick, R., & Jenkinson, C. (1993). Tacit models of disability underlying health status instruments. *Social Science and Medicine, 37,* 69–75.

CHAPTER 6

The Concept of Handicap in Rehabilitation and Research

Barry Willer, Jennifer Button, and John D. Corrigan

The success of the World Health Organization (WHO) in the development of diagnostic codes and common language for medical rehabilitation provided a significant improvement in the definition and research potential of rehabilitation outcomes. The primary product of the WHO review of definitions in rehabilitation was the *International Classification of Impairments, Disabilities and Handicaps* (ICIDH), which was published in 1980. This document and its definitions of impairments and disabilities are described throughout this book. The concept of handicap, however, is the subject of this chapter and probably represents the greatest challenge to researchers and rehabilitation practitioners, both as a concept warranting further definition and research and as a statement of purpose for rehabilitation services.

The ICIDH presents definitions and also a model of rehabilitation. Badley (1993) referred to the ICIDH as a conceptual framework for the consequence of disease. As with most authors on the subject, Badley refers to the conceptual framework as the disablement model. For the purpose of explaining the conceptualization of handicap within the disablement model, this chapter describes the model within the context of several models originally presented by Minaire (1992). Some of the research and measurement issues of the disablement model are then reviewed. A literature search on rehabilitation research that uses the word *handicap* reveals the usage and inconsistent definition of *handicap*.

In addition to a discussion of the meaning and measurement of the concept of handicap and the discussion of the disablement model, this chapter reviews two assessment instruments. Both instruments were specifically designed to assess handicap, and both have undergone evaluation for reliability and validity. Both instruments were designed with the ICIDH definition of *handicap* and the disablement model in mind. Research on the two instruments has been instructive regarding the meaning of *handicap* and the relationship of handicap to impairments and disabilities. The chapter concludes with the issues of definition of ICIDH components and presents an alternative to the disablement model, called the enablement model.

MODELS OF REHABILITATION

Minaire (1992) provided a succinct discussion of four models used to provide a conceptual framework for rehabilitation. Each of these models assumes that an individual has had a disease or injury that has led to a permanent or semipermanent alteration of function. The first model, the biomedical model, assumes a simple linear relationship between etiology, pathology, and manifestation (impairments). As Minaire pointed out, there is little room in the biomedical model for consideration of how the patient is affected by the disease. In the origin of the biomedical model, the Greek philosophers (e.g., Hippocrates) and religious leaders agreed that issues of the mind and spirit would remain the purview of religion, and physicians would confine their attention to the physical aspects of illness. The application of the biomedical model to ongoing health condition or long-term impairment is problematic because of the obvious overlay of emotional and social aspects of adjustment.

An example of the application of the biomedical model to the business of providing health and rehabilitation services is the effort to predict the number of hospital days required to treat a specific illness or injury type. Such predictions do not account for family or personal variables that might influence the need for hospitalization. Minaire pointed out that the biomedical model is essentially concerned with three variables: diagnosis (e.g., lesions), symptoms, and related physiologic factors (e.g., glucose levels, respiratory or cardiac parameters). The biomedical model does not view personality factors, emotional responses, or family issues as part of the symptom picture unless these can be clearly linked to the original pathology. Health is viewed as the mere absence of disease. Rehabilitation is focused first on the pathology and second on the symptoms.

There are numerous problems with the application of the biomedical model to rehabilitation, including that biomedical diseases or injuries are neither invariable nor universal. For example, efforts to predict length of hospital stay on the basis of diagnoses such as spinal cord injury or multiple sclerosis have been largely unsuccessful. However, it must be recognized that the biomedical model is still the most accepted approach to the provision of hospital-based rehabilitation services. According to Minaire, all other models are derived from the biomedical model, regardless of its apparent weaknesses. An underlying assumption of the biomedical model is that disease is independent of the person affected by the disease. This assumption interferes with the development of models of rehabilitation that reflect the perspective of the individual involved in rehabilitation (Peters, 1995).

The disablement model, based on the efforts of the WHO to define impairments, disabilities, and handicaps, is a conceptual model that Minaire (1992) described as similar to the biomedical model in terms of linearity. The model assumes that something abnormal occurs within an individual (impairment), someone becomes aware of this occurrence (diagnosis), the performance or behavior of the individual is altered as a result (disabilities), and the diagnosis or disabilities may place the individual at a disadvantage relative to others (handicap). The disablement model is considered an improvement over the biomedical model because it allows for a more complete picture of the needs and services received by individuals with disabilities. The disablement model also is described as superior to the biomedical model as the basis for research into the course and outcomes of rehabilitation.

Minaire and others stated that the disablement model greatly expanded the research and rehabilitation parameters. At minimum, research generated by the disablement model is devoted to the assessment of both performance (disabilities) and disadvantage (handicap). The model has expanded the range of interventions and goals of rehabilitation. The biomedical model tends to restrict the interventions to those that confront the disease or the injured part of the body, whereas the disablement model legitimizes interventions that increase performance (reduce disabilities) or that decrease disadvantage (reduce handicap). Minaire also highlighted that the disablement model applies equally well to individual assessment and population surveys.

The primary criticism of the disablement model, according to Minaire, is the excessive emphasis placed on the individual experience as a source of the disablement process (similarly to the biomedical model) and the limited emphasis placed on the role of the environment in creating disadvantage. In addition, Minaire suggested that confusion still exists regarding the dividing lines between the various conceptual elements, especially between disabilities and handicap. Furthermore, Peters (1995) pointed out that the disablement model is guilty of ignoring the perception of impairment and disabilities held by the individual, in much the same manner that the biomedical model ignores the role of individual perceptions. The disablement model also rejects the concepts of psychological well-being or quality of life and has little room for consideration of personality or emotional issues, a carryover from its roots in the biomedical model.

The biomedical and disablement models are described by Minaire as static, whereas the situational handicap model recognizes that disablement varies according to life circumstances, which tend to vary greatly over time. The situational handicap model, according to Minaire, divides life into microsituations (e.g., opening doors, moving from one place to another) and macrosituations (e.g., housing, school, employment, family life). Handicap is the result of the encounter between inabilities (in performance in microsituations) and environmental situations, which presumably influence macrosituations. The individual is thus viewed within an open system, in terms of both time and circumstance. Analysis of the situational handicap involves measurement of impairment, disabilities, handicaps, and the environment of the system. Environmental factors (sometimes referred to as barriers) include physical, economic, religious, cultural, administrative, and other aspects of the individual's life circumstances.

The situational handicap model implies that the interventions of the rehabilitation experts should be aimed at integrating the individual into the environment of choice. The model suggests that efforts to remove barriers or increase environmental compatibility are legitimate activities for interventionists. However, the situational handicap model described by Minaire (1992) does not offer a strategy for assessing the environmental barriers that interfere with integration.

The fourth model, which Minaire calls the quality of life model, is immediately weakened by the array of perceptions and definitions of the concept of quality of life. Some perceive quality of life as an extension of the WHO definition of *handicap*, that is, performance of roles that are age-appropriate and culturally appropriate. Most, however, view quality of life as representing the subjective experience of the individual, including the perception of personal health and social functioning. Although issues of definition and measurement plague each of the models, definition and measurement of quality of life are perhaps the most critical weaknesses in the continuum represented by the quality of life model.

The four models described by Minaire are presented in Figure 1 as an evolution of rehabilitation approaches. The components of these models are assumed to be linear in relationship, with the exception of environmental barriers, which interact specifically with disabilities to produce handicaps. It is further theorized that the relationship between most components in each of the models is interactive. In other words, it is suggested that impairment can cause further injury or disease (e.g., vascular problems for an individual who is nonambulatory), disabilities can cause impairment (e.g., limited range of motion, leading to contractures), and handicap can cause disabilities (e.g., isolation from family and friends, leading to depression). A stronger interaction effect is proposed for the relationship between disabilities and environmental barriers.

Fougeyrollas (1995) criticized the linearity of the models presented by Minaire (1992), suggesting that environmental factors influence all as-

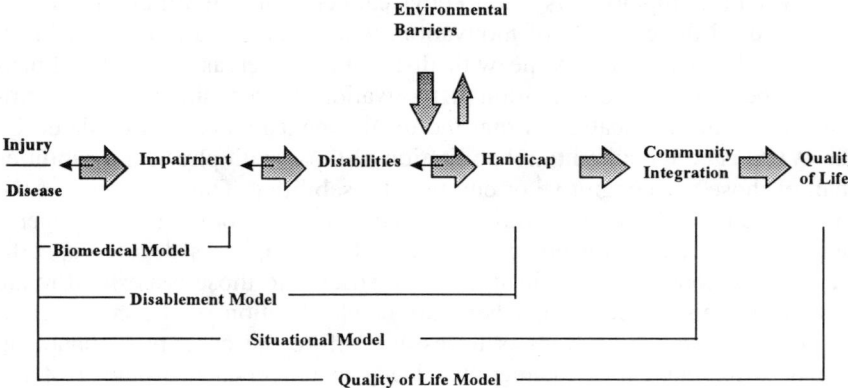

Figure 1. Four models of rehabilitation. (Based on a description by Minaire, P. [1992]. Disease, illness and health: Theoretical models of the disablement process. *Bulletin of the World Health Organization, 70*[3], 373–379.)

pects from impairment to quality of life and are not adequately represented in any of the models. The oversight of important environmental determinants of disablement is made more prominent by the problems of definition that exist in each of the models, particularly between disabilities and handicaps. Fougeyrollas suggested that the WHO description of handicap dimensions is essentially indistinguishable from the disability dimensions. The environmental context of disablement, according to Fougeyrollas, has been essentially overlooked.

MEASUREMENT AND RESEARCH ISSUES

As the development of models of rehabilitation has progressed outward from the biomedical model, so, too, has research and measurement precision. Assessment, research, and measurement of disease and impairment have greatly outweighed research and measurement of disabilities, and research and measurement of disabilities have greatly outweighed the research and measurement of handicap. Systematic assessment of environmental barriers and quality of life is even further behind as a subject of research within rehabilitation. The future of the models is dependent in many respects on the conceptual clarity that is often one result of research. Of particular importance in the relatively early stage of this model is research into measures of key components of the models, such as research on handicap.

Mooney (1987) suggested that rehabilitation practitioners confuse impairment with disabilities. In discussing the applicability of the disablement model to those with mental illness, Ustun et al. (1995) pointed out that the confusion between impairment and disabilities is even more pronounced than when the impairments lead to physical performance difficulties. These authors used the example of motivation, which may be a factor that influences performance of anyone with disabilities, whereas in mental illness (and other neurologic conditions), motivation relates directly to the impairment. The implication is that the disablement model as articulated by the WHO is better suited to rehabilitation of those with physical disabilities than of those with cognitive or emotional disabilities. This weakness of the disablement model is even more pronounced when looking at the operationalization of the concept of handicap. This chapter is devoted specifically to the concept of handicap and is restricted to those issues that relate directly to this concept; however, further clarification of the concepts of impairments and disabilities is necessary before the concept of handicap can be articulated in a manner that leads to universal acceptance of the concept.

Handicap is defined by the WHO as a "disadvantage for a given individual resulting from an impairment or disability, that limits or prevents the fulfillment of a role that is normal (depending on age, sex, and social and cultural factors) for that individual"(WHO, 1980, p. 183). Handicap is concerned with the individual as a member of a social structure and is characterized by a discordance between the individual's status or performance and the expectations of the individual or of the particular group of which he or she is a member (de Klein-de Vrankrijker, 1995). Impairment is described as existing at the organ level, disability at the person level, and handicap at the person in society level.

The operational dimensions of handicap, outlined by the WHO, include the following:

- *Orientation:* Understand where individual is in time and in place with respect to surroundings
- *Physical independence:* Maintain independence with respect to immediate needs, including feeding and personal hygiene
- *Mobility:* Move around effectively within the environment
- *Occupation:* Effective use of time and energy in home, school, or recreation
- *Social integration:* Participate in and maintain social relationships
- *Socioeconomic independence:* Employment

These dimensions of handicap are described as survival roles and are to be distinguished from life roles in general. An individual who is unable to fulfill one of these survival roles as a result of impairments or disabilities is therefore considered disadvantaged or handicapped in relation to peers. However, it is readily apparent that the dimensions of handicap are easily confused with the dimensions of disability. Badley (1995) suggested that the confusion exists primarily for the first three dimensions of handicap. For example, an individual who is unable to transfer from bed to wheelchair (disability) is likely to have short-interval dependence and therefore is regarded as handicapped on the physical independence dimension. The question, according to Badley, is whether an individual is handicapped when assistance in transfer is required or is merely disabled and therefore requires assistance and is handicapped only when assistance is not provided.

The confusion between disability and handicap dimensions is particularly evident with the dimension of orientation. If an individual has neurologic impairment (e.g., mental illness, brain injury, Alzheimer's disease) that interferes with spatial or temporal awareness, the individual's disabilities would presumably be described as disorientation. If the individual is accompanied by others and therefore spatial disorientation is not restricting the individual, then the individual is no longer disadvantaged and therefore is not handicapped on this dimension. This type of confusion over cognitive factors in the ICIDH format interferes with the facile application of ICIDH to mental illness and mental retardation services.

Badley (1995) suggested that the confusion about the concept of handicap is largely explained by ambiguity with the concept of social role. Disabilities refer to reduced performance in instrumental activities. Some instrumental activities (e.g., laundry, cooking, mobility) also reflect social roles. Badley suggested that a solution might be to view disabilities as activities that an individual cannot perform and to view handicap as the consequence of the inability to perform the activity.

The confusion surrounding the definition of *handicap* is more apparent when assessing handicap. Research obviously requires carefully defined and measurable concepts. However, research into handicap or any other concept can also assist in the further clarification of the concept. The goal of clarifying handicap as a concept is added to a list of research questions, presented in the following paragraphs, being addressed in rehabilitation outcomes research.

First, how do disabilities relate to handicap? The concept of handicap indicates that the presence of disabilities is a prerequisite for handicap, although handicap is considered to be on a different plane or axis from disabilities. In addition, factors such as demographic characteristics and environmental conditions are expected to relate to handicap, given that handicap refers to performance of the individual as a member of a social group.

Second, is handicap a singular concept made up of various dimensions, or do the various dimensions of handicap stand alone? Furthermore, do the dimensions of handicap, as articulated by the WHO, capture the gestalt of handicap as defined by interference with social role performance? Related questions reflect on the comparison of the role performance among those with disabilities and those who do not have apparent disabilities.

Third, how does handicap relate to aspects of other models presented by Minaire (1992), such as community integration and quality of life? Is there research support for the continuum from impairment to disabilities, handicap, community integration, and quality of life? These research questions are dependent on the development of valid measures of each concept, including community integration and quality of life.

Use of *Handicap* in the Literature

The authors of this chapter reviewed all articles published since 1980 in the medical rehabilitation literature that used the word *handicap* or any of its derivations in the title or abstract. We were interested in literature that included some form of research so that the words *measure* or *assess* or any of their derivations were also included. This review was conducted using Medline and was limited to articles written in English and dealing with humans. As such, the review was not intended to be comprehensive, but rather to give a general impression of the use and definitions of *handicap* within the professional literature. The first level of screen revealed 159 articles published since 1980 that relate to handicap.

Despite the efforts of the WHO to have universal agreement on the definitions and use of the terms in the ICIDH, the authors' review of the literature revealed considerable disagreement regarding the term *handicap*. In the majority of cases, *handicap* as a term used in the professional rehabilitation literature is used interchangeably with impairment and disabilities. We identified only 72 research publications that looked at handicap as an aspect of disablement independent of disabilities and impairment, although the definition of *handicap* was rarely consistent with the WHO definition. A number of authors described handicap assessment scales that were specific to an impairment group. For example, there are handicap assessments specific to those with hearing impairment (e.g., Newman, Weinstein, Jacobson, & Hug, 1990; Schow, Smedley, & Longhurst, 1990; Tannahill, 1979), oral impairment (Fiske, Gelbier, & Watson, 1990), vertigo or dizziness (Jacobson & Newman, 1990; Jacobson, Newman, Hunter, & Balzer, 1991; Yardley & Putman, 1992), and arthritis (Koepcke, Hasford, Weber Falkensammer, & Zwingers, 1984). In most instances, researchers have assessed handicap as limitations in role function but have focused on those limitations that relate to the specific impairment. Although this literature is instructive, handicap as a concept should relate to impairments and disabilities but should not be limited to specific impairment groups.

There is another body of literature that focuses on a broader range of impairment groups but limits the attention to specific aspects of handicap.

For example, there are numerous articles that focus on employment or educational outcomes as an important aspect of handicap (Costa, Scriver, & Childs, 1985; Elwes, Marshall, Beattie, & Newman, 1991; Floyd & Kettl, 1991; Kuldau & Dirks, 1987; Mooney, 1987). There are other studies that focus on employment and social participation or on social participation alone (Borgel et al., 1992; Bruininks, McGrew, & Maruyama, 1988; Helzer, Brockington, & Kendell, 1981; Lequesne, 1991; Segal & Everett-Dille, 1980; Sergl, Ruppenthal, & Schmitt, 1992). Several investigators examined employment, marital status, and housing as aspects of handicap (see Anderman & Anderman, 1992). Other measures of handicap have focused on physical independence (Badley & Tennant, 1991, 1993; Badley, Tennant, & Wood, 1990) and activities of daily living (Angeleri, Angeleri, Foschi, Giaquinto, & Nolfe, 1993; Wolfe, Taub, Woodrow, & Burney, 1991; Wolfe et al., 1993). Each of these approaches to handicap assessment has limited its focus to one or just a few components of handicap rather than a comprehensive assessment of the range of survival roles specified by the WHO (1980).

There is also a body of literature on the disablement model and assessment of disablement that relates to handicap assessment. There are authors who describe the use of ICIDH taxonomy directly to evaluate impairments, disabilities, and handicap (Badley, 1993; Beckung & Uvebran, 1993; Harper et al., 1992; Roy, Hunter, Arthurs, & Prescott, 1992; Talo, Puuka, Rytokoski, Ronnemaa, & Kallio, 1994; Verloove et al., 1994). Although these efforts to use the ICIDH taxonomy may prove useful as a clinical assessment approach, the lack of reliability of the assessment process renders this approach of limited value to research. There are a number of other broad-based instruments that purport to measure disablement, but again they suffer from a lack of scientific rigor sufficient to answer some of the important research questions posed earlier in this chapter (Mattison, Aitken, & Prescott, 1991, 1992; Schuling, de Haan, Limburg, & Groener, 1993; Truelle et al., 1992).

To summarize, the literature on handicap has been limited by the tendency to fit the concept of handicap within the biomedical model, that is, to look at impairment- or disability-specific handicap rather than a concept of handicap relatively independent of impairments or disabilities. The majority of research that looks at handicap does not distinguish handicap from impairments or disabilities. Of the 72 research articles found to appropriately distinguish the various components of the ICIDH model, most looked at impairment-specific measures or limited the focus to one or two aspects of handicap. There are eight research articles that describe and evaluate handicap using the Craig Handicap Assessment and Reporting Technique (CHART) and six research articles that describe and evaluate handicap using the Community Integration Questionnaire (CIQ). These two instruments are the only broad-based instruments that assess handicap and community integration in a manner consistent with the WHO definition. These two instruments are presented as having psychometric properties that have been evaluated with sufficient scientific rigor, so that conclusions may be drawn from the research about the appropriateness of the disablement model and the situational handicap model presented by Minaire (1992). The CHART and CIQ literature are reviewed separately.

The Craig Handicap Assessment and Reporting Technique

The CHART was designed by Whiteneck, Charlifue, Gerhart, Overholser, and Richardson (1992) to quantify the extent of handicap experienced by individuals with disabilities. The CHART is a direct behavioral assessment of the operational dimensions of handicap identified and described by the WHO (1980) with the exception that the CHART does not contain a measure of orientation, although a measure of this dimension is in development. Thus, the CHART does have measures of physical independence, mobility, occupation, social integration, and economic self-sufficiency.

Although the CHART heeded the WHO definitions of each dimension, the development of specific items for each dimension required careful attention to social variability in determining the acceptability of role fulfillment. For example, *occupation* is defined by the WHO as an ability to occupy time in a manner customary to the individual's sex, age, and culture. Whiteneck et al. (1992) concluded that there are a multitude of ways in which an individual can spend time in a meaningful and acceptable fashion but ended up with a measure of hours spent in employment, educational pursuits, home maintenance, volunteer work, recreation, and self-improvement. The influence of social values on the measurement of role fulfillment is considerably more complex than the social valuation of disabilities and impairments. In creating the measure of occupation, Whiteneck et al. excluded activities that are generally considered nonproductive, such as watching television or sleeping.

The attempt by the authors to avoid the influence of social values on assessment of role fulfillment is further evidenced by the manner in which items within scales are weighted. Because the goal of the CHART is to measure deviation from the norm, it was assumed that people without disabilities would score the maximum (100 points) on each of the dimensions. Individuals who scored less than 100 would therefore be considered to have a handicap. Individuals who scored 100 were considered not to have a handicap, regardless of the level of disabilities. Thus, physical independence, which assesses the number of hours a helper is paid to assist with independence, has a maximum of 100 points for individuals who do not have a paid helper. Mobility assesses the number of hours per day spent out of bed and out of the house. Social integration assesses the number of people who have contact with the individual but also gives points for living arrangement and romantic involvement. Economic self-sufficiency is an assessment of total household income and anyone living with an income equal to or greater than the designated poverty level obtains a score of 100.

Several pilot studies were conducted to determine the psychometric properties of the CHART. Test–retest reliability for the CHART, over a 1-week period, produced highly acceptable reliability coefficients ranging from .95 for mobility to .81 for social integration. When CHART scores were obtained from a family member or proxy and compared with those obtained through interview with the individual with spinal cord injury, the scores were similar but the subscales varied greatly in how they correlated. Subject–proxy correlations ranged from .84 for mobility to .28 for social integration. These results are reported by Whiteneck et al. (1992) for a population of individuals with spinal cord injury with primarily motoric disabilities; therefore, it cannot be assumed that the results can be generalized to individuals with cognitive disabilities.

A 1995 study by Segal and Schall set out to validate the CHART with individuals with stroke, whose disabilities included cognitive and physical limitations. Although the study sample was small ($N = 38$), the findings are instructive to the understanding of the concept of handicap as it is represented by the CHART. Segal and Schall (1995) found that there was a very low correlation between individuals with stroke and their family members on the assessment of social integration. This is not surprising, because the same low correlation was found by Whiteneck et al. (1992) in their original description of the scale. In addition, Segal and Schall (1995) found they were unable to obtain a reliable estimate of family income (economic self-sufficiency). The authors also questioned whether family income was a legitimate concern in the assessment of handicap. Segal and Schall found a high correlation between measures of physical disabilities (using the Functional Independence Measure [FIM; State University of New York at Buffalo, 1993]) and CHART subscales of physical independence, mobility, and occupation, but not between social integration and economic self-sufficiency. They also found that cognitive disabilities (using FIM) did not correlate to any significant degree with any of the subscales of the CHART. They concluded that the CHART and FIM are both suited more to individuals with physical limitations than to those with cognitive limitations. The results of this study also raise concerns about the reliability of the social integration assessment within the CHART.

The CHART has been used as a measure of handicap in a number of studies that assessed the relationship of handicap to various physical and emotional aspects of disability. Menter et al. (1991) examined data on 205 subjects with spinal cord injury and found that impairment levels were associated with handicap as represented by the CHART. Measures of impairment were negatively correlated with CHART scores. Rintala, Hart, and Fuhrer (1993) reported that disability, as measured by the FIM, was significantly related to mobility, occupation, and social integration. Another group of studies examined the relationship of depression to handicap. Depression (whether a factor of impairment or disability) was associated with less mobility and less social integration, as assessed by the CHART (Fuhrer, Rintala, Hart, Clearman, & Young, 1993). In another study, Tate, Forchheimer, Maynard, and Dijkers (1994) found similar results demonstrating that physical independence and social integration when assessed by the CHART were associated with depression. Each of these studies focused on individuals with spinal cord injury.

Community Integration Questionnaire

Minaire (1992) suggested that handicap results from the encounter between disabilities and environmental situations. The goal of rehabilitation, according to Minaire, is the successful integration of the individual into his or her environment and the integration of the environment into the personal experience of the individual. Willer and Corrigan (1994) suggested that community integration is composed of three areas of community functioning: 1) control over home environment, 2) integration into a social support network, and 3) integration into productive activities. Willer, Linn, and Allen (1993) developed a questionnaire to assess community integration along these three dimensions, called the CIQ. They brought together a group of rehabilitation experts and consumers to develop a pilot instrument to assess community integration along these three dimensions. The pilot instrument was assessed on a pilot sample and, through various statistical procedures, pared down to a brief but reliable assessment instrument named the CIQ. The authors defined community integration in terms of role performance and therefore regarded community integration as the converse of handicap. The authors did not make a distinction between survival roles and roles that serve to define the person as a successful member of society.

Willer, Rosenthal, Kreutzer, Gordon, and Rempel (1993) compared three populations on the CIQ: 1) individuals with brain injury who received rehabilitation services from model programs ($N = 94$); 2) individuals with brain injury who did not receive rehabilitation services ($N = 352$); and 3) individuals who do not have recognized disabilities ($N = 237$). Individuals without disabilities clearly had higher levels of integration than those with disabilities, especially in the area of productive activity. Individuals with brain injury who received rehabilitation from the model programs had higher levels of integration than individuals who did not receive these services. Willer, Rosenthal, et al. (1993) also reported that test–retest reliability of the CIQ was high, at .91 for individuals with brain injury and

.97 for family members. Correlations across subscales between family members and individuals with disabilities ranged from .74 for social integration to .96 for productive activity. Indicators of internal consistency point to highly adequate psychometric properties.

Willer, Ottenbacher, and Coad (1994) analyzed the same data on this large sample of individuals with brain injury and demonstrated that the phenomenon of community integration is clearly related to an individual's living situation. Individuals living in institutions were significantly less integrated than individuals living independently. In addition, the authors demonstrated that the phenomenon of community integration may be different for individuals who have disabilities and individuals who do not. An individual with disabilities may be limited in one area of integration, but those individuals who cope effectively compensate by increased integration in other areas. Individuals without disabilities tend to be integrated in some areas (e.g., employment) at the expense of integration into other areas (e.g., social network). Individuals with disabilities were, on average, integrated into a broader range of community activities but overall were considerably less integrated than their peers without disabilities.

Corrigan and Deming (1995) conducted an extensive replication of the CIQ psychometric evaluation and found virtually identical results. This replication study included individuals with brain injury as well as a sizable sample of individuals with disabilities from other impairments. Internal consistency was found to be adequate for social integration and home integration, but integration into productive activities showed some problems with internal consistency. Corrigan and Deming also assessed individuals' preinjury community integration scores on a retrospective basis. On the whole, individuals with disabilities showed a marked decline in integration after injury compared with before the injury. Preinjury integration scores were largely similar to the integration scores for the population without disabilities in the studies by Willer, Rosenthal, et al. (1993). Community integration, and the CIQ specifically, was found to be applicable to all populations of individuals with disabilities, regardless of the impairments or etiology.

Schmidt, Garvin, Heinemann, and Kelly (1995) examined age and gender differences in the resumption of roles, as assessed by the CIQ. The large sample ($N = 716$) was drawn from a multicenter study of individuals with acquired brain injury. The study found that women had slightly better integration scores following rehabilitation than men. However, people of all ages reported reduced integration following injury and resulting disabilities, with the exception of those ages 16–19 who reported greater integration after injury. Heinemann and Whiteneck (1995) examined the same multicenter sample of individuals with acquired brain injury as Schmidt et al. (1995). Heinemann and Whiteneck found that levels of disabilities account for approximately one fourth of the variance of the integration into the community. A measure of disabilities (defined in this instance as limitations in activities of daily living) was found to be a better predictor of handicap (defined as community integration) than indicators of impairment and demographic factors such as age, education, and gender.

Willer, Rosenthal, et al. (1993) compared the CIQ with the CHART on the same sample of individuals with brain injury, including assessments by both the individual and a family member. The home integration subscale of the CIQ did not have a counterpart in the CHART. The occupation subscale of the CHART was very similar in intent and items to the CIQ's productive activity subscale, and the correlation between the two was .55 when the respondent was the individual and .72 for family members serving as proxies for the individual. The social integration subscale of the CHART and CIQ also have similar intent but approach assessment differently. Correlations between the two scales were .35 and .25 for individual and family member respondents, respectively. These correlations were not only nonsignificant but also considerably below the expected scores. The authors explained that the CHART social integration scores for those individuals with brain injury were close to or at the maximum of 100; therefore, there was very little variance in the scores. Willer, Rosenthal, et al. (1993) raised important questions about the appropriateness of the social integration subscale of CHART for assessment of individuals with cognitive limitations. Their concerns echo those of Segal and Schall (1995). Questions from the CHART (e.g., "How many relatives, business associates, or friends do you visit, phone, or write to at least once a month?") posed considerable difficulty for those with cognitive limitations and for many proxies. There was even more difficulty with the question about how many strangers the individuals had engaged in conversation within the past month. For individuals with brain injury, initiating conversation with strangers can often reflect a problem with executive function and a high score generally would not reflect greater integration.

HANDICAP, COMMUNITY INTEGRATION, AND LIFE SATISFACTION

In describing the quality of life model, Minaire (1992) outlined the difficulty in defining quality of life. He suggested that quality of life in the ICIDH disablement model appears to be encompassed within the broad definition of *handicap.* Minaire further suggested that quality of life should be reserved for the subjective assessment of health and well-being by individuals. Fuhrer, Rintala, Hart, Clearman, and Young (1992) adopted this definition of quality of life and suggested that certain constructs are especially important: life satisfaction, happiness, and morale. Fuhrer et al. (1992) focused their attention on life satisfaction and used a 12-point scale representing life domains that individuals rated as important aspects of life satisfaction. The domains of life satisfaction represented are instructive to the discussion of whether life satisfaction or quality of life is separate from the concept of handicap. The highest-ranked domain was satisfaction with family relationships, second was spiritual life, third was daily living tasks, fourth was housing, and fifth was transportation. Many of these domains of life satisfaction are subsumed under the general definition of *handicap* but reflect the individual's perspective rather than the perspective of the health care provider.

Fuhrer and his colleagues (1992) also researched the relationship of the life satisfaction index (Version A) to measures of disability (FIM) and handicap (CHART) among individuals with physical disabilities, primarily as a result of spinal cord injury. The researchers found that individuals with disabilities were, on average, significantly less satisfied with life than those with no disabilities. There were no statistically significant relationships between life satisfaction and impairment indicators (level of paralysis) and between life satisfaction and disability measures. There was a relationship between life satisfaction and three domains of the CHART—namely, social integration, mobility, and occupation. A stepwise regression analysis demonstrated that the best predictors of life satisfaction were other subjective appraisals of quality of life, such as self-assessment of health status, perceived control, and perceived social support. The addition of the handicap-related variables from the CHART actually contributed to a slight decrease in the amount of variance accounted for in the regression equation.

Heinemann and Whiteneck (1995) also evaluated life satisfaction within the disablement model. They studied individuals with acquired brain injury and used a disability assessment that primarily measured activities of daily living. The measure of handicap was the CIQ, which purports to assess community integration. Life satisfaction was assessed using a single item: "Overall, how do you feel about the quality of your life in the last month or so?" The strongest relationship to life satisfaction was with the measures of community integration: the social integration and productivity subscales. There was a weak statistical relationship between life satisfaction and disability and no apparent relationship with impairment.

THE DISABLEMENT MODEL REVISITED

The WHO model (1980) for rehabilitation, variously called ICIDH, disablement, and sometimes enablement, is a long way from universal acceptance, as evidenced by the frequent confusion about the terms used in rehabilitation research. Perhaps no term is more regularly misused or confused than the term *handicap*. Furthermore, the model's components of impairments, disabilities, and handicap are still in need of conceptual clarity and research, and, until this clarity is provided, confusion over the terms is likely to continue.

The process of clarification is likely to inspire additional research, but the additional research is just as likely to add further clarification. This is especially true of research on the concept of handicap. This chapter presented two measures of handicap that have been evaluated for reliability and validity and therefore have added significantly to the potential for research on handicap. The CHART, developed by Whiteneck and colleagues (1992) at Craig Hospital in Denver, Colorado, was intended as a direct assessment of the components of handicap articulated by the WHO. The CIQ was developed by Willer and colleagues at the State University of New York at Buffalo as a measure of community integration, and it defined *handicap* in terms of role performance in the community. The CIQ assesses the spirit of handicap by assessing role function whereas the CHART assesses the survival roles specified by WHO. Both measures of handicap have led to important research on the relationship of impairments, disabilities, and handicap. There has also been research into the relationship of handicap to life satisfaction.

Research on the CHART and CIQ has produced relatively similar findings on the relationship between the components of the ICIDH, although the measures have somewhat different theoretical bases and have generally been used with different impairment groups. The CHART has been used primarily in the study of people with spinal cord injury, and the CIQ has been used primarily with people who have an acquired brain injury. However, with both measures, there is a relatively weak relationship between impairment and handicap. Individuals who are not impaired show significantly less handicap and therefore significantly greater community integration than individuals who are impaired. However, the degree to which an individual experiences role interference (handicap) does not vary substantially on the basis of level of impairment. It would appear that impairment represents a threshold and that anyone who is impaired sufficiently to warrant diagnosis and rehabilitation is impaired enough to experience handicap; however, more or less impairment may not affect the extent of handicap. This observation on the relationship of impairment to handicap is not inconsistent with the WHO model of disablement.

The relationship of disabilities to handicap is more pronounced than the relationship of impairments to disabilities. This is the expected finding, according to Fuhrer et al. (1992), because the linearity of the model represented by ICIDH implies that handicap is more distant from impairment in the causal flow. The research on the CHART and its relationship to disabilities is not as complete as the research on the CIQ; however, it is speculated that CHART measures would be more closely aligned to measures of disabilities. The CHART has several components that closely relate to disability because the definitions provided by the WHO also relate to disabilities. Mobility, for example, is presented as a role by the WHO, and therefore as a component of handicap, and would naturally be expected to have a strong relationship to indicators of gross motor skills or ambulation.

Measures of disabilities appear to account for about one quarter of the variance of those measures of handicap that are not direct measures of one or more aspects of disabilities. Some of the unexplained variance is the direct result of errors of measurement. Problems of reliability in all forms of assessment persist. Some of the variance is accounted for by environmental factors. Dawson and Chapman (1995) conducted a population-based study of individuals with brain injury and looked specifically at the disablement model and the relationship between disabilities and handicap. The authors added two important environmental factors to the analysis: living situation (living alone versus living with others) and barriers to mobility. The three areas of handicap defined for the population were physical independence, occupation, and social integration. Physical independence was considerably less problematic than occupation or social integration handicaps for individuals with brain injury. Environmental factors as assessed in this study accounted for a greater proportion of variance for each of the areas of handicap than did the various measures of disabilities. The study also pointed out the significant role of age, gender, and education in determining handicap.

The study of Dawson and Chapman (1995) also highlighted further issues of measurement. The measure of mobility barriers, considered a measure of environmental constraints, is very similar to the measure of mobility in the CHART. The measure of living situation as an environmental factor is incorporated as an important component of the measure of social integration in the CHART. The measure of economic self-sufficiency in the CHART merely asks about family income and could be considered an indicator of financial environment. The question thus becomes "Is the concept of handicap independent of the concept of environmental barriers?"

The relationship of handicap, whether assessed by the CIQ or CHART, to life satisfaction begins to address the larger issue of the place of quality of life within the disablement model. The quality of life model presented by Minaire (1992) appears workable. Handicap is somewhat predictive of life satisfaction, at least based on the two studies reviewed in this chapter (Fuhrer et al., 1992; Heinemann & Whiteneck, 1995). However, the studies of depression and its association with handicap add a source of confusion (Fuhrer et al., 1993; Tate et al., 1994). According to this research, depression correlates with measures of handicap in much the same manner as other measures of impairment or disability. However, satisfaction with life or the lack thereof is an important component of depression. Therefore, is life satisfaction a component at the end of the causal model, as proposed by Minaire, or is it merely a component of depression (disability)?

The confusion over depressive symptoms and life satisfaction is related to confusion over a number of components of the ICIDH model. The CHART, whose developers carefully attended to the articulation of handicap presented by the WHO, was unable to assess orientation. In the mental health field, orientation is generally considered an important factor in cognitive abilities along with planning, problem solving, and awareness. Each of these abilities can be restricted by mental illness and other neurologic impairments. In most instances, the limitations of these abilities are viewed as important disabilities and not as handicap. Orientation is not considered a survival role any more than any other cognitive abilities. Any definition or measure of disabilities or handicap has to be applicable to all impairment groups, and the ICIDH will gain greater clarity and applicability by attending to individuals with mental illness and other cognitive and emotional disabilities, as well as to those with physical limitations.

PROPOSAL FOR REVISION OF THE DISABLEMENT MODEL: THE ENABLEMENT MODEL

Fuhrer (1987) suggested that discussion of the ICIDH and disablement model is important for consideration of the purpose of rehabilitation. The purpose of rehabilitation is also important for the consideration of the disablement model and its alternatives. At the risk of oversimplifying the models, the following are proposed as statements of purpose for rehabilitation, based on Minaire's (1992) presentation on the components of each model:

- *Biomedical model:* To restore the individual to good health by eliminating the disease and impairment
- *Disablement model:* To restore the individual to life roles by reducing impairment, decreasing disabilities, and reducing environmental barriers
- *Situational model:* To assist the individual to become an active, integrated person within the community by assisting the individual to return to life roles, by reducing impairments, by decreasing disabilities, and by decreasing environmental barriers
- *Quality of life model:* To restore the individual to a suitable quality of life, by assisting the individual to be integrated within the community, by assisting the individual to fulfill life roles, by reducing impairments and decreasing disabilities, and by decreasing environmental barriers

The primary criticisms of the disablement model become more apparent in this presentation format:

- As in the biomedical model, *health* is defined as the absence of disease rather than the presence of function.
- There is confusion over the definition of *handicap,* as distinct from disabilities.
- The perspective of the individual with disabilities is left out of the equation.

The authors of this chapter propose a slight variation of the disablement model, which we are calling the enablement model. Rehabilitation should emphasize the development of strengths and not just the reduction of disabilities. In presenting the enablement model, we believe we can consider a broad, multifaceted purpose of rehabilitation that reflects the needs and perspective of the individual with disabilities:

1. To reduce the impairment experienced after a trauma or disease that is disabling. In addition, rehabilitation is committed to prevention of further impairment through early intervention.
2. To increase the level and types of abilities of the individual, to reduce the disabilities experienced as a result of impairments, to prevent the exacerbation of disabilities, and to find ways to assist individuals to adjust to disabilities that cannot be eliminated or prevented from deterioration. Adjustment is assisted through various means, including education, use of assistive or prosthetic devices, or environmental modification.
3. To increase the extent to which an individual with disabilities is integrated into a home, family, and friendship network and productive activities that are appropriate to age, gender, and personal choice, or, for those individuals who have declining abilities, that maintain the individual as closely as possible to existing levels of integration. This goal includes an assessment and promotion of environmental supports necessary for successful integration or maintenance of integration, including sufficient financial and personal resources and reduction of physical barriers and prejudice or discrimination.

The goals of rehabilitation should relate directly to the model of rehabilitation. We believe that the enablement model and its components do relate directly to the purpose of rehabilitation as previously described. The concept of handicap as defined in the enablement model and as expressed in the previous statement of goals is phrased in the language of community integration. Previously stated goals do not include economic self-sufficiency of the individual as part of the concept of handicap, because we believe economic factors are part of the environmental support structure. Mobility as a component of handicap within the disablement model is either subsumed within the category of disabilities or is part of the concern for environmental barriers within the enablement model. Orientation is clearly part of the disabilities associated with cognitive impairments and is not part of community integration and therefore is not part of handicap within the enablement model.

Thus, the enablement model is slightly different from the disablement model. The enablement model is a product of the theoretical underpinnings provided by the WHO (1980), Minaire (1992), and Fougeyrollas (1995). It is also enhanced by the practical research opportunities provided by the development of two measures of handicap, the CIQ and the CHART. Figure 2 presents the enablement model (and its similarity to the disablement model is apparent). The enablement model is more consistent with available research on handicap and is more applicable to all populations with disabilities, including those whose impairments are emotional or cognitive in nature. The model does not include any aspects of quality of life or life satisfaction, essentially because these concepts are not considered to be sufficiently operationalized. However, the concept of quality of life should eventually be added as a component of the enablement model to enhance both the model and the statement of purpose of rehabilitation.

Problems of definition of disabilities and handicap have interfered with the development of the conceptual scheme of the disablement model. The success of the two measures of handicap, the CIQ and CHART, has served to further identify the problems of definition. However, on the basis of research, principles of the disablement model can be delineated and the model can be strengthened for further research. We have chosen to call the revised model the *enablement model*. The word *enablement* is preferred because it presents a more positive view of the rehabilitation process and

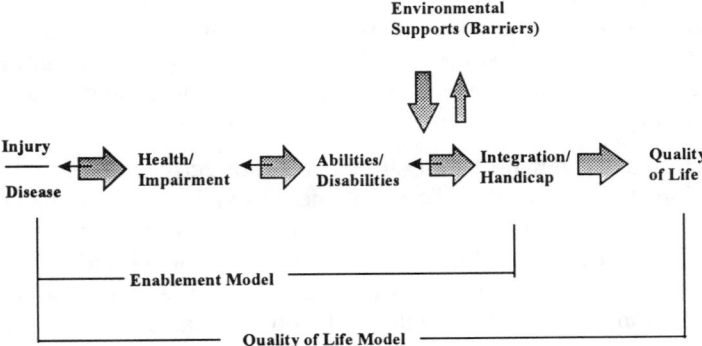

Figure 2. Proposed enablement model for rehabilitation.

moves the rehabilitation process further away from the biomedical model and the emphasis in that model on disease, diagnosis, and symptoms.

In the enablement model, the concept of handicap is differentiated from that of disabilities on the basis of interaction with others. Disabilities, according to the WHO, occur at the personal level, whereas handicap occurs at the level of interaction between the individual with disabilities and the rest of society. If this is the case, orientation (or, more accurately, disorientation) belongs with disabilities along with other cognitive and emotional consequences of impairment. Thus, any measure of handicap must clearly indicate the interactive nature of the behavior in question in relation to the society within which the behavior is expressed.

The concept of handicap representing interference with role function is a useful concept and should not be abandoned. The difference between social roles and survival roles is artificial, in the opinion of the authors of this chapter. Social roles, such as those carried out within a family setting, may not affect survival as directly as occupation, but they are certainly as critical to self-esteem and psychological well-being. The description of roles represented by the CIQ as integration in a home-like setting, integration into a social network, and integration into meaningful and productive activities seems defensible and consistent with the WHO's description of social integration and occupation. In the enablement model, handicap is seen as the converse of community integration; that is, handicap represents the lack of full integration into society. Integration is reduced through the presence of disabilities and the presence of environmental barriers.

CONCLUSIONS

Most of the observations and conclusions the authors of this chapter have reached regarding the strengths and weaknesses of the disablement model are consistent with the conclusions of Fougeyrollas (1995). Fougeyrollas insisted that handicap is the result of an interaction between disabilities and the environment. Environmental factors include all of the sociocultural or physical obstacles an individual with disabilities faces in assuming life roles. Fougeyrollas also included employment and recreation as environmental factors; however, we regard these as outcomes of the interaction and therefore more as a part of handicap. Regardless, the enablement model proposed in this chapter is greatly enhanced by the consideration of environmental factors—both the supportive factors and the environmental barriers. In consideration of barriers, most are drawn to the obvious barriers in the physical environment, such as narrow doorways, curbs, and inaccessible transportation. We hope that, when the WHO operationalizes the environment concept, more subtle barriers such as discriminatory practices are considered. In addition, individuals with cognitive and emotional disabilities face very different barriers from individuals with physical limitations. To an individual with cognitive disabilities, a crowded room or high noise levels can serve as major barriers to community integration.

The efforts of the WHO to develop the common nomenclature, and more specifically the ICIDH, have allowed for the development of measures of the various concepts. The development of these measures has led to important research on process and outcomes of rehabilitation. The efforts of the WHO also have allowed for the development of alternate models of rehabilitation. Most important, the ICIDH has forced the field of medical rehabilitation to examine and reexamine the purpose of rehabilitation.

REFERENCES

Anderman, L., & Anderman, F. (1992). University student with epilepsy: A study of social aspects. *Seizure, 1*(3), 173–176.

Angeleri, F., Angeleri, V.A., Foschi, N., Giaquinto, S., & Nolfe, G. (1993). The influence of depression, social activity, and family stress on functional outcome after stroke. *Stroke, 24*(10), 1478–1483.

Badley, E.M. (1993). An introduction to the concepts and classifications of the International Classification of Impairments, Disabilities, and Handicaps. *Disability and Rehabilitation, 15*(4), 161–178.

Badley, E.M. (1995). The genesis of handicap: Definition, models of disablement, and role of external factors. *Disability and Rehabilitation, 17*(2), 53–62.

Badley, E.M., & Tennant, A. (1991). A survey of disablement in a British population using an action-orientated measure, physical independence handicap: Problems with activities of daily living and level of support. *International Disability Studies, 13*(3), 91–98.

Badley, E.M., & Tennant, A. (1993). Disablement associated with rheumatic disorders in a British population: Problems with activities of daily living and level of support. *British Journal of Rheumatology, 32*(7), 601–608.

Badley, E.M., Tennant, A., & Wood, P.H. (1990). The assessment of physical independence handicap: Experience in a community disablement survey. *International Disability Studies, 12*(2), 47–53.

Beckung, E., & Uvebran, P. (1993). Motor and sensory impairments in children with intractable epilepsy. *Epilepsia, 34*(5), 924–929.

Borgel, F., Benhamo, P.Y., Zmirou, D., Balducci, F., Halimi, S., & Cordonnier, D. (1992). Assessment of handicap in chronic dialysis diabetic patients (Uremidiab section study). *Scandinavian Journal of Rehabilitation Medicine, 24*(4), 203–208.

Bruininks, R., McGrew, K., & Maruyama, G. (1988). Structure of adaptive behavior in samples with and without mental retardation. *American Journal on Mental Retardation, 93*(3), 265–272.

Corrigan, J.D., & Deming, R. (1995). Psychometric characteristics of the Community Integration Questionnaire: Replication and extension. *Journal of Head Trauma Rehabilitation, 10*(4), 41–53.

Costa, T., Scriver, C.R., & Childs, B. (1985). The effect of Mendelian disease on human health: A measurement. *American Journal of Medical Genetics, 21*(2), 231–242.

Dawson, D.D., & Chapman, M. (1995). The disablement experienced by traumatically brain-injured adults living in the community. *Brain Injury, 9*(4), 339–353.

de Klein-de Vrankrijker, M.W. (1995). Editorial: The International Classification of Impairments, Disabilities, and Handicaps (ICIDH): Perspectives and developments (Part 1). *Disability and Rehabilitation, 17*(3), 109–111.

Elwes, R.D., Marshall, J., Beattie, A., & Newman, P.K. (1991). Epilepsy and employment: A community based survey in an area of high unemployment. *Journal of Neurology, Neurosurgery and Psychiatry, 54*(3), 200–203.

Fiske, J., Gelbier, S., & Watson, R.M. (1990). The benefit of dental care to an elderly population assessed using a sociodental measure of oral handicap. *British Dental Journal, 168*(4), 153–156.

Floyd, M., & Kettl, M. (1991). A computer-based approach to measurement of employment handicap. *International Journal of Rehabilitation Research, 14*(1), 37–47.

Fougeyrollas, P. (1995). Documenting environmental factors for preventing the handicap creation process: Quebec contributions relating to ICIDH and social participation of people with functional differences. *Disability and Rehabilitation, 17*(3), 145–153.

Fuhrer, M.J. (1987). Overview of outcome analysis in rehabilitation. In M. Fuhrer (Ed.), *Rehabilitation outcomes: Analysis and measurement* (pp. 1–18). Baltimore: Paul H. Brookes Publishing Co.

Fuhrer, M.J., Rintala, D.H., Hart, K.A., Clearman, R., & Young, M.E. (1992). Relationship of life satisfaction to impairment, disability, and handicap among persons with spinal cord injury living in the community. *Archives of Physical Medicine and Rehabilitation, 73*(6), 552–557.

Fuhrer, M.J., Rintala, D.H., Hart, K.A., Clearman, R., & Young, M.E. (1993). Depressive symptomatology in persons with spinal cord injury who reside in the community. *Archives of Physical Medicine and Rehabilitation, 74*(3), 255–260.

Harper, A.C., Harper, D.A., Lambert, L.J., Andrews, H.B., Lo, S.K., Ross, F.M., & Straker, L.M. (1992). Symptoms of impairment, disability and handicap in low back pain: A taxonomy. *Pain, 50*(2), 189–195.

Heinemann, A.W., & Whiteneck, G.G. (1995). Relationships among impairment, disability, handicap, and life satisfaction in persons with traumatic brain injury. *Journal of Head Trauma Rehabilitation, 10*(4), 54–63.

Helzer, J.E., Brockington, I.F., & Kendell, R.E. (1981). Predictive validity of DSM-III and Feighner definitions of schizophrenia. A comparison with research diagnosis criteria and CATEGO. *Archives of General Psychiatry, 38*(7), 791–797.

Jacobson, G.P., & Newman, C.W. (1990). The development of the Dizziness Handicap Inventory. *Archives of Otolaryngology—Head and Neck Surgery, 116*(4), 424–427.

Jacobson, G.P., Newman, C.W., Hunter, L., & Balzer, G.K. (1991). Balance function test correlates of the Dizziness Handicap Inventory. *Journal of the American Academy of Audiology, 2*(4), 253–260.

Koepcke, W., Hasford, J., Weber Falkensammer, H., & Zwingers, T. (1984). Rheumatology trials: Selection of adequate response variables and their evaluation. *Revue du Epidemiologie et de Sante Publique, 32*(3–4), 237–242.

Kuldau, J.M., & Dirks, S.J. (1987). Controlled evaluation of a hospital-originated community transitional system. *Archives of General Psychiatry, 34*(11), 1331–1340.

Lequesne, M. (1991). Indices of severity and disease activity for osteoarthritis. [Review]. *Seminars in Arthritis and Rheumatism, 20*(6 Suppl 2), 48–54.

Mattison, P.G., Aitken, R.C., & Prescott, R.J. (1991). Rehabilitation status—The relationship between the Edinburgh Rehabilitation Status Scale (ERSS), Barthel Index, and PULSES profile. *International Disability Studies, 13*(1), 9–11.

Mattison, P.G., Aitken, R.C., & Prescott, R.J. (1992). Rehabilitation status in multiple handicap. *Archives of Physical Medicine and Rehabilitation, 73*(10), 926–929.

Menter, R.R., Whiteneck, G.G., Charlifue, S.W., Gerhart, K., Solnick, S.J., Brooks, C.A., & Hughes, L. (1991). Impairment, disability, handicap and medical expenses of persons aging with spinal cord injury. *Paraplegia, 29*(9), 613–619.

Minaire, P. (1992). Disease, illness and health: Theoretical models of the disablement process. *Bulletin of the World Health Organization, 70*(3), 373–379.

Mooney, V. (1987). Impairment, disability, and handicap. *Clinical Orthopaedics and Related Research, 221,* 14–25.

Newman, C.W., Weinstein, B.E., Jacobson, G.P., & Hug, G.A. (1990). The Hearing Handicap Inventory for Adults: Psychometric adequacy and audiometric correlates. *Ear and Hearing, 11*(6) 430–433.

Peters, J.D. (1995). Human experience in disablement: The imperative of the ICIDH. *Disability and Rehabilitation, 17*(3), 135–144.

Rintala, D.H., Hart, K.A., & Fuhrer, M.J. (1993). *Handicap and spinal cord injury: Levels and correlates of the mobility, occupation and social integration dimensions.* Paper presented at the American Spinal Injury Association meeting, San Diego, CA.

Roy, C.W., Hunter, J., Arthurs, Y., & Prescott, R.J. (1992). Is "handicap" affected by a hospital based rehabilitation programme? *Scandinavian Journal of Rehabilitation Medicine, 24*(2), 105–112.

Schmidt, M.F., Garvin, L.J., Heinemann, A.W., & Kelly, J.P. (1995). Gender- and age-related role changes following brain injury. *Journal of Head Trauma Rehabilitation, 10*(4), 14–27.

Schow, R.L., Smedley, T.C., & Longhurst, T.M. (1990). Self-assessment and impairment in adult-elderly hearing screening: Recent data and new perspectives. *Ear and Hearing, 11*(5 Suppl), 17S–27S.

Schuling, J., de Haan, R., Limburg, M., & Groener, K.H. (1993). The Frenchay Activities Index. Assessment of functional status in stroke patients. *Stroke, 24*(8), 1173–1177.

Segal, M.E., & Schall, R.R. (1995). Assessing handicap of stroke survivors: A validation study of the Craig Handicap Assessment and Reporting Technique. *American Journal of Physical Medicine and Rehabilitation, 74*(4), 276–286.

Segal, S.P., & Everett-Dille, L. (1980). Coping styles and factors in male-female social integration. *Acta Psychiatrica Scandinavia, 61*(1), 8–20.

Sergl, H.G., Ruppenthal, T., & Schmitt, H.G. (1992). Disfigurement and psychosocial handicap of adults with extreme mandibular prognathism. *International Journal of Adult Orthodontics and Orthognathic Surgery, 7*(1), 31–35.

State University of New York at Buffalo. (1993). *Guide for the Uniform Data Set for Medical Rehabilitation (Adult FIM), version 4.0.* Buffalo, NY: Author.

Talo, S., Puuka, P., Rytokoski, U., Ronnemaa, T., & Kallio, V. (1994). Can treatment outcome of chronic low back pain be predicted? Psychological disease consequences clarifying the issue. *Clinical Journal of Pain, 10*(2), 107–121.

Tannahill, J.C. (1979). The Hearing Handicap Scale as a measure of hearing aid benefit. *Journal of Speech and Hearing Disorders, 44*(1), 91–99.

Tate, D., Forchheimer, M., Maynard, F., & Dijkers, M. (1994). Predicting depression and psychological distress in persons with spinal cord injury based on indicators of handicap. *American Journal of Physical Medicine and Rehabilitation, 73*(3), 175–183.

Truelle, J.L., Van Zomeren, A.D., de Barsy, T., Brooks, D.N., Janzik, H.H., & Lay, W. (1992). A European head injury evaluation chart. *Scandinavian Journal of Rehabilitation Medicine, 26*(Suppl.), 115–125.

Ustun, T.B., Cooper, J.E., van Duuren-Kristen, S., Kennedy, C., Hendershot, G., & Sartorius, J.E. (1995). Revision of the ICIDH: Mental health aspects. *Disability and Rehabilitation, 17*(3), 202–209.

Verloove, J., Vanhorick, S.P., Veen, S., Ens Dokkum, M.H., Schreuder, A.M., Brand, R., & Ruys, J.H. (1994). Sex difference in disability and handicap at five years of age in children born at very short gestation. *Pediatrics, 93*(4), 576–579.

Whiteneck, G.G., Charlifue, S.W., Gerhart, K.A., Overholser, J.D., & Richardson, G.N. (1992). Quantifying handicap: A new measure of long-term rehabilitation outcomes. *Archives of Physical Medicine and Rehabilitation, 73*(6), 519–526.

Willer, B., & Corrigan, J.D. (1994). Whatever it takes: A model for community-based services. *Brain Injury, 8*(7), 647–659.

Willer, B., Linn, R., & Allen, K. (1993). Community integration and barriers to integration for individuals with brain injury. M.A.J. Finlayson & S.H. Garner (Eds.), *Brain injury rehabilitation: Clinical considerations* (pp. 355–375). Baltimore: Williams & Wilkins.

Willer, B., Ottenbacher, K.J., & Coad, M.L. (1994). The Community Integration Questionnaire: A comparative examination. *American Journal of Physical Medicine and Rehabilitation, 73*(2), 103–111.

Willer, B., Rosenthal, M., Kreutzer, J.S., Gordon, W.A., & Rempel, R. (1993). Assessment of community integration following rehabilitation for traumatic brain injury. *Journal of Head Trauma and Rehabilitation, 8*(2), 75–88.

Wolfe, C.D., Taub, N.A., Woodrow, E.J., & Burney, P.G. (1991). Assessment of scales of disability and handicap for stroke patients [see comments]. *Stroke, 22*(10), 1242–1244.

Wolfe, C.D., Taub, N.A., Woodrow, E.J., Richardson, E., Warburton, F.G., & Burney, P.G. (1993). Patterns of acute stroke care in three districts of southern England. *Journal of Epidemiology and Community Health, 47*(2), 144–148.

World Health Organization (WHO). (1980). *International classification of impairments, disabilities, and handicaps.* Geneva, Switzerland: Author.

Yardley, L., & Putman, J. (1992). Quantitative analysis of factors contributing to handicap and distress in vertiginous patients: A questionnaire study. *Clinical Otolaryngology, 17*(3), 231–236.

CHAPTER 7

Measuring Quality of Life

Marcel Dijkers

The increase in the latter half of the 20th century in the number of people with chronic diseases such as heart disease, stroke, and arthritis has been cited as the reason behind the emergence of quality of life as a major concern in the health care field (Levine, 1987). There is no cure for these diseases, but pain and discomfort can be relieved, function can be enhanced, adjustment can be supported, and mental health can be improved. In all areas of health care where chronic disorders are treated, enhancement (or at least maintenance) of quality of life has become of paramount concern (Wenger, Mattson, Furberg, & Elinson, 1984).

Where does rehabilitation, and more specifically medical rehabilitation, fit in? In a sense, rehabilitation has been ahead of its time and ahead of the other health care specialties in that it has had from its inception a unique concern for patients' function (e.g., activities of daily living [ADL], communication, mobility), as well as for their emotional and social well-being. Many U.S. rehabilitation facilities have some variation of "adding life to years" as their slogan, which may be contrasted with the "years added to life" characteristic of many other branches of health care.

Although the field of medical rehabilitation is in the forefront of concern for life's quality, the term *quality of life* is not used frequently. Other areas of health care, such as cardiovascular disease (Wenger et al., 1984), oncology (Aaronson, 1991), clinical trials science (Spilker, 1990), and health services research (Stewart & Ware, 1992), tend to be further advanced in the conceptualization and measurement of quality of life. In addition, rehabilitationists tend to be unfamiliar with developments in these other fields (cf. Keith, 1994).

It would be fair to say that momentum was lost in the 1980s. The theme of the 1979 annual meeting of the American Congress of Rehabilitation Medicine was the quality of life of the person with a disability. This was followed by discussions by a number of prominent rehabilitation practitioners (Anderson, 1982; Freed, 1984; Kottke, 1982). Alexander and Willems (1981) discussed measurement requirements based on their conceptualization of quality of life, and Cardus, Fuhrer, and Thrall (1981) indicated the need for inclusion of quality of life in rehabilitation research cost–benefit analyses. Finally, in what should have been a seminal article, Flanagan (1982) presented the state of the art in quality-of-life measurement for the general population and suggested ways in which these procedures can be used to develop instruments for measurement of the life quality of people with disabilities.

Since then, developments have been limited. A 1988 Rehab Brief published by the National Institute on Disability and Rehabilitation Research reported that the National Rehabilitation Information Center held 100 documents classified under both "quality of life" and "rehabilitation." Only one quarter of these were inquiries into quality of life per se, and, of these, only half were research or methodologic reports. Most of these, and the ones published since 1988, concern descriptive analyses of quality of life in specific subgroups (e.g., Fuhrer, Rintala, Hart, Clearman, & Young, 1992; Siösteen, Lundqvist, Blomstrand, Sullivan, & Sullivan, 1990).

No study by rehabilitation researchers was identified to follow Flanagan's (1982) suggestion to develop a quality-of-life instrument specifically attuned to the situation of people with disabilities. Other purely methodologic studies, for example, into the domains of life relevant to quality of life for people with disabilities or into measures useful with subjects who have cognitive or communicative deficits, are also lacking. There is little systematic consideration of how *quality of life* should be defined and conceptualized and what measures are useful in assessing the unique life quality of rehabilitation patients. (Compare Wood-Dauphinee and Kuechler [1992] for a similar conclusion and Day [1993] for an opposing viewpoint.) If in rehabilitation little solid scholarship exists on quality of life, it is useful to review what has been accomplished in other areas of research.

CONCEPTUALIZATION AND MEASUREMENT OF QUALITY OF LIFE

Campbell, Converse, and Rodgers (1976), who constitute one group of pioneers of studies on quality of life, noted that "quality of life is a vague and ethereal entity, something that many people talk about, but which nobody very clearly knows what to do about" (p. 471). That has not stopped researchers and clinicians from using, defining, and operationalizing the construct. The result is claims that quality of life has been given so many definitions and operationalizations and has become so fashionable that it has lost its usefulness as a concept (cf. Bergner, 1989; Taylor, 1994).

A more common criticism in papers reviewing quality-of-life measurement is that definitions of quality of life are missing, that authors disagree as to what quality of life is, and that measurement instruments or batteries are developed and used with limited or no underlying conceptualization (e.g., Bergner, 1989; Bowling, 1991; de Haes & van Knippenberg, 1985; Dossa, 1989; Gill & Feinstein, 1994; Mor & Guadagnoli, 1988; Sutcliffe & Holmes, 1991; van Dam, 1986; van Knippenberg & de Haes, 1988). This poor state of development is not surprising, given the relative newness of the field, the existence of three separate research traditions, and the diverse interests of the people who create and use quality-of-life measures. This includes researchers in areas as diverse as economics, gerontology, political science, and rheumatology; politicians and policy makers; clinicians and other service providers; and human services and health care administrators and regulators. However, enough study and comparison of approaches and instruments has been performed that it is possible to group conceptualizations, definitions, and measurements (cf. Croog, n.d.; Schipper, Clinch, & Powell, 1990).

The major dividing lines coincide with three traditions that can be distinguished. The first, social indicators research, locates quality of life in the availability to aggregates of people of the natural, economic, social, and other resources that are needed to obtain or that constitute the goods and services required for better living. Indicators of quality of life of countries or other political divisions typically used in these studies include per capita energy consumption, life expectancy, percentage of children in the labor force, physicians per 1,000 population, and gross domestic product. This area of research is not considered here, because individual practitioners or the field of rehabilitation as a whole has little or no capacity to affect the supply of these resources.

The second tradition, the subjective tradition (also designated as the evaluative or internal determinants school), defines *quality of life* as the congruence between aspirations and accomplishments, as perceived or experienced by the person involved. Reactions to congruence and disparity can be either predominantly *cognitive,* the approach taken by the life satisfaction school (e.g., Cantril, 1965; Zhan, 1992), or *emotional* in nature, the approach of those who focus on happiness or positive and negative affect (e.g., Bradburn, 1969). Measures used by researchers in the latter tradition tend to shade over in instruments of mental health (e.g., self-esteem, depression); however, the latter tend to lack the reflective component that is unique to subjective quality-of-life conceptualizations. A combination of approaches is not uncommon; for example, Fabian (1990) defined quality of life as "a measure of subjective well-being, an abstract and multifaceted concept which subsumes related, but structurally different concepts such as happiness and life satisfaction" (p. 161).

Within the cognitive group, a distinction may be made between those who use a concept of quality of life as a global entity (e.g., Diener, 1984) and those who define and delineate various domains of life, all of which are evaluated separately (e.g., Flanagan, 1982). An overall score may then be based on explicit importance rankings of domains by the subject (e.g., Ferrans & Powers, 1992) or developed by the investigator based on either personal judgment or the results of sophisticated statistical analysis methods, such as factor analysis.

In the third tradition, the objective tradition, *quality of life* is defined as the sum total of a person's scores on measures of characteristics that can be objectively determined. This is exemplified most by health care research, but this approach also can be found in developmental disabilities studies (e.g., Goode, 1994) and gerontology (e.g., George & Bearon, 1980). The components of quality of life are simple things such as income level, the number of television sets in the home, and the desirability of the neighborhood in which the home is located. These tend to be items that presumably are valuated with a high level of consensus by members of a society and that consequently have easily established "best" and "worst" extremes. For instance, well-educated is better than poorly educated and having few symptoms of a chronic disorder is better than having many.

How the person involved feels about things is generally not considered; at best, the instrument designer's personal judgment of item scaling and relative weights of the items in an index is replaced by the consensus judgment of groups (of professionals or patients, in the case of health measures). For example, this is the approach taken by the developers of the General Health Policy Model and the associated method of measuring health state utilities, the Quality of Well-Being Scale (Kaplan & Anderson, 1990). The increasingly used Quality-Adjusted Life Years (QALY) technique is an extension of this approach, combining life quantity (years remaining until death) and quality, defined as the mean of the utility (quality) ratings that groups of respondents give to various health states.

However, in most instances, it is the researcher developing the quality-of-life instrument (or the clinician administering it) who defines and determines what factors affect quality of life. The assumption is made that, for example, performing many activities is better than being involved in few activities, and that by definition subjects (patients) who report engaging in many activities have a better quality of life. Wolfensberger (1994) is one of several authors who pointed out that such definitions easily accommodate the prejudices of a particular culture or ruling class.

McCullough (1984) noted that the use of objective measures of health-related quality of life by care providers and researchers fits into a beneficence model of health care: The professional knows best what is good for the patient. Subjective measures fit into an autonomy model: Patients are the specialists who know what is in their best interest. Gill and Feinstein (1994) complained that investigators tend to specify what are important issues for quality of life instead of asking patients or clients. Only a limited number of studies have used a more qualitative methodology that allows for specification of domains and their importance by the people whose quality of life is under study (e.g., Bach & McDaniel, 1993).

HEALTH-RELATED QUALITY OF LIFE

Health-related quality-of-life (HRQOL) conceptualizations and measures deserve greater attention. *Conceptualization* in many instances is too grand a term. Bowling (1991) noted that "it is becoming fashionable to equate all non-clinical data with 'quality of life,' which is likely to be a source of conceptual confusion" (p. 9). Several reviewers (e.g., Aaronson, 1991) remarked that health-related quality-of-life research is lacking in theory; however, that is slowly changing (see, e.g., Wilson & Cleary, 1995).

In the term *health related, health* should be understood in the broadest sense of the term (for instance, as in the World Health Organization's definition of *health* as physical, mental, and social well-being). The variables considered range from symptoms to side effects of treatment to impairments, disabilities, and handicaps (as defined by the WHO, 1980), fatigue and pain, social and physical activities, bed or home restriction days, neuropsychologic function, and even available social supports. Many writers appear to equate HRQOL with (comprehensive) health status, and many HRQOL measures are indistinguishable from health-status measures or at best have somewhat less emphasis on negative health components (cf. Keith, 1994; see also Chapter 8 of this book for a discussion of health status measures).

A broad definition is offered by Patrick and Erickson (1993). *Health-related quality of life* is "the value assigned to duration of life as modified by the impairments, functional states, perceptions, and social opportunities that are influenced by disease, injury, treatment, or policy" (p. 22). For illustrative purposes, Patrick and Erickson's concepts and domains are presented in Table 1. It should be noted that the definition explicitly refers to a time period rather than a point and that the domains include satisfaction with health as well as well-being and happiness. Other investigators also include mental and emotional well-being and other aspects of adjustment, and even direct questions on satisfaction (with health, with functioning, or with life in general), in their definitions or measures (cf. Jette, 1993). This suggests that, in HRQOL measures, the objective and subjective approaches are sometimes combined, often without much attention to the crucial differences between the two classes of items.

Based on the way HRQOL is conceptualized and measured, a number of approaches can be distinguished. There are disease-specific measures, for instance, for throat cancer, and more generic instruments, applicable to

Table 1. Domains of health-related quality of life

Opportunity
  Social or cultural handicap (including disadvantage because of health)
  Individual resilience (capacity for health, physical/mental reserve)
Health perceptions
  Satisfaction with health (physical, psychologic, and social)
  General health perceptions (self-rating of health, health concerns)
Functional status—social
  Acute or chronic limitations in usual social roles
  Social integration (community participation)
  Contact with others
  Intimacy and closeness (sexual and other)
Functional status—psychologic
  Affective (distress, general well-being, happiness)
  Cognitive (e.g., alertness, orientation, reasoning, memory, communication)
Functional status—physical
  Acute or chronic limitations in physical activity (e.g., mobility, self-care)
  Fitness (performance of vigorous activities)
Impairment
  Subjective complaints (reports of physical and psychologic symptoms,
    sensations, pain, health problems)
  Signs (evidence of defect or abnormality observable upon physical
    examination)
  Self-reported disease or impairments
  Physiologic measures (laboratory data, records)
  Tissue alterations (pathologic evidence)
  Diagnoses (clinical judgments based on any of the above)
Death and duration of life (mortality, survival, longevity)

Adapted from Patrick and Erickson (1993).

all types of cancers or even to all chronic disorders (cf. Aaronson, 1991). What specific items (e.g., symptoms, side effects, functions) are included depends on the underlying conceptualization of health-related quality of life. (It should be noted that some characteristics included in an index of objective health-related measures can be assessed only by asking the subject, for instance, a patient's amount of pain and discomfort. However, patient report does not equate with patient evaluation. The subject is not asked whether, for instance, he or she is happy with the level of pain because it is less than before or less than expected.)

The many existing health-related quality-of-life measures also differ in psychometric characteristics. Some investigators are more interested in developing a battery of the best available instruments, whereas others focus on combining items relevant to all QOL aspects that are of interest into a single instrument, with or without subscores (e.g., Ware & Sherbourne, 1992; Wood-Dauphinee, Opzoomer, Williams, Marchand, & Spitzer, 1988). A few instruments consist of a single item, for example, the Glasgow Outcome Scale (Jennett & Bond, 1975).

Another methodologic distinction between measurement approaches is based on who provides information. Although that normally is the patient, in some instances, such as cases of mental or emotional incompetence, a proxy is used, either a family member or significant other or a health professional. However, experience has shown that there generally is a poor correspondence between reports of patients and those of proxies, even for behaviors that are open to observation by others, such as functional status (cf. Slevin, Plant, Lynch, Drinkwater, & Gregory, 1988). Patients tend to report higher quality of life (e.g., less impairment, more social support) and rate as more satisfactory a given objective constellation of characteristics. When people without disabilities estimate the subjective quality of life of people with disabilities as a group, the discrepancy may be even larger than when the quality of life of specific people is the focal point (Bach, 1992; Bach & Campagnolo, 1992).

Usually, the quality of life at a particular point in time is assessed, but some investigators are interested in future and long-term quality of life, estimated to be forthcoming, given certain present patient characteristics and likely or possible health care interventions. The investigators may focus on developing a single index number that expresses quality and quantity of life (Kaplan & Anderson, 1990).

Overviews of HRQOL and its components, and reviews of specific measures, were provided by Bell, Bombardier, and Tugwell (1990); Bowling (1991); Bungay and Ware (1993); Gill and Feinstein (1994); McDowell and Newell (1996); Patrick and Deyo (1989); Spilker (1990); Stewart and Ware (1992); and van Knippenberg and de Haes (1988).

Utility Approaches and QALY

A marriage of objective quality-of-life measurement and decision-making theory has resulted in what is termed the *utility approach* to measuring HRQOL, which more recently has given birth to the QALY approach. Utility quality-of-life instruments give a quantitative measure of the value or utility people attach to various health states along the death-to-perfect-health continuum. A variety of methods (e.g., time trade-off, willingness to pay, standard gamble) are available to develop such utilities. The values used in health policy or administrative decisions generally are the means of ratings made by specific groups or by a sample representative of the general public. The goal is to maximize utility per dollar spent, for example, on patients selected for costly treatments and on reimbursable interventions. (For a more detailed discussion on utility approaches, see Chapter 9 of this book.)

Combining life expectancy with utility score provides QALY. For instance, Treatment A for a particular disease will result in death in 6 years, with each year estimated to carry a utility of 0.564. Treatment B will provide only 4 years of life, with a score of 0.973 each. Treatment B (QALY score of $4 \times 0.973 = 3.892$) is preferred over Treatment A (QALY score of $6 \times 0.564 = 3.384$).

That the utility derived is a cardinal measure of the strength of preferences of individuals (singly or in aggregate) makes it possible for the QALY approach to be used to reach decisions concerning benefits and costs–benefits of alternative treatments or alternative programs for patients, groups of patients, or whole communities. An overview of the various approaches to the development of utilities is provided in Kane and Kane (1982); Patrick and Erickson (1993); Pliskin, Shepard, and Weinstein (1980); and Torrance (1987).

Selected Quality-of-Life Instruments

The total number of instruments designed as measures of quality of life or used by researchers other than the instruments' developers as measures of quality of life or one of its components runs in the hundreds. For most, few tests of psychometric qualities have been performed, and their applicability to a population with physical disability is generally unknown. Some of the best-known and more adequate instruments are described in this section. More detail on the content and practicality, reliability, validity, and sensitivity of these and other measures may be found in Bell et al. (1990); Bowling (1991); Bungay and Ware (1993); de Haan, Aaronson, van Limburg, Langton Hewer, and van Crewel (1993); Gill and Feinstein (1994); Jette (1993); McDowell and Newell (1996); and Spilker (1990).

Quality-of-life instruments are reviewed here in four categories: 1) generic health-related, 2) disease- or disorder-specific, 3) life satisfaction, and 4) emotional or mental well-being. These reviews do not aim to provide an exhaustive description or a complete evaluation of clinicometric properties based on published evidence. The major purpose is to suggest the spectrum of QOL instruments and the variety of conceptualizations, measurement approaches, and content areas represented.

Generic Health-Related Instruments The Nottingham Health Profile (NHP) (Hunt & McEwen, 1980) was developed based on lay, rather than professional, concepts of health. It reflects how people behave and feel when they experience various states of health. Subjects indicate with "Yes" or "No" the applicability to their daily life of each of 38 statements (e.g., "I feel I am a burden to people," "I'm tired all the time") in six dimensions: mobility, pain, sleep, social isolation, emotional reactions, and energy level. The number of affirmed "departures from normal functioning" constitutes the total score; a weighted version is also available. NHP dimension subscores may be used as a profile. Internal consistency and test–retest reliability of all dimensional scores are good to excellent. Profile scores discriminate adequately between various diagnostic groups. Because the NHP (like many other health-related life quality measures) covers only negative aspects of health, it cannot discriminate among relatively healthy people. It is useful as a research and clinical instrument and is popular in Great Britain, where it was developed.

The (Spitzer) Quality of Life Index was formulated to encompass the major components of quality of life as identified by people with chronic diseases (especially cancer), their families, and health professionals (Spitzer et al., 1981). Single items, each reflecting one of five dimensions of quality of life (health, social support, outlook, daily living, and activity, that is, occupation), are summed to give an overall score. The instrument is completed by the treating physician, although a self-report version also is available. Correlations between physician and patient ratings have been reported to be moderate (0.61). Internal consistency and interrater reliability are adequate. Evaluation of treatment and palliative care of patients is the purpose of this brief and easy-to-administer instrument.

The Sickness Impact Profile (SIP) was developed in the United States to measure sickness, conceived as illness as experienced by the individual in terms of its impact on daily behavior. As a health status measure, it was designed to be broadly applicable across types and severities of illness, as well as across ethnic and other subgroups (Bergner, Bobbitt, Carter, & Gelson, 1981). The SIP focuses on performance rather than on capacity in 12 categories, which can be summarized in two dimensions: physical and psychosocial. Physical encompasses ambulation, mobility, body care, and movement (e.g., "I do not bathe myself at all, but am bathed by someone else"). Psychosocial includes social interaction, communication, alertness behavior, and emotional behavior (e.g., "I laugh or cry suddenly"). There are self- and interviewer-administered versions. Completing the 136 items takes 20–30 minutes, which many researchers and patients consider excessive. The SIP has been used widely in the United States but also in translations in many Western languages. The SIP is sensitive to change (and for this reason has been used in clinical trials), and many studies have indicated high test–retest reliability and internal consistency. Validity has been demonstrated through substantial correlations with many other health status and functional assessment measures.

The MOS 36-Item Short-Form Health Survey (SF-36) was constructed to represent the health status components most commonly used in survey research. Experience and actual items from prior research (especially the Rand studies [e.g., Ware et al., 1980]) were used to extract a maximum amount of information from a minimum number of questions (Ware & Sherbourne, 1992). Proper use of the SF-36 results in a profile of eight concepts or dimensions: 1) physical functioning (10 items) (e.g., "Does your health now limit you in . . . bending, kneeling, or stooping: a lot, a little or none?"); 2) role limitations due to physical problems (4 items); 3) role limitations due to emotional problems (3 items); 4) social functioning (2 items); 5) bodily pain (2 items); 6) general mental health (5 items); 7) vitality (4 items); and 8) general health perceptions (5 items) (e.g., "In general, would you say your health is excellent/very good/good/fair/poor?").

Likert scaling of these items, each with from two to six answer categories, is used to score the dimensions, providing greater sensitivity than do measures that count only health effects on behavior. Because of its heritage in two major health services research projects (the Rand Health Insurance Study [Ware et al., 1980] and the Medical Outcomes Study [Stewart & Ware, 1992]) and the involvement of eminent researchers who have published extensive clinicometric data, the SF-36 in a short time has become the health outcomes measure of choice. The limited time needed to complete the measure through personal, telephone, or self-administration (5–10 minutes) also is a reason. The SF-36 may have a ceiling effect when used with healthy subjects and a floor effect (for some dimensions) when used with people with severe disability.

The Quality of Well-Being Scale (QWBS) (formerly called the Health Status Index and the Index of Well-Being) was formulated for use in cost–benefit evaluations of all types of health programs and interventions. The investigators (Fanshel & Bush, 1970), by permutation of three basic health or functional status dimensions (mobility or confinement, physical activity, social activity), each with four or five categories, derived 43 separate statuses. A population sample employed an equal-appearing interval scaling procedure to develop weights for each of the statuses. The weights reflect desirability or utility and social preferences or judgments of relative value that people give to each status (e.g., death = 0.0 [reference point]; in hospital, in bed or chair, and receiving help with self-care = 0.47; fully mobile in community, walk with physical limitations, do self-care but not work or school or housework = 0.63; "normal" = 1.00 [reference point]).

In evaluating a health intervention, patients involved are interviewed to determine their status. Value ratings corresponding to these statuses can be averaged over cases and over programs (or clinical trial arms) to assess outcomes. Utilities may be further refined by taking into account 36 symptoms or problems that likely limit function or at least detract from complete well-being. The presence of these symptoms also is established by interviewing, and their values are based on population sample ratings. Because the QWBS ratings are interval-scale based, an extension to QALY is easily made: Time spent in each of a series of statuses can be multiplied with the corresponding utilities and added for a total value (e.g., from the time of diagnosis to death). A further step is often taken to calculate the cost of the interventions considered per (adjusted) year. The General Health Policy Model (Kaplan, Bush, & Berry, 1976) incorporates the QWBS into a formal system of cost–benefit evaluation. Most of the applications of the instrument have been in this area. It has also inspired other, less complicated utility measures that are used in research.

Disease- or Disorder-Specific Instruments The Glasgow Outcome Scale (GOS) was designed by Jennett and Bond (1975) as a simple scale for describing overall outcome after traumatic or nontraumatic brain injury. The original scale classifies patients into five categories, based on extensive definitions and descriptions: 1) death, 2) vegetative state, 3) severe disability, 4) moderate disability, and 5) good recovery. Versions with finer gradations within the last three categories have been proposed to improve the sensitivity of the measure. Good to excellent interrater agreement on classification of patients has been reported. Applications of the GOS have been limited almost exclusively to people with traumatic brain injury and stroke.

The Arthritis Impact Measurement Scale (AIMS) was created by Meenan, Gertman, and Mason (1980) to assess patient outcomes in arthritis. The AIMS consists of 45 items (some of them adapted from earlier instruments) in nine categories: 1) mobility, 2) dexterity, 3) physical activity, 4) activities of daily living, 5) household activities, 6) social activities, 7) depression, 8) anxiety, and 9) pain.

Self-administered or interviewer-administered versions of AIMS take about 15 minutes to complete. Guttman reproducibility and test–retest reliability coefficients for all scales are adequate. Validity is indicated by correlations with arthritis activity scores, self-rated health, and other relevant measures. Most questions are not specific to arthritis (e.g., "Can you easily turn a key in a lock?") and do not mention this disorder or its unique symptoms. With modification of the questions specific to arthritis (e.g., "During the past month, how long has your morning stiffness usually lasted from the time you woke up?"), the instrument has been applied to other diagnostic groups.

The Craig Handicap Assessment and Reporting Technique (CHART) (Whiteneck, Charlifue, Gerhart, Overholser, & Richardson, 1992) was designed to measure five of the WHO's (1980) six dimensions of handicap in people with spinal cord injury: 1) physical independence, 2) mobility, 3) activity (occupation), 4) social integration, and 5) economic self-sufficiency. Orientation, the sixth dimension, was omitted because typically it does not constitute a problem in this population. For each dimension, between two and five questions are used. An example is, "How many relatives (not in your household) do you visit, phone or write to at least once a month?" Scoring has been based on normative expectations for members of society without disabilities, that is, a typical person without a disability will obtain maximum scores on all dimensions; but, depending on a number of factors, including impairment and disability, someone with spinal cord injury likely will not. None of the items included in CHART are specific to spinal cord injury, but the instrument has not been used with other disability groups. Test–retest reliability of the CHART dimensions is excellent, as is the correlation of subject and caregiver responses (except for social integration). Validity is supported by findings that CHART scores discriminate between people identified as high or low on handicap by professionals and between people with varying levels of impairment.

Life Satisfaction Instruments The Satisfaction with Life Scale (SWLS) (Diener, Emmons, Larsen, & Griffin, 1985) is a measure of global life satisfaction consisting of five items (e.g., "In most ways, my life is close to my ideal," "The conditions of my life are excellent"). Diener et al. (1985) reported that the scale has satisfactory reliability and validity, despite its limited number of items. They also found that the social desirability response set was not a problem with the SWLS. Other research also found high internal consistency, high test–retest reliability, high convergent validity, and encouraging correlations (> 0.50) between self-reported and peer-reported satisfaction with life, both for a geriatric sample and for a student sample.

Flanagan's Quality of Life Scale (Flanagan, 1982) presents respondents with a listing of 16 domains, for each of which they indicate importance and need satisfaction. Selection of the domains was based on interviews with small groups using the critical incident technique. Domains cover material and physical well-being; relations with other people; social, community, and civic activities; personal development and fulfillment; and recreation. Importance ratings are made on a 5-point Likert scale (from "very important" to "very unimportant"); satisfaction of wants and needs in each domain is also rated on a 5-point scale (from "very well met" to "not at all well met"). The products of importance and satisfaction ratings are added to obtain a total score. Psychometric information is not clearly reported; however, other research using a similar approach (Andrews & Withey, 1976; Campbell et al., 1976) has found good internal consistency and adequate test–retest reliability if the time frame of reference is not too narrow. The Quality of Life Scale has been used with people with spinal cord injury.

Emotional and Mental Well-Being Instruments Bradburn (1969) designed the Affect-Balance Scale (ABS) as a measure of happiness or general psychological well-being. Positive and negative affect are seen as independent dimensions, and well-being is considered the balance of these two. The scale includes 10 items to which subjects reply "Yes" or "No," 5 items for positive affect (e.g., "Pleased about having accomplished something," "Excited, interested in something"), and 5 for negative (e.g.,

"Bored," "Upset because someone criticized you"), all referring to the past few weeks. Calculation of the ABS score is a rather complex procedure. Internal consistency for both the negative and the positive items is adequate, and test–retest reliability is excellent. The ABS is sensitive to change and has been shown to correlate well with morale scales. It is easily administered and is considered by some the best measure of affect available.

The General Well-Being Schedule (GWBS) is a broad but brief measure of feelings of well-being and distress (Fazio, 1977). Six dimensions are included: 1) self-control, 2) vitality, 3) positive well-being, 4) general health worries, 5) anxiety, and 6) depression. Both positively phrased (e.g., "Have you been in firm control of your behavior, thoughts, emotions, or feelings?") and negatively phrased (e.g., "Have you felt downhearted and blue?") items are included, all referring to the past month. The GWBS has been used mostly in government surveys, for example, the Health and Nutrition Examination Surveys. Data from these studies indicate moderate test–retest reliability and high internal consistency. Correlations of GWBS with depression and anxiety instruments and with health and health services use data suggest adequate validity. Factor analysis has in some cases replicated the six dimensions incorporated by the developers, but in other instances suggested three factors: 1) anxiety, tension, and depression; 2) health and energy; and 3) life satisfaction or positive well-being.

The Life Satisfaction Index (LSI) is best characterized as a measure of morale designed specifically for use with older adults. It encompasses items reflective of five dimensions of morale: 1) zest, 2) resolution and fortitude, 3) mood tone, 4) positive self-concept, and 5) congruence between desired and achieved goals (Neugarten, Havighurst, & Tobin, 1961). The original LSI (designated LSI-A) consisted of 20 items, 12 positive (e.g., "I've gotten pretty much what I expected out of life") and 8 negative (e.g., "This is the dreariest time of my life"). For each statement, respondents indicate whether they agree, disagree, or are not sure. Later versions included the LSI-B, with 12 items, and the LSI-Z, with 13 items. An 18-item version, also called the LSI-A, is most popular. Internal consistency is the most commonly reported reliability measure and tends to be adequate for a measure designed to incorporate five dimensions. (However, empirical studies have failed to demonstrate a five-factor structure; three factors have been consistently found: mood, zest for life, and congruence of goals.) Correlations with objective quality-of-life measures (health, wealth) have not consistently been found. LSI scores do correlate highly with other subjective rating instruments and with ratings of morale by a professional. That some of the items seem appropriate only for elderly subjects (e.g., "I feel my age, but it does not bother me") has not stopped investigators from using the LSI with younger groups.

Quality of Life of People with Disabilities

As previously stated, the field of medical rehabilitation is lagging behind other areas of health care in the conceptualization and measurement of quality of life. Since the mid-1980s, there have been many sophisticated developments in rehabilitation outcomes measurement (e.g., Rasch analysis of measures of disability); however, these generally have not extended to the area of quality of life. Most rehabilitation outcomes research does not explicitly refer to quality of life and at best fits in the conceptual category of objective quality-of-life research. Alexander and Willems (1981) explicitly took the position that quality of life consists of objectively determinable characteristics. It would appear that most other authors seem to assume that their own judgments (about what the most important aspects of disablement or health status or quality of life are, and how they should be measured or weighted) are shared by others, including people with disabilities (see, e.g., DeVivo & Richards, 1992). They assume that the ability to dress oneself or the absence of bed restriction days constitutes quality of life by itself. Only a few studies have taken a systematic approach to the development of measures of satisfaction of people with disabilities in specific domains of life (e.g., Kinney & Coyle, 1992). The sophistication of utility weighting has been applied, on a limited scale, to measurement of disability (Wolfson, Sinclair, Bombardier, & McGear, 1982) and handicap (Dijkers, 1991; Whiteneck et al., 1992), again without the benefit of a specific quality-of-life perspective.

People with disabilities have a lower (health-related) quality of life than people without disabilities, if objective quality-of-life measures are considered. They have impairments that almost always impose activity restrictions and frequently have an effect on cognitive and affective functioning. They very likely have a major chronic illness with various signs, symptoms, and sometimes treatment side effects. If healthy, they often have a razor-thin margin of health and frequently struggle with various acute illnesses. Activity restrictions and other forced lifestyle modifications often lead to secondary disabilities. Although mortality has declined for most disability groups, it is still higher than for age- and gender-matched people without disabilities. All of this has been documented extensively in the literature, both for all people with major disability combined and for specific groups.

Not as well known to most medical rehabilitation specialists and researchers are data documenting that, as a group, people with disabilities rank lower than their counterparts without disabilities in almost all objective measures of quality of life that are not, or are not directly, related to health (Thompson-Hoffman & Storck, 1991). Impairments and disabilities rob them of educational, vocational, and other opportunities, or at least severely restrict chances to enjoy such things as community participation, contacts with others, parenting, and sexual intimacy. Statistics show that people with disabilities are less educated, more often are not working, and have lower incomes.

Research has shown that frequently there is a large discrepancy between objective conditions such as material well-being or health and satisfaction with these conditions (Campbell et al., 1976; Diener, 1984). Very often the discrepancy, whether it is satisfaction with what are meager accomplishments or dissatisfaction with above-average circumstances, can be explained by reference to the standards the person uses. These standards may flow from the values held by the person or the group to which he or she belongs, or, more simply, they may be the result of comparisons with what others have or what the person used to have or expected to have. Several authors have argued that, without exploration of such standards, goals, and values, subjective quality-of-life research is handicapped because it does not provide a true understanding of why a person reports a particular quality-of-life level (Rapkin & Fisher, 1992; Thomas & Chambers, 1989). Fabian (1990) reviewed some of the theories that have been developed to explain gaps between objective circumstances and subjective evaluations.

The same phenomenon of unexplainable discrepancies also has been noted in the area of disability. Weinberg (1984) noted that various studies have documented that many people see individuals with disabilities as less happy and less satisfied with life, as well as unable to attain a worthwhile existence. However, Weinberg found that the 30 people with physical disabilities she interviewed rated their quality of life very highly and that most would not be willing to undergo a no-risk surgery that would completely cure their disability. The major reason behind this was that the disability had become part of their self-image and social identity. Most had struggled to adapt to their disability, fighting loneliness and depression as well as negative stereotypes on the part of others; but, once having won that struggle, they did not want to disturb the harmony that now existed in their social activities and in their "improved" selves.

These findings do not mean that the subjective, self-assessed quality of life of people with disabilities is never affected by their impairment or disability. Some obviously report diminished quality of life compared with their peers without disabilities or compared with themselves before onset of disability (cf. Ahlsio, Britton, Murray, & Theorell, 1984; Osberg, McGinnis, DeJong, & Seward, 1987). Reviewing the literature on spinal cord injury, Buda Abela and Dijkers (1994) found that compared with their peers without disabilities, people with a spinal injury report consistently less life satisfaction. They also found a trend toward a negative correlation of severity of impairment and disability with life satisfaction (cf. also Evans et al., 1994). Bränholm, Eklund, Fugl-Meyer, and Fugl-Meyer (1991) reported a low life satisfaction of people with disabilities (compared with controls without disabilities) on admission to vocational rehabilitation. Reported quality of life improved significantly for those who were successfully rehabilitated.

People with disabilities may derive satisfaction from the same things as those without disabilities do (e.g., material well-being, successful marriage) and to the same degree, and their overall level of life satisfaction is not necessarily lower than that of their peers without disability. Cameron, Titus, Kostin, and Kostin (1973) found that there were no differences on ratings of life satisfaction, frustration with life, or mood between their subjects with and without disabilities. Stensman (1985) reported that 36 people with severe disabilities (all wheelchair users in need of daily personal care assistance services) and a control group of people without disabilities did not differ in overall life satisfaction ratings. The two groups also did not differ much in the rank order in which they sorted 30 domains in terms of their value to the quality and meaningfulness of life (e.g., loving and being loved, family and friends, driving a car). However, given the diminished opportunity people with disabilities have to obtain common sources of satisfaction and happiness (e.g., material wealth, health, family life) because of limitations imposed by the disability or by society, it is not surprising that the *average* person with a disability has lower subjective quality of life than a person without a disability, unless compensatory psychological mechanisms are in effect.

RECOMMENDATIONS

The degree of life satisfaction or subjective quality of life enjoyed by people with disabilities is an empirical question. Research is needed on the specific deficits in objective quality-of-life domains (the impairment or disability itself or social achievement deficits due to the disability per se or due to social discrimination) that are of concern to people with disabilities. Research also is needed on the mechanisms they employ to make and change judgments about their subjective quality of life. However, before such research is initiated, both theoretical perspectives and measurement instruments need to be developed. Several suggestions for improving medical rehabilitation outcomes research may be made.

First, in a modification of a specification provided by Calman (1984), *subjective quality of life* should be defined as the gap between a person's expectations and achievements as experienced by the person in the perspective of time (see Figure 1). *Expectations* is a label for the way the person feels or thinks life should be, for example, goals, values, standards of comparison, desires, or life plans. Achievements, what the person ac-

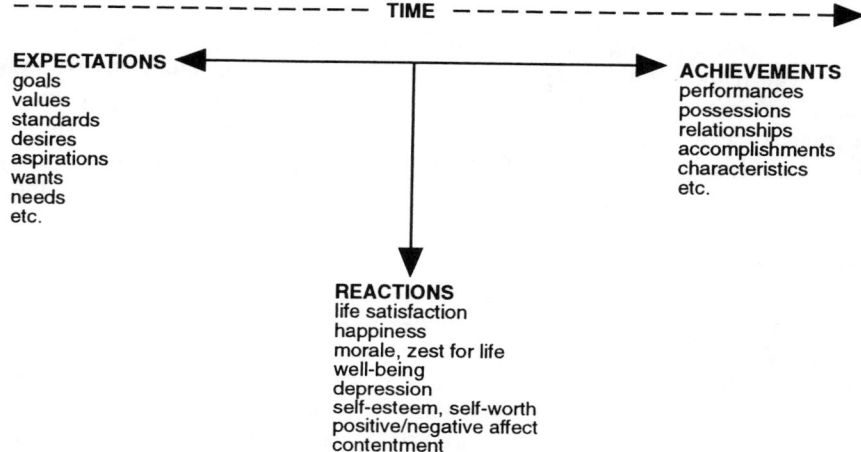

Figure 1. A model of quality of life.

tually has, is, owns, or controls, are held up to those standards. Depending on the congruence between expectations and achievements, the cognitive or emotional reaction is one of satisfaction or dissatisfaction, happiness or depression, and so forth. Time is a significant element because the duration of a particular status or the time expected to elapse before a certain achievement is accomplished plays a major role in the subjective reactions to the gap between what is desired and what is reality.

A full understanding of quality of life, of a person with a disability and others alike, requires investigation of all three components shown in Figure 1. The objective tradition of quality-of-life research has investigated achievements, such as income level, size of residence, ADL capability, and number of bed restriction days, and the subjective tradition has studied personal reactions, such as marital satisfaction, emotional well-being, and zest for life. A few investigators have combined expectations and achievements in a single instrument, and even sometimes into a single index. Very few, however, have explicitly considered expectations as well as achievements and reactions. (The exceptions include Rapkin and Fisher [1992] and Thomas and Chambers [1989].)

One possible reason why investigators have disregarded expectations may be that they assume that all people want the same out of life (or at least want the same as researchers do). It may indeed be true that most people want pretty much the same things—for example, good health, a satisfying job, an attractive spouse, and well-behaved children. It may even be true that people have more or less the same notions of what successive levels of health and beauty are. Presumably, interindividual differences come into play when trade-offs must be made, for instance, when a choice must be made between achievements in one area or another.

Even if the standards and goals people use were the same, that would not necessarily mean that all people would react in the same way. It may be that some are better able to deceive themselves about the lack of fit between what they want out of life and what they are getting. Cognitive and emotional mechanisms for evaluating achievements and resolving the cognitive dissonance created by the gap between goals and realities constitute a neglected field of study.

If consideration of all three elements (expectations, achievements, and experiences) is not feasible, presumably it is best for rehabilitation clinicians and researchers to focus on experiences, the end result of the process of evaluating one's life. Life satisfaction, morale, and emotional well-being are the determinants of, or at least the predictors of, many behaviors and states, including morbidity and mortality (Fava, 1990; Ganz, Lee, & Siau, 1991; McClellan, Anson, Birkell, & Tuttle, 1991).

Second, the domains of life traditionally considered by students of health-related quality of life (see Table 1) are too narrow a selection for research on disablement and on the results of rehabilitation interventions. Because of the links among impairment, disability, and handicap, and because of social processes such as discrimination against people with disabilities and economic realities, the effects of disabling impairments cascade to affect much broader areas of life. Figure 2 shows some of the consequences, direct and indirect, of an illness or injury that results in significant, permanent impairment (e.g., a spinal cord injury).

Because of the potential importance the components of disablement (impairment, and especially the resulting disability and handicap) have in evaluation of quality of life by people with disabilities, it is necessary to include these components in studies of their quality of life. The domains-of-life approach developed by the subjective tradition of quality-of-life research is a suitable model; however, it has to be expanded because, in these studies, health is just a single domain to be rated among 15 (Flanagan, 1982) or 60 (Andrews & Withey, 1976) other domains. It is an empirical question whether people with disabilities differentiate health from disability and give either one or both significant weight in evaluating their overall quality of life. Depending on the nature and severity of disability, each of a number of disablement components (e.g., impairments, disabilities, various handicaps) needs to be evaluated in addition to, for example, overall health status.

However, it would be erroneous not to measure satisfaction with those domains that contribute to overall quality-of-life judgments by the population at large (e.g., material possessions). This is a mistake often made by researchers working in HRQOL measurement. Disability has, directly or

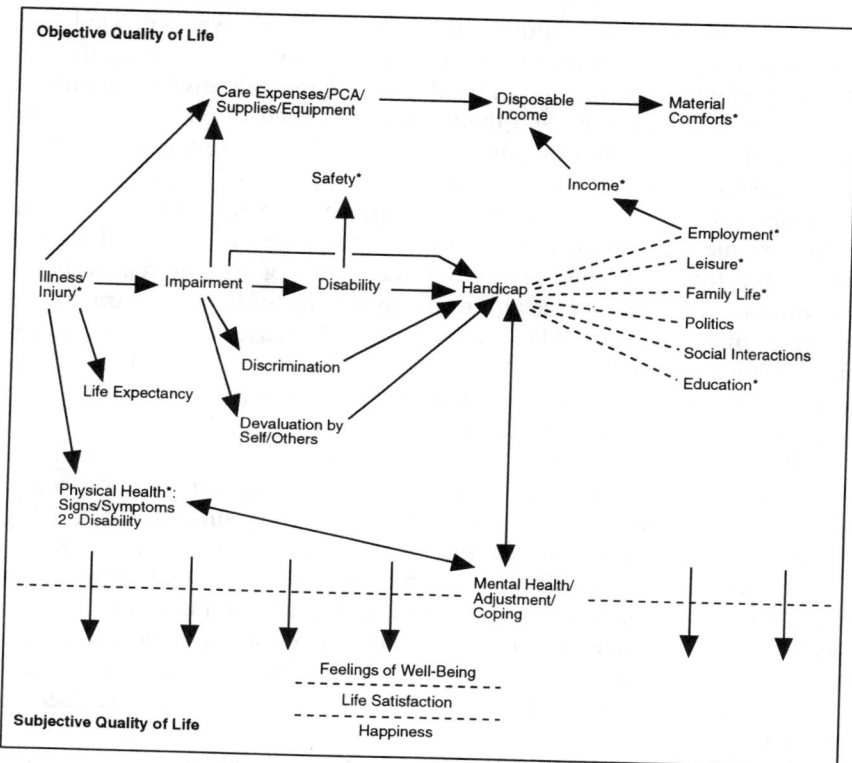

Figure 2. The cascade of effects of impairment. (* = Domains commonly included in studies of life satisfaction of the population without disabilities—presumably areas that are crucial in determining overall quality of life of the average person, - - - - = Specifications, ⟶ = Presumed causal effects.)

indirectly, effects on most components of life (Figure 2), and, depending on the purposes of a particular study, measurements of indirect effects and satisfactions with them are useful if not absolutely necessary. For instance, disability often affects the standard of living, because the person cannot return to employment, a family member needs to stop working in order to become a caregiver, or impairment-related expenditures take a large bite out of the family income. In most studies of the general population, material comforts are one of the most important influences on overall life quality judgments. Although people who have made a good adjustment to their disability may not discount their quality of life because of the disability per se, their reduced standard of living likely will have such an effect. Thus, it is important that studies evaluating the quality of life of people with disabilities measure a wide array of domains of life that may be affected directly or indirectly by the disablement.

The field of rehabilitation lacks scientifically derived knowledge of how commonly used treatments affect objective and subjective quality-of-life components. Randomized clinical trials of rehabilitative interventions are still fairly uncommon, and their end points tend to be limited to molecular rather than global outcomes. Knowledge of what tends to make a stroke patient happier—restoration of speech or elimination of gait problems—is missing. Satisfaction and happiness are not standard program evaluation measures. Fuhrer (1994) noted that there is a lack of studies using subjective well-being to measure the results of specific rehabilitation interventions and that there is almost no knowledge of how more traditional outcomes measures (e.g., ADL independence, decreased complications) relate to subjective well-being. "The picture is similarly incomplete regarding how subjective well-being changes during the course of learning to live with an acquired physical disability" (Fuhrer, 1994, p. 362).

Third, many researchers in the objective tradition of quality-of-life measurement tend to aggregate several conventionally agreed-upon health indices into a single score reflecting health-related quality of life. Quality of life is a complex concept reflecting the confrontation of a person's ideals with reality and the reaction to the results. Hyland (1992) argued that quality of life is a causal sequence resulting from the interaction among objective disability, health and other circumstances, and psychological factors and that information about causal processes is lost if aggregate measures or single-item measures of one aspect of quality of life are used in research.

The conceptualization set forth in Figure 2 not only is comprehensive but also suggests the need for separate measurement of various components of quality of life, which allows for testing of specific hypotheses regarding the quality of life of people with various types, severities, and durations of disabilities. For instance, it may be hypothesized that, over the months and years after a sudden-onset disability (e.g., stroke), issues of impairment initially affect subjective quality of life most, matters of disability are of overarching concern in a later stage, and issues of handicap last. There is also a body of evidence to suggest that quality of life plays a major role in the development of secondary disabilities (e.g., Fava, 1990); it may be hypothesized that those who have a poor objective quality of life develop more secondary disabilities, but that the individuals' evaluations of life's quality play an independent role.

Fourth, when asked to rate the quality of life of people with disabilities, people without disabilities, almost without exception, come up with estimates that are significantly lower than the self-ratings made by the individuals involved. This holds true even for those who, by virtue of occupation, have sufficient opportunities to become familiar with the life of representatives of the group involved (Bach, 1992; Bach & Campagnolo,

1992). The paradoxical situation exists that, before a disabling disease or injury, people think that such disablement will result in poor quality of life but afterward have a completely different opinion. Selection processes cannot explain the discrepancy, and it is concluded that, over time, people who incur a severe impairment change the criteria they use to evaluate their quality of life or change the relative weights of criteria or use some other mechanism to resolve the contradiction between expectations and achievements.

Research is lacking on the nature, pace, and outcomes of this process. Autobiographies and other anecdotal materials can be used to develop hypotheses regarding the phases, components, and determinants of this process and the external (e.g., social support systems) and internal (e.g., personality) factors that guarantee positive or negative outcomes. But prospective longitudinal research using both qualitative and quantitative methods is needed to test them.

Lack of longitudinal research into quality of life is a problem in all areas, not just medical rehabilitation (cf. Fuhrer, 1994). The QALY approaches purport to give a summary index of quality of life from a specific point onward through the end of life or some other defined end point. These estimates are derived by adding up the quality–quantity product for each segment of that period with a different quality-of-life utility than the previous segment. Such a reconstituted utility of remaining life is not really longitudinal but cross-sectional and is completely different from the subjective experiences of the people involved. Although subjective quality of life may decrease over time with the progression of an ongoing health condition, it would appear that it declines much more slowly than objective quality of life, precisely because of the ability of human beings to continuously adjust the criteria they use to measure their achievements. Research is needed into the mechanisms of this process, especially the amount of "stretch" people's criteria can take and the factors that limit its operation, such as in cases of suicide after a severe disabling condition.

CONCLUSIONS

Implicitly or explicitly, the quality of life of people with an ongoing health condition and their families has always been a major concern of the field of medical rehabilitation. The relative emphasis on various components may have changed with shifts in the values in the overall society that affect rehabilitation recipients as well as the rehabilitation system as a whole, with changes in technology and expertise available, and with changing economic pressures. However, in the management and evaluation of an individual patient's rehabilitation, in the development of new programs in local institutions, in the management of national rehabilitation policy, and even in research, quality of life often has not been adequately conceptualized, let alone quantified. In those instances in which quality of life was an explicit consideration, the emphasis tended to be on the objective components (e.g., the disability level, return to work or school) rather than on the subjective and evaluative ones, that is, the opinions and feelings of patients and families regarding what changes in function actually mean to them. This holds true for research as much as for day-to-day practice; for example, a major volume on rehabilitation outcomes measurement (Fuhrer, 1987) does not have a chapter on quality of life, and the term is also absent from the index.

Research and program evaluation in rehabilitation have made great strides in the development of better outcomes measures (especially measures of impairment and functional status or disability). However, explicit adoption of the perspective of quality of life and use of information on patients' and families' evaluations and opinions about what the changes in their statuses mean to them will dramatically enhance the usefulness of these measures. It will have a significant impact on descriptive research of patients and their change over time; on interpretation of the results of clinical trials of rehabilitation interventions; on clinical management; and on program development at institutional, state, and national levels. As stated in the Rehab Brief of the National Institute on Disability and Rehabilitation Research (1988), failure to solve the methodologic problems involved in measuring personal satisfaction and other subjective reactions "condones the exclusion of the people being assessed from actively participating in decisions that affect their lives" (p. 4).

REFERENCES

Aaronson, N. (1991). Methodologic issues in assessing the quality of life of cancer patients. *Cancer, 67*(Suppl. 3), 844–850.

Ahlsio, B., Britton, M., Murray, V., & Theorell, T. (1984). Disablement and quality of life after stroke. *Stroke, 15*(5), 886–890.

Alexander, J., & Willems, E. (1981). Quality of life: Some measurement requirements. *Archives of Physical Medicine and Rehabilitation, 62,* 261–265.

Anderson, T.P. (1982). Quality of life of the individual with a disability. *Archives of Physical Medicine and Rehabilitation, 63,* 55.

Andrews, F., & Withey, S. (1976). *Social indicators of well-being: Americans' perceptions of life quality.* New York: Plenum.

Bach, C.A., & McDaniel, R.W. (1993). Quality of life in quadriplegic adults: A focus group study. *Rehabilitation Nursing, 18,* 364–367.

Bach, J.R. (1992). Ventilator use by Muscular Dystrophy Association patients. *Archives of Physical Medicine and Rehabilitation, 73,* 179–183.

Bach, J.R., & Campagnolo, D.I. (1992). Psychosocial adjustment of post-poliomyelitis ventilator assisted individuals. *Archives of Physical Medicine and Rehabilitation, 73,* 934–939.

Bell, M.J., Bombardier, C., & Tugwell, P. (1990). Measurement of functional status, quality of life, and utility in rheumatoid arthritis. *Arthritis and Rheumatism, 33,* 591–601.

Bergner, M. (1989). Quality of life, health status, and clinical research. *Medical Care, 27*(Suppl. 3), 148–156.

Bergner, M., Bobbitt, R., Carter, W., & Gelson, B. (1981). The Sickness Impact Profile: Development and final revision of a health status measure. *Medical Care, 19,* 955–962.

Bowling, A. (1991). *Measuring health. A review of quality of life measurement scales.* Philadelphia: Open University Press.

Bradburn, N. (1969). *The structure of psychological well-being.* Chicago: Aldine.

Bränholm, I., Eklund, M., Fugl-Meyer, K.S., & Fugl-Meyer, A. (1991). On work and life satisfaction. *Journal of Rehabilitation Sciences, 4*(2), 29–34.

Buda Abela, M., & Dijkers, M. (1994, April). *Predicting life satisfaction among spinal cord injured patients one to three years post-injury.* Paper presented at the Annual Meeting of the American Spinal Injury Association, Philadelphia, PA.

Bungay, K.M., & Ware, J.E. (1993). *Measuring and monitoring health-related quality of life.* Kalamazoo, MI: Upjohn Co.

Calman, K.C. (1984). Quality of life in cancer patients—an hypothesis. *Journal of Medical Ethics, 10,* 124–127.

Cameron, P., Titus, D.G., Kostin, J., & Kostin, M. (1973). The life satisfaction of non-normal persons. *Journal of Consulting and Clinical Psychology, 41,* 207–214.

Campbell, A., Converse, P., & Rodgers, W. (1976). *The quality of American life.* New York: Russell Sage.

Cantril, H. (1965). *The pattern of human concerns.* New Brunswick, NJ: Rutgers University Press.

Cardus, D., Fuhrer, M.J., & Thrall, R.M. (1981). Quality of life in benefit-cost analyses of rehabilitation research. *Archives of Physical Medicine and Rehabilitation, 62,* 209–211.

Croog, S.H. (n.d.). Current issues in conceptualizing and measuring quality of life. In National Institutes of Health, *Quality of life assessment: Practice, problems and promise* (pp. 11–20). Bethesda, MD: National Institutes of Health.

Day, H. (1993). Quality of life: Counterpoint. *Canadian Journal of Rehabilitation, 6,* 135–142.

de Haan, R., Aaronson, N., van Limburg, M., Langton Hewer, R., & van Crewel, H. (1993). Measuring quality of life in stroke. *Stroke, 24,* 320–327.

de Haes, J.C.J.M., & van Knippenberg, F.C.E. (1985). The quality of life of cancer patients: A review of the literature. *Social Science and Medicine, 20*(8), 809–817.

DeVivo, M., & Richards, J.S. (1992). Community reintegration and quality of life following spinal cord injury. *Paraplegia, 30,* 108–112.

Diener, E. (1984). Subjective well-being. *Psychological Bulletin, 95,* 542–575.

Diener, E., Emmons, R., Larsen, R., & Griffin, S. (1985). The Satisfaction With Life Scale. *Journal of Personality Assessment, 49*(1), 71–75.

Dijkers, M. (1991). Scoring CHART: Survey and sensitivity analysis. *Journal of the American Paraplegia Society, 14,* 85–86.

Dossa, P.A. (1989). Quality of life: Individualism or holism? A critical review of the literature. *International Journal of Rehabilitation Research, 12*(2), 121–136.

Evans, R.L., Hendricks, R.D., Connis, R.T., Haselkorn, J.K., Ries, K.R., & Mennet, T.E. (1994). Quality of life after spinal cord injury: A literature critique and meta-analysis (1983–1992). *Journal of the American Paraplegia Society, 17,* 60–66.

Fabian, E.S. (1990). Quality of life: A review of theory and practice implications for individuals with long-term mental illness. *Rehabilitation Psychology, 35*(3), 161–170.

Fanshel, S., & Bush, J.W. (1970). A Health-Status Index and its application to health-services outcomes. *Operations Research, 18,* 1021–1065.

Fava, G.A. (1990). Methodological and conceptual issues in research on quality of life. *Psychotherapy and Psychosomatics, 54,* 70–76.

Fazio, A.F. (1977). A concurrent validational study of the NCHS *General Well-Being Schedule* (Vital and Health Statistics Series 2, No. 73) (DHEW Publication No. [HRA] 78-1347). Hyattsville, MD: U.S. Department of Health, Education and Welfare, National Center for Health Statistics.

Ferrans, C.E., & Powers, M.J. (1992). Psychometric assessment of the Quality of Life Index. *Research in Nursing and Health, 15,* 29–38.

Flanagan, J. (1982). Measurement of quality of life: Current state of the art. *Archives of Physical Medicine and Rehabilitation, 63,* 56–59.

Freed, M.M. (1984). Quality of life: The physician's dilemma. *Archives of Physical Medicine and Rehabilitation, 65,* 109–111.

Fuhrer, M.J. (Ed.). (1987). *Rehabilitation outcomes: Analysis and measurement.* Baltimore: Paul H. Brookes Publishing Co.

Fuhrer, M.J. (1994). Subjective well-being: Implications for medical rehabilitation outcomes and models of disablement. *American Journal of Physical Medicine and Rehabilitation, 73,* 358–364.

Fuhrer, M., Rintala, D., Hart, K., Clearman, R., & Young, M. (1992). Relationship of life satisfaction to impairment, disability, and handicap among persons with spinal cord injury living in the community. *Archives of Physical Medicine and Rehabilitation, 73,* 552–557.

Ganz, P.A., Lee, J.J., & Siau, J. (1991). Quality of life assessment: An independent prognostic variable for survival in lung cancer. *Cancer, 67,* 3131–3135.

George, L., & Bearon, L. (1980). *Quality of life in older persons: Meaning and measurement.* New York: Human Sciences Press.

Gill, T.M., & Feinstein, A.R. (1994). A critical appraisal of the quality of quality-of-life measurements. *Journal of the American Medical Association, 272,* 619–626.

Goode, D. (Ed.). (1994). *Quality of life for persons with disabilities: International perspectives and issues.* Cambridge, MA: Brookline Books.

Hunt, S.M., & McEwen, J. (1980). The development of a subjective health indicator. *Sociology of Health and Illness, 2,* 231–246.

Hyland, M. (1992). A reformulation of quality of life for medical science. *Quality of Life Research, 1,* 267–272.

Jennett, B., & Bond, M. (1975). Assessment of outcome after severe brain damage. *Lancet, 1,* 480–484.

Jette, A.M. (1993). Using health-related quality of life measures in physical therapy outcomes research. *Physical Therapy, 73,* 528–537.

Kane, R., & Kane, R. (Eds.). (1982). *Values and long-term care.* Lexington, MA: Lexington Books.

Kaplan, R.M., & Anderson, J.P. (1990). The General Health Policy Model: An integrated approach. In B. Spilker (Ed.), *Quality of life assessment in clinical trials* (pp. 131–151). New York: Raven Press.

Kaplan, R.M., Bush, J.W., & Berry, C.C. (1976). Health status: Types of validity and the Index of Well-Being. *Health Services Research, 11,* 478–507.

Keith, R.A. (1994). Functional status and health status. *Archives of Physical Medicine and Rehabilitation, 75,* 478–483.

Kinney, W.B., & Coyle, C.P. (1992). Predicting life satisfaction among adults with physical disabilities. *Archives of Physical Medicine and Rehabilitation, 73,* 863–869.

Kottke, F.J. (1982). Philosophic considerations of quality of life for the disabled. *Archives of Physical Medicine and Rehabilitation, 63,* 60–62.

Levine, S. (1987). The changing terrains in medical sociology: Emergent concern with quality of life. *Journal of Health and Social Behavior, 28,* 1–6.

McClellan, W.M., Anson, C., Birkell, K., & Tuttle, E. (1991). Functional status and quality of life: Predictors of early mortality among patients entering treatment for end stage renal disease. *Journal of Clinical Epidemiology, 44,* 83–89.

McCullough, L.B. (1984). The concept of quality of life: A philosophical analysis. In N.K. Wenger, M.E. Mattson, C.D. Furberg, & J. Elinson (Eds.), *Assessment of quality of life in clinical trials of cardiovascular therapies* (pp. 25–45). New York: Le Jacq.

McDowell, I., & Newell, C. (1996). *Measuring health: A guide to rating scales and questionnaires* (2nd ed.). New York: Oxford University Press.

Meenan, R.F., Gertman, P.M., & Mason, J.H. (1980). Measuring health status in arthritis: The Arthritis Impact Measurement Scales. *Arthritis and Rheumatism, 23,* 146–152.

Mor, V., & Guadagnoli, E. (1988). Quality of life measurement: A psychometric Tower of Babel. *Journal of Clinical Epidemiology, 41,* 1055–1058.

National Institute on Disability and Rehabilitation Research. (1988). *Quality-of-life research in rehabilitation* [Rehab Brief]. *7*(1), 1–4.

Neugarten, B.L., Havighurst, R.J., & Tobin, S.S. (1961). The measurement of life satisfaction. *Journal of Gerontology, 16,* 134–143.

Osberg, J.S., McGinnis, G.E., DeJong, G., & Seward, M.L. (1987). Life satisfaction and quality of life among disabled elderly adults. *Journal of Gerontology, 42*(2), 228–230.

Patrick, D.L., & Deyo, R.A. (1989). Generic and disease-specific measures in assessing health status and quality of life. *Medical Care, 27*(Suppl. 3), S217–S232.

Patrick, D.L., & Erickson, P. (1993). *Health status and health policy. Quality of life in health care evaluation and resource allocation.* New York: Oxford University Press.

Pliskin, J., Shepard, D., & Weinstein, M. (1980). Utility functions for life years and health status. *Operations Research, 28,* 206–224.

Rapkin, B.D., & Fisher, K. (1992). Framing the construct of life satisfaction in terms of older adults' personal goals. *Psychology and Aging, 7,* 138–149.

Schipper, H., Clinch, J., & Powell, V. (1990). Definitions and conceptual issues. In B. Spilker (Ed.), *Quality of life assessment in clinical trials* (pp. 11–24). New York: Raven Press.

Siösteen, A., Lundqvist, C., Blomstrand, C., Sullivan, L., & Sullivan, M. (1990). The quality of life of three functional spinal cord injury subgroups in a Swedish community. *Paraplegia, 28,* 476–485.

Slevin, M.L., Plant, H., Lynch, D., Drinkwater, J., & Gregory, W.M. (1988). Who should measure quality of life, the doctor or the patient? *British Journal of Cancer, 57,* 109–112.

Spilker, B. (Ed.). (1990). *Quality of life assessment in clinical trials.* New York: Raven Press.

Spitzer, W.O., Dobson, A.J., Hall, J., Chesterman, E., Levi, J., Shepherd, R., Battista, R.N., & Catchlove, B.R. (1981). Measuring the quality of life of cancer patients: A concise QL-Index for use by physicians. *Journal of Chronic Disease, 34,* 585–597.

Stensman, R. (1985). Severely mobility-disabled people assess the quality of their lives. *Scandinavian Journal of Rehabilitation Medicine, 17,* 87–99.

Stewart, A.L., & Ware, J.E. (Eds.). (1992). *Measuring functioning and well-being: The Medical Outcomes Study approach.* Durham, NC: Duke University Press.

Sutcliffe, J., & Holmes, S. (1991). Quality of life: Verification and use of a self-assessment scale in two patient populations. *Journal of Advanced Nursing, 16,* 490–498.

Taylor, S.J. (1994). In support of research on quality of life, but against QOL. In D. Goode (Ed.), *Quality of life for persons with disabilities: International perspectives and issues* (pp. 260–265). Cambridge, MA: Brookline Books.

Thomas, L.E., & Chambers, K.O. (1989). Phenomenology of life satisfaction among elderly men: Quantitative and qualitative views. *Psychology and Aging, 4,* 284–289.

Thompson-Hoffman, S., & Storck, I.F. (Eds.). (1991). *Disability in the United States: A portrait from national data.* New York: Springer-Verlag.

Torrance, G.W. (1987). Utility approach to measuring health-related quality of life. *Journal of Chronic Disease, 40*(6), 593–600.

van Dam, F. (1986). Quality of life: Methodological aspects. *Bulletin du Cancer, 73,* 607–613.

van Knippenberg, F.C.E., & de Haes, J.D.J.M. (1988). Measuring the quality of life of cancer patients: Psychometric properties of instruments. *Journal of Clinical Epidemiology, 41*(11), 1043–1053.

Ware, J.E., Brook, R.H., Davies-Avery, A., Williams, K.N., Stewart, A.L., Rogers, W.H., Donald, C.A., & Johnston, S.A. (1980). *Conceptualization and measurement of health for adults in the health insurance study: Vol. I. Model of health and methodology.* (Pub. No. R-1987/1-HEW). Santa Monica, CA: Rand Corp.

Ware, J.E., & Sherbourne, C.D. (1992). The MOS 36-Item Short-Form Health Survey (SF-36). I. Conceptual framework and item selection. *Medical Care, 30,* 473–483.

Weinberg, N. (1984). Physically disabled people assess the quality of their lives. *Rehabilitation Literature, 45,* 12–15.

Wenger, N.K., Mattson, M.E., Furberg, C.D., & Elinson, J. (Eds.). (1984). *Assessment of quality of life in clinical trials of cardiovascular therapies.* New York: Le Jacq.

Whiteneck, G., Charlifue, S., Gerhart, K., Overholser, J., & Richardson, G. (1992). Quantifying handicap: A new measure of long-term rehabilitation outcomes. *Archives of Physical Medicine and Rehabilitation, 73,* 519–526.

Wilson, I.B., & Cleary, P.D. (1995). Linking clinical variables with health-related quality of life. A conceptual model of patient outcomes. *Journal of the American Medical Association, 273,* 59–65.

Wolfensberger, W. (1994). Let's hang up "quality of life" as a hopeless term. In D. Goode (Ed.), *Quality of life for persons with disabilities: International perspectives and issues* (pp. 286–319). Cambridge, MA: Brookline Books.

Wolfson, A., Sinclair, A., Bombardier, C., & McGear, A., (1982). A reference measurement for functional status in stroke patients: Interrater and intertechnique comparisons. In R.L. Kane & R. Kane (Eds.), *Values and long-term care* (pp. 191–214). Lexington, MA: Lexington Books.

Wood-Dauphinee, S., & Kuechler, T. (1992). Quality of life as a rehabilitation outcome: Are we missing the boat? *Canadian Journal of Rehabilitation, 1,* 3–12.

Wood-Dauphinee, S., Opzoomer, M.A., Williams, J.I., Marchand, B., & Spitzer, W.O. (1988). Assessment of global function: The Reintegration to Normal Living Index. *Archives of Physical Medicine and Rehabilitation, 69,* 583–590.

World Health Organization (WHO). (1980). *International classification of impairments, disabilities, and handicaps: A manual of classification relating to the consequences of disease.* Geneva, Switzerland: Author.

Zhan, L. (1992). Quality of life: Conceptual and measurement issues. *Journal of Advanced Nursing, 17,* 795–800.

CHAPTER 8

Assessing Health Status Outcomes in Rehabilitation

Alan M. Jette and Diane U. Jette

It is troubling to note the degree to which the research and subsequent literature on functional assessment in rehabilitation (Fuhrer, 1987; Granger & Gresham, 1984) and health status assessment in general medicine (McDowell & Newell, 1996) have evolved largely independently of each other. Although the origins and conceptual roots of the functional and health status outcomes traditions are quite distinct and different, they share common goals and face similar challenges that would lend themselves to cross-fertilization (Jette, 1993; Keith, 1994). There has been so little communication across these fields of inquiry that researchers in rehabilitation have begun to develop new instruments to assess concepts such as community integration, seemingly without building on existing health status instruments that cover the same conceptual territory (Willer, Ottenbacher, & Coad, 1994). Rather than inventing new language and instruments, rehabilitation researchers might do well to look to the health status literature for measures that have been well tested and might prove useful for assessing rehabilitation intervention outcomes. Both fields would be enriched by sharing methods and ideas to address common challenges. An example of this type of collaboration is the application of Rasch analysis (Haley, McHorney, & Ware, 1994) to the evaluation of a prominent health status instrument.

This chapter defines the traditional meaning of the term *health status* as applied in medical outcomes research, reviews briefly the conceptual roots of health status assessment, and discusses their applicability for evaluating the achievement of desired goals within the rehabilitation field. Two investigations in rehabilitation are highlighted that have used health status outcome instruments, and some of the challenges are discussed that will be faced in applying health status methodology more widely within rehabilitation.

EVOLUTION OF HEALTH STATUS INSTRUMENTS

Measurement of health status, one type of social indicator, is based on aggregated data intended to provide a profile of the health state of specific subpopulations or groups of individuals. Indicators of the health status of individuals were principally developed and used initially in social science research aimed at studying differences in health, and the causes and consequences thereof, within specific cohorts or study populations (Andrews & Withey, 1976; Elinson & Siegmann, 1979; Moriyama, 1968; Ware, Brook, Davies, & Lohr, 1981). Health status instruments have been adapted and used to evaluate the outcomes of health care interventions. Many authors mark the rising interest in health status instruments as corresponding to the declining use of more traditional outcomes indicators of mortality and morbidity, which are of limited value in making decisions about the outcomes of providing care to patients with chronic conditions (Ellwood, 1988; Lansky, Butler, & Waller, 1992).

As the goals of health care have changed to meet the evolving needs of the U.S. population, so too have the indicators used to evaluate the achievement of those goals (Epstein, 1990; Relman, 1988). With the U.S. population living longer than in the past, more people are likely to develop the clinical manifestation of a chronic health condition, and outcomes indicators in medicine have changed in response to these trends. Health status measurement is considered important not only in determining the effectiveness of treatment but also in evaluating quality of care, determining the health needs of large populations, improving provider decision making, and elucidating the causes and consequences of differing levels of health in populations (Ware et al., 1981).

In treating patients with chiefly chronic conditions, rehabilitation professionals have long recognized the need to assess patients' health beyond morbidity. An empirical approach to assessing patients' functioning has been used in the clinical setting in an effort to document patients' progress toward independent living, ability to function in the home and work settings, and requirement for assistance in activities needed for daily function. Those working with patients in the rehabilitation setting realized the necessity of identifying practical goals consistent with their patients' needs and wishes and used progress toward those goals as indicators of the success of the rehabilitation program. This awareness resulted in many "homegrown" tools designed simply to describe patients' function, particularly in the areas of basic activities of daily living, mobility, and locomotion. Measurement of health has greatly benefited from the development of conceptual frameworks for describing health and theories of disablement, as well as the application of psychometric principles to the development of measurement tools. Thus, measurement of health status has moved beyond an empirical approach to describing patients' function and making assumptions concerning the effects of intervention.

The conceptual roots of health status instruments can be traced to the 1950s, when the World Health Organization (WHO) first defined *health* in terms of "physical, mental, and social well-being, and not merely the absence of disease and infirmity" (WHO, 1958). When it was first introduced, many criticized the concept as unmeasurable and overly subjective, but, as subsequent methodologic development reveals, researchers have been heavily influenced by this early conceptual foundation provided by the WHO.

Engel's biopsychosocial model provides a useful framework for relating the various dimensions of health status (Engel, 1980). This model, which is based on a systems theory, views nature as being arranged in a hierarchy ranging from less complex, smaller systems (e.g., specific organs) to the more complex, larger social systems (e.g., the family). Within Engel's framework, overall health status dimensions can be viewed as consisting of the following four basic dimensions:

1. The biologic component, which looks at subindividual components, includes the combined functioning of cells, specific organs, and organ systems. This is the objective component of health included in most traditional clinical research, wherein various biochemical or physiologic indices are assessed to evaluate the effectiveness of medical and other health interventions. This component is rarely included in health status instruments of the type discussed in this chapter.
2. The physical function component encompasses the individual's performance of activities of daily living (ADL). Examples include performance of basic life activities (basic ADL), such as dressing, bathing, and walking, and more complex life activities (called instrumental ADL) such as meal preparation, shopping, and transportation.
3. The psychological component consists of various cognitive, perceptual, and personality traits of the individual.
4. The social component, with the individual at its base, is viewed as the interaction of the individual within a larger social context or structure.

Examples of the type of elements included in each of the four components are illustrated in Figure 1.

Within Engel's conceptual framework, an individual's overall health status can be described as a composition of various biologic, physical function, psychological, and social capabilities with the importance of various elements within each component differing among individuals and within individuals over time. All four components may interact with others in the framework; alterations in one component will affect the others within the hierarchy.

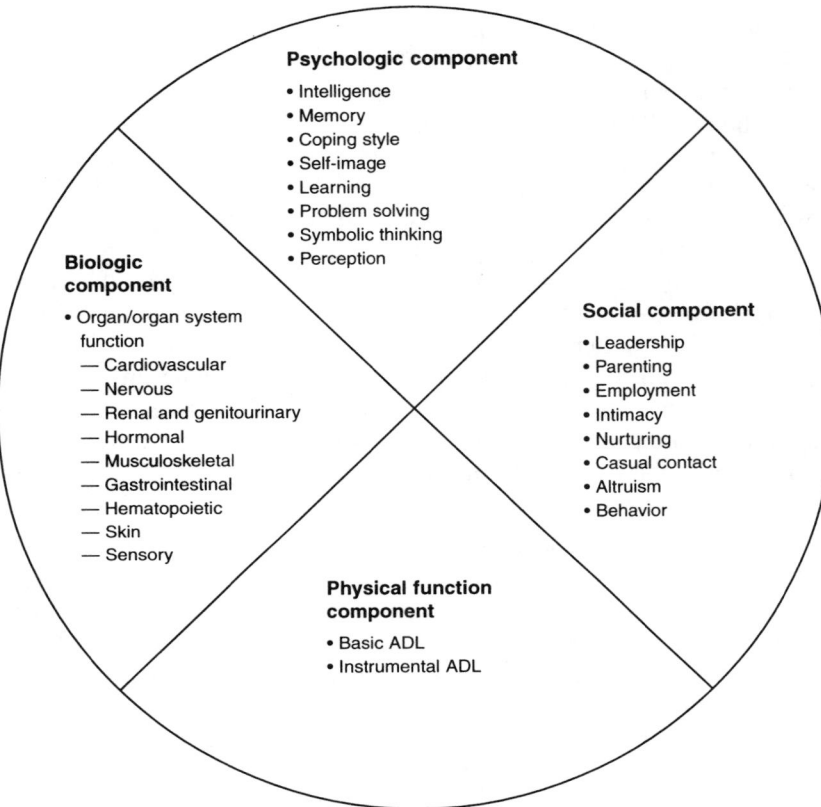

Figure 1. Components of the biopsychosocial framework.

The biopsychosocial framework provides an approach for discussing and measuring various components of health status for rehabilitation outcomes research. The focus of health status measurement varies from study to study, depending on the magnitude and direction of the intervention's effect on health status. In traditional clinical research, health outcomes have been defined very narrowly, focusing primarily on traditional clinical indices that measured elements within the biologic component of the biopsychosocial model. However, there is growing recognition of the need to go beyond traditional physiologic parameters to include broader health status components based primarily on data from patients. The health status dimensions in most health status instruments available in the 1990s include signs and symptoms of disease, performance of basic life activities, performance of social roles, emotional state or affect, intellectual functioning, and general satisfaction with life or well-being.

Health status instruments require either the assessor or the person being assessed to make a judgment that forms the basis of the indicator of that person's health status. Although similar to data collected in taking a traditional medical history, information on subjective dimensions of health status differs in that it is collected in a standardized fashion and converted to numerical scores that can be manipulated mathematically. Assessment and scaling techniques originally developed and applied by social psychologists in the measurement of attitudes have found general application in health status instruments (McDowell & Newell, 1996). Because questionnaires and instruments of this nature are not inherently quantitative, various forms of rating systems have been developed to translate responses such as "limited in walking" to a form suitable for statistical manipulation. Psychological rating and scaling techniques have had a major impact on methods used in the field of health status measurement (Stevens, 1962).

HEALTH STATUS INSTRUMENTS

A number of health status instruments have been designed for clinical use. Several available instruments are summarized in Table 1 to illustrate the range available to the rehabilitation professional.

Scoring systems for health status instruments vary widely, ranging from the very crude (e.g., COOP Charts) to multidimensional profiles designed to detect small differences in health status (e.g., Medical Outcome Study [MOS] instrument, Functional Status Questionnaire [FSQ], Nottingham Health Profile). Most approaches use simple sums as the method of scoring, yet others offer more complex scoring algorithms. Length of available instruments ranges from a few minutes (e.g., COOP Charts) to 30 minutes or more (e.g., Sickness Impact Profile). Fortunately, some of the newer instruments provide computer algorithms (e.g., FSQ) to facilitate scoring and interpretation.

The computer is quickly becoming a major asset for the storage, integration, and easy retrieval of complex health status information in clinical practice (Barnett, 1984). Using a computer algorithm, the clinician not only can score and review health status information on a particular patient at one point in time but also can place the findings from one assessment in the context of previous assessments of health status. The computer can easily display trends in health status, permitting the clinician to compare a patient's health status with past data to detect improvement, deterioration, or lack of change. Such a feature is particularly useful when monitoring high-volume practices. A number of health status instruments have computer algorithms that facilitate the scoring, interpretation, and retrieval of serial health status information (e.g., FSQ, MOS instrument).

Issues in Choosing Measures of Health-Related Quality of Life

Most clinicians have general impressions about the health status of their patients, yet most are unsure of what specific dimensions require systematic

Table 1. Several health status instruments

Measure	Content area	Length (items)	Mode	Time (min)
MOS 36-Item Short-Form Health Survey (SF-36) (Ware & Sherbourne, 1992)	Physical Role limitations due to physical and emotional problems Social functioning General mental health Bodily pain Energy/fatigue General health perceptions	36	Self-report	10
COOP Charts (Nelson, Wasson, & Kirk, 1987)	Physical Mental Role Social Pain Overall health change Social resources Life quality	9	Self-report or clinical rating	< 10
Duke–UNC Health Profile (Parkerson et al., 1981)	Symptom status Physical function Emotional function Social function	64	Self-report	15–20
Sickness Impact Profile (SIP) (Bergner, Bobbitt, Carter, & Gelson, 1981)	Physical: Ambulation, mobility, body care Psychosocial: Social interaction, communication, alertness, emotional behavior Other: Sleep and rest, eating, work, home management, recreational pastimes	136	Self-report	30

Instrument	Domains	Items	Method	Time
McMaster Health Index Questionnaire (MHIQ) (Chambers, MacDonald, Tugwell, Buchanan, & Kraag, 1982)	Physical: Mobility, self-care, communication, global physical function Social: General well-being, work or social role, performance, social support and participation, global self-function Emotional: Self-esteem, personal relationships, critical life events, global emotional function	59	Self-report	20
Nottingham Health Profile (NHP) (Hunt, McEwen, & McKenna, 1985)	Six domains of experience: Pain, physical mobility, sleep, emotional reactions, energy, social isolation Seven domains of daily life: Employment, household work, relationships, personal life, sex, hobbies, vacations	45	Self-report	10
Quality of Well-Being Scale (QWB) (Fanshel & Bush, 1970)	Functional performance: Self-care, mobility, institutionalization, social activities Symptoms and problems	50	Self-report	12
Functional Status Questionnaire (FSQ) (Jette et al., 1986)	Physical: Basic and instrumental activities of daily living Emotional function: Anxiety and depression, quality of social interaction Social performance: Occupational function, social activities Other: Sexual, global disability, global health satisfaction, social contacts	34	Self-report	10

assessment, how to measure them, and how to gauge the extent to which they are affected by therapeutic intervention. A number of authors (Feinstein, 1992; Kirshner & Guyatt, 1985; McDowell & Newell, 1996; Nelson & Berwick, 1989) have provided guidelines for the review and selection of available test scales or questionnaires designed to measure health status. The proper selection of a standardized instrument depends on several important factors, including selecting which dimensions to measure, psychometric properties, and practicality. Selection of a health status instrument requires that the clinician carefully delineate the appropriate dimensions of health status likely to be affected by specific conditions and those likely to be altered by the intervention. This selection is based foremost on the clinical judgment and experience of the professional in addition to a thorough review of the existing literature on the topic under investigation.

In reviewing the literature on existing instruments, the appropriate target populations (e.g., age group) should be clearly identified and the diseases for which the instrument was developed (if relevant) should be clearly outlined. The items in the instrument and the scales used to quantify responses would be appropriate to that of the disease or target group under study. A number of reviews of various health status instruments are available (Jenkinson, 1994; McDowell & Newell, 1996; Patrick & Bergner, 1990; Patrick & Erickson, 1993). The following section of this chapter illustrates the use of two different health status instruments in two different rehabilitation patient populations.

The SF-36 Health Survey and the Functional Status Questionnaire

The authors of this chapter have used both the Short Form 36-item (SF-36) health status instrument (Ware & Sherbourne, 1992) developed for the MOS and the FSQ (Jette et al., 1986) developed by researchers at Boston's Beth Israel Hospital and the University of California at Los Angeles in outpatient rehabilitation outcomes studies (Jette & Jette, 1996, in press; Jette et al., 1996). Both instruments have been designed for use in the ambulatory care setting and have been evaluated for their psychometric properties and usefulness.

The SF-36 is a generic, multidimensional health status instrument that measures eight health concepts: 1) physical functioning (10 items), 2) social functioning (2 items), 3) role limitations due to physical problems (4 items), 4) role limitations due to emotional problems (3 items), 5) mental health (5 items), 6) energy/fatigue (4 items), 7) bodily pain (2 items), and 8) general health perception (5 items). A single item evaluates the patient's perception of change in health over the past year and is not included in scoring any of the dimensions (see Figure 2).

The FSQ is a generic, multidimensional health status instrument containing 37 questions that are the basis for six scale scores and six single

SF-36 Health Survey

1. In general, would you say your health is:
2. *Compared to one year ago,* how would you rate your health in general *now?*
3. The following items are about activities you might do during a typical day. Does *your health now limit you* in these activities? If so, how much?
   a. *Vigorous activities,* such as running, lifting heavy objects, participating in strenuous sports
   b. *Moderate activities,* such as moving a table, pushing a vacuum cleaner, bowling, or playing golf
   c. Lifting or carrying groceries
   d. Climbing *several* flights of stairs
   e. Climbing *one* flight of stairs
   f. Bending, kneeling, or stooping
   g. Walking *more than a mile*
   h. Walking *several blocks*
   i. Walking *one block*
   j. Bathing or dressing yourself
4. During the *past 4 weeks,* have you had any of the following problems with your work or other regular daily activities *as a result of your physical health?*
   a. Cut down the *amount of time* you spent on work or other activities
   b. *Accomplished less* than you would like
   c. Were limited in the kind of work or other activities
   d. Had *difficulty* performing the work or other activities (for example, it took extra effort)
5. During the *past 4 weeks,* have you had any of the following problems with your work or other regular daily activities *as a result of any emotional problems* (such as feeling depressed or anxious)?
   a. Cut down the *amount of time* you spent on work or other activities
   b. *Accomplished less* than you would like
   c. Didn't do work or other activities as *carefully* as usual
6. During the *past 4 weeks,* to what extent has your physical health or emotional problems interfered with your normal social activities with family, friends, neighbors, or groups?
7. How much *bodily* pain have you had during the *past 4 weeks?*
8. During *the past 4 weeks,* how much did *pain* interfere with your normal work (including both work outside the home and housework)?
9. The questions are about how you feel and how things have been with you *during the past 4 weeks.* For each question, please give the one answer that comes closest to the way you have been feeling. How much of the time during the past four weeks
   a. Did you feel full of pep?
   b. Have you been a nervous person?
   c. Have you felt so down in the dumps that nothing could cheer you up?
   d. Have you felt calm and peaceful?
   e. Did you have a lot of pep and energy?
   f. Have you felt downhearted and blue?
   g. Did you feel worn out?
   h. Have you been a happy person?
   i. Did you feel tired?

(continued)

Figure 2. SF-36 Health Survey. (Copyright © 1992 by Medical Outcomes Trust. All rights reserved. Reproduced with permission of the Medical Outcomes Trust. Survey Available from the Medical Outcomes Trust, 20 Park Plaza, Suite 1014, Boston, Massachusetts 02116 (617) 426-4046.)

Figure 2. *(continued)*

10. During the past 4 weeks, how much of the time has your *physical health or emotional problems* interfered with your social activities (like visiting with friends, relatives, etc.)?
11. How TRUE or FALSE is *each* of the following statements for you?
    a. I seem to get sick a little easier than other people.
    b. I am as healthy as anybody I know.
    c. I expect my health to get worse.
    d. My health is excellent.

SF-36 Response Choices

1. Excellent, Very Good, Good, Fair, Poor
2. Much better now than one year ago, Somewhat better now than one year ago, About the same now as one year ago, Somewhat worse now than one year ago, Much worse now than one year ago
3. Yes, Limited a lot; Yes, Limited a little; No, Not limited at all
4. a–d. Yes, No
5. a–c. Yes, No
6. Not at all, Slightly, Moderately, Quite a bit, Extremely
7. None, Very mild, Mild, Moderate, Severe, Very severe
8. Not at all, A little bit, Moderately, Quite a bit, Extremely
9. All of the time, Most of the time, A good bit of the time, Some of the time, A little of the time, None of the time
10. All of the time, Most of the time, Some of the time, A little of the time, None of the time
11. Definitely true, Mostly true, Don't know, Mostly false, Definitely false

items. Scales include basic ADL, instrumental ADL, social activities, mental health, quality of interaction, and work performance. The single items include employment status, frequency of social contact, bed days, restricted activity days, sexual relationships, and satisfaction with health (see Figure 3).

The standardized form of each instrument assesses the individual's health status over the past month. Standardized response choices using Likert scales allow the individual to indicate the extent of various limitations due to his or her health. Scale scores are then determined by transforming the data to obtain a score ranging from 0 to 100 as a percentage of the total possible score for each scale. In each scale, higher scores indicate better health status, with a score of 100 indicating maximum ability. Scores across the scales provide a profile of the health status of an individual; neither instrument provides a summary score.

Several criteria are recommended for evaluating the quality of any health status instrument and its usefulness for a specific outcomes research application. The degree to which the SF-36 and FSQ meet these criteria is reviewed briefly.

Validity *Validity* refers to the degree to which a health status instrument actually measures the health dimensions it purports to assess. Many

Functional Status Questionnaire

Category	Item
Physical function	*During the past month, have you had difficulty:*
Basic activities of daily living	Taking care of yourself, that is, eating, dressing, or bathing?
	Moving in and out of a bed or chair?
	Walking indoors, such as around your home?
Instrumental activities of daily living	Walking several blocks?
	Walking one block or climbing one flight of stairs?
	Doing work around the house, such as cleaning, light yard work, and home maintenance?
	Doing errands, such as grocery shopping?
	Driving a car or using public transportation?
	Doing vigorous activities, such as running, lifting heavy objects, or participating in strenuous sports?

Responses: Usually did with no difficulty (4), usually did with some difficulty (3), usually did not do because of health (1), usually did not do for other reasons (0).

Psychologic function	*During the past month:*
Mental health	Have you been a very nervous person?
	Have you felt calm and peaceful?*
	Have you felt downhearted and blue?
	Were you a happy person?*
	Did you feel so down in the dumps that nothing could cheer you up?

Responses: All of the time (1), most of the time (2), a good bit of the time (3), some of the time (4), a little of the time (5), none of the time (6).

Social-role function	*During the past month, have you:*
Work performance (for those employed during the previous month)	Done as much work as others in similar jobs?*
	Worked for short periods of time or taken frequent rests because of your health?
	Feared losing your job because of your health?

Responses: All of the time (1), most of the time (2), some of the time (3), none of the time (4).

Social activity	*During the past month, have you had difficulty:*
	Visiting with relatives or friends?
	Participating in community activities, such as religious services, social activities, or volunteer work?
	Taking care of other people, such as family members?

Responses: Usually did with no difficulty (4), usually did with some difficulty (3), usually did with much difficulty (2), usually did not do because of health (1), usually did not do for other reasons (0).

(continued)

Figure 3. Functional Status Questionnaire. (* = Scores are reversed.) (Adapted from Jette et al., 1986.)

Figure 3. *(continued)*

Category	Item
Quality of interaction	*During the past month, did you:* Isolate yourself from people around you? Act affectionately toward others?* Act irritably toward those around you? Make unreasonable demands on your family and friends? Get along well with other people?*

Responses: All of the time (1), most of the time (2), a good bit of the time (3), some of the time (4), a little of the time (5), none of the time (6).

Single-item questions:

Which of the following statements best describes your work situation during the past month? Responses: Working full-time, working part-time, unemployed, looking for work, unemployed because of my health, retired for some other reason.

During the past month, how many days did illness or injury keep you in bed all or most of the day? Response: 0–31 days.

During the past month, how many days did you cut down on the things you usually do for one-half day or more because of your illness or injury? Response: 0–31 days.

During the past month, how satisfied were you with your sexual relationships? Responses: Very satisfied, satisfied, not sure, dissatisfied, very dissatisfied, did not have any sexual relationships.

How do you feel about your own health? Responses: Very satisfied, satisfied, not sure, dissatisfied, very dissatisfied.

During the past month, how often did you socialize with friends or relatives, that is, go out together, visit in each other's homes, or talk on the telephone? Responses: Every day, several times a week, about once a week, two or three times a month, about once a month, not at all.

techniques are available for the determination of instrument validity. At the very least, an instrument is valid if it measures fully the dimensions of a particular concept. Both the FSQ and the SF-36 measure dimensions that are generally considered to be related to health, although there may be some disagreement about the inclusion of some concepts or the exclusion of others. Depth of measurement is accomplished by including more than one item to assess each dimension. The validity of each instrument also has been evaluated through lengthy processes of psychometric testing. For example, the SF-36 has been evaluated by using a factor analysis in which the scales were shown to be related to one of two factors that represent generally accepted physical and mental dimensions of health (McHorney, Ware, & Raczek, 1993). The unidimensionality of the physical functioning scale has been validated by using Rasch item analysis (Haley et al., 1994). Validity of the FSQ has been evaluated by showing the relationship of its scales to factors generally accepted to be related to health in a general population, such as age and reported number of days of disability (Jette et al., 1986), and poor performance on the instrumental ADL scale has been shown to be predictive of subsequent mortality (Reuben, Rubenstein, Hirsch, & Hays, 1992).

Reliability As with measurement of any phenomenon, a health status indicator based on perceptions of the individual or clinician can be susceptible to measurement bias. To be useful, health status indicators must minimize the extent to which their scores are influenced by the feelings of the assessor, the testing instrument itself, or extraneous characteristics of the individual being tested.

A health status instrument's reliability represents the degree to which extraneous factors have introduced error into the health status measurement. Although error cannot be completely eliminated from measurement, to the extent that random error is slight, health status instrument scores can be said to be stable, reproducible, or reliable. To be meaningful, a health status instrument must demonstrate that the measurements of individuals assessed on different occasions or by similar or parallel tests produce the same or similar results. In evaluating reliability, determination of internal consistency is important when an index contains several items that evaluate the same phenomenon. Cronbach's (1951) alpha is commonly used to quantitatively express the intercorrelation of items within the same scale. The internal consistency of items can be expected to vary with instrument administration to different groups (Cronbach, 1951).

Internal consistency reliabilities of the scales of the SF-36 were reported to be between 0.80 and 0.92 when administered to a group of ambulatory patients seen by general practitioners (Garratt, Ruta, Abdalla, Buckingham, & Russell, 1993). Similarly, the internal consistency of the FSQ scales has been determined for its use with a group of ambulatory patients seen in internal medicine practices (Jette et al., 1986) and ranged from 0.64 to 0.82. Similar levels of reliability for the FSQ scales have been reported for a Swedish-language version of the instrument (Einarsson & Grimby, 1990). Test–retest reliability has not been reported for either instrument.

Responsiveness and Sensitivity Kirshner and Guyatt (1985) have defined *responsiveness* as the degree to which a health status instrument detects clinically meaningful change within individuals to whom it is applied. In this sense, responsiveness of an instrument is determined by the extent to which the health indicator yields more or less the same scores when subjects are stable (referred to previously as instrument reliability) and by the degree to which the instrument registers change when the subject's health has been altered. The method of measurement of responsiveness of health status instruments is still controversial. A common method has been to equate responsiveness with improvement in health status scores when an intervention of known efficacy is applied. Improvement of scores on the health status instrument is considered evidence of its responsiveness.

The responsiveness of the SF-36 and FSQ has been reported (Katz, Larson, Phillips, Fossel, & Liang, 1992) for patients undergoing total hip arthroplasty. Standardized response means (mean change divided by the standard deviation of the change) ranged from 0.31 to 1.28 for the SF-36 and from 0.55 to 1.10 for the FSQ.

For an instrument to be useful for a particular group, its sensitivity must be sufficient to detect differences in health state among the individuals in the group being assessed. Instruments designed for use in one group may not be able to detect subtle differences in health status among individuals in another group. Lack of sensitivity of an instrument can lead to "floor" or "ceiling" effects. Sensitivity of an instrument can be evaluated by examining the difference in health status scores of groups of individuals known to differ according to a common biomedical assessment of health (Chambers, Haight, Norman, & MacDonald, 1987).

The sensitivity of the SF-36 has been reported by McHorney et al. (1993). They found statistically significant mean differences in SF-36 scores between groups of patients with medical versus psychiatric conditions and between groups of patients with severe versus minor ongoing health conditions.

Feasibility Other criteria being fulfilled, the feasibility of using a health status instrument in a particular clinical context frequently makes the difference in whether it is used. Instrument feasibility is determined by the mode in which it is administered (e.g., self- versus interviewer administration), the time it takes to complete it, whether it requires the use of props or other equipment, requirements for special training of the assessors, respondent burden, and the complexity of the subsequent scoring. In evaluating a health status instrument's feasibility, how an instrument has been field-tested also should be considered. Has the instrument been tested under conditions similar to its proposed use? Has it been used in a population similar to the target group? What have been response rates in previous applications of the instrument? What are rates of missing data? On average, how long did it take to administer the instrument? Both the SF-36 and FSQ can be self-administered or administered by face-to-face or telephone interviews and can be completed in approximately 10 minutes. The surveys have been used in a variety of settings, including ambulatory settings and hospital settings, and with a variety of groups of patients, including those with total hip arthroplasty (Lansky et al., 1992), postpolio syndrome (Einarsson & Grimby, 1990), asthma (Bousquet et al., 1994), atrial fibrillation (Ganiats, Palinkas, & Kaplan, 1992), coronary artery bypass graft

(Cleary et al., 1991), and peptic ulcer (Garratt et al., 1993). The FSQ also was designed to be clinically useful to a health practitioner. A simple computer-based assessment of the questionnaire can provide a printed interpretation for practicing clinicians, similar to that provided for other laboratory tests. Warning zones, indicating levels below which an individual can be expected to be significantly limited, are included in the assessment along with the patient's actual score for each scale and a brief narrative.

Application of Health Status Assessment in the Rehabilitation Setting

There are unanswered questions about the extent to which health status instruments are appropriate and relevant for rehabilitation outcomes research. Are the health status dimensions relevant to rehabilitation outcomes included within health status instruments? Do they have validity for use in rehabilitation? Are they responsive to the level of change in outcomes anticipated within outpatient rehabilitation contexts? The following section describes the application of the SF-36 and FSQ in two different outpatient rehabilitation settings. Each illustrates the potential usefulness and challenges of applying these tools in a rehabilitation research context.

Focus on Therapeutic Outcomes The SF-36 instrument has been applied in an outpatient rehabilitation outcomes project called Focus on Therapeutic Outcomes (FOTO). The FOTO database network, initiated in 1993 by a consortium of six outpatient rehabilitation companies, was developed in response to the need for an outcomes-oriented, standardized outpatient rehabilitation database network. The initial objective of FOTO was to document and track the health outcomes of patients receiving outpatient physical therapy services for lumbar, cervical, and knee impairments and to compare outcomes for specific practices and groups of practices across the country with outcomes achieved by all practices in the FOTO network.

Member practices in the FOTO network provided information on the characteristics of their practice; background data on therapists in the network; and a core set of data, including SF-36 scores, on eligible patients entered into the network on admission and discharge from their episode of outpatient physical therapy. Information about practices, therapists, and patient episodes was recorded on preprinted "bubble forms" that were subsequently scanned and entered into a consolidated FOTO database.

On a much smaller scale, the FSQ has been included as part of admission and follow-up evaluations of patients seen in a small outpatient pulmonary rehabilitation setting. Patients seen in this practice have a wide range of chronic pulmonary diseases. FSQ profiles are computer generated for each patient. In addition to the FSQ, data concerning patients' impairments are collected in a systematic manner and can be linked to the health status profiles.

Health status scores obtained in each of these applications have been used in a number of ways. Health status data in both projects have been used to describe and characterize the general health status of individuals seeking rehabilitation care, to describe the type and degree of health status changes observed over time, and to identify factors related to change in health status. Such data can be useful to clinicians for understanding the impact of their services and extraneous factors on overall health and prognosis of their patients, for screening and triaging patients for certain types of services, for recognizing unusual patterns for further investigation, and for focusing their treatment goals.

For example, in the FOTO network, standardized health status admission profiles across the eight SF-36 dimensions were calculated for knee, cervical, and low-back impairment groupings for all patients who completed their episodes of care. These admission profiles were generated periodically and shared with each company participating in the FOTO network. These reports allowed each participating rehabilitation company to compare the admission status of their patients with admission SF-36 scores for all patients with that impairment in the overall FOTO network. It also allowed them to compare the health status of their patients with adult population norms generated by the developers of the SF-36 (Ware & Sherbourne, 1992).

Figure 4 illustrates a typical FOTO admission profile using data from one practice in the FOTO network of patients with a lumbar impairment who completed their episodes of care during the first 6 months of 1994. The figure also shows the admission profile for the entire FOTO network. As the data in Figure 4 reveal, there were substantial reductions in physical function and social functioning, and increases in role limitation due to physical problems, bodily pain, and energy fatigue for these patients with low-back impairments on admission to physical therapy.

In the pulmonary rehabilitation setting, individual admission profiles ($n = 108$) were compared with the critical values for each scale (see Figure 5). The critical levels for each scale were developed based on consensus of clinicians and serve to warn clinicians of major limitations. On average, patients with pulmonary impairment fall below the critical levels in three of the five scales. Their most severe limitation is in the area of instrumental ADL. Social activities are also problematic.

Use of Health Status Data   Health status data were also used to quantitatively document the type and amount of change in health status occurring over a rehabilitation episode of care. These change data provide some evidence of effectiveness of rehabilitation interventions and may help justify third-party reimbursement. For example, in both the FOTO network and the pulmonary rehabilitation project, health status outcomes profiles

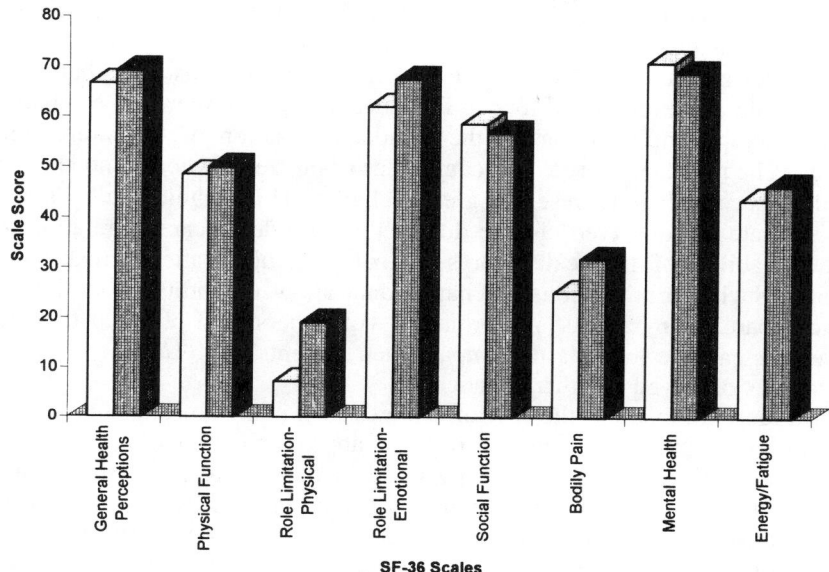

Figure 4. Admission profiles for patients with lumbar impairments. (□ = Practice X, ■ = FOTO network.)

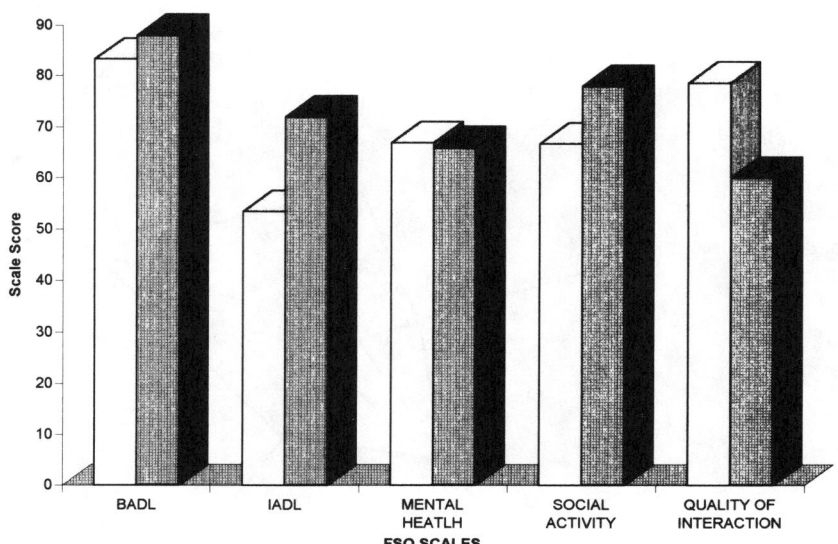

Figure 5. Admission profile for patients with pulmonary impairment. (BADL = Basic activities of daily living, IADL = Instrumental activities of daily living, □ = Patients with pulmonary disease, ■ = Critical level.)

were generated by using the method recommended by Kazis, Anderson, and Meanan (1989) for assessing change in health status. An outcomes profile for all patients was generated by calculating the absolute change in each scale score of the SF-36 or FSQ between admission and discharge from therapy and dividing by the standard deviation of that admission score. The resultant score was a coefficient where zero indicated no change and higher numbers represented greater change. This technique allows one to evaluate the observed change during the episode of care in relation to the variability of the scale scores in that particular patient impairment group. Such representations of change data allow individual practitioners to compare their patients' performance with others, and physical therapy practices can use the data to compare their patients' performance with the outcomes observed in other practices.

Figure 6 illustrates the type of changes seen in health status in patients with chronic pulmonary disease over an approximately 1-month episode of rehabilitation. The data are illustrated in this figure in a radar graph format where no change in each health status dimension is in the center of the axis and the outermost point on each axis represents a full standard deviation of change for that health dimension. The greatest amount of improvement in this group of patients is in the area of IADL, with a change of slightly greater than 1 standard deviation.

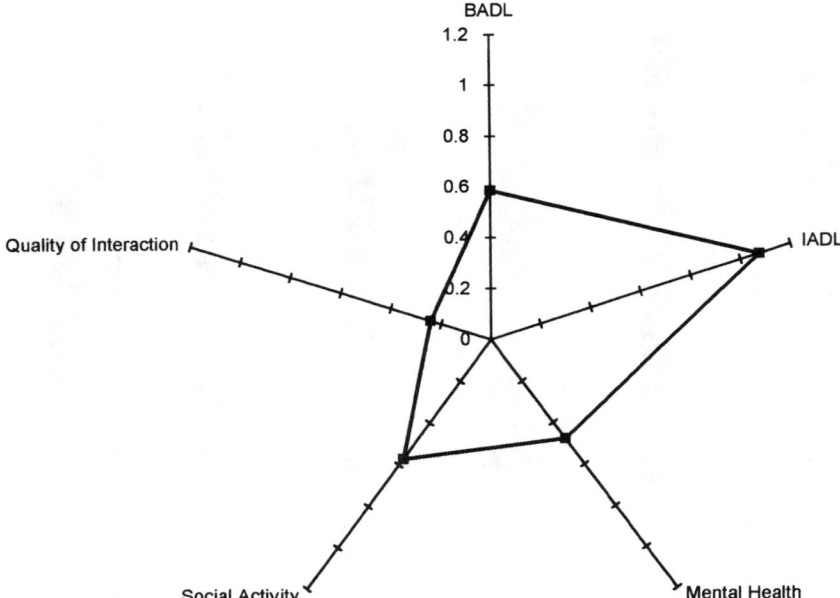

Figure 6. Outcomes profile for patients with pulmonary impairment. (BADL = Basic activities of daily living, IADL = Instrumental activities of daily living.)

Figure 7 illustrates a FOTO outcomes profile using data from the same patients with a lumbar impairment illustrated in Figure 4. In the outcomes profile for the total FOTO network, the greatest degree of improvement was achieved in the dimensions of physical function and pain relief, approximately three quarters of a standard deviation for each. Less change was seen in the other SF-36 dimensions. The outcomes profile illustrated in Figure 7 also allows one to compare the pattern and magnitude of change for one practice ($n = 34$) (Practice X) versus the total FOTO network ($n = 518$). In comparison with the total FOTO network, patients seen by Practice X achieved substantially more improvement in the areas of role performance and social functioning.

Factors associated with improvement, such as type and severity of disease, type of treatment provided, length of treatment, and characteristics of the patient and practitioner, may also be examined using health status indicator data. For example, Figures 8(a) and 8(b) provide illustrations of the pattern of health status improvement seen in the FOTO network for two different types of musculoskeletal impairments. These data, which compare patients with lumbar impairments versus those with cervical impairments, come from all episodes completed during the first 6 months of 1994. Very different patterns of change are revealed across the two outcomes profile illustrations. For patients with a lumbar impairment, health status improvement is concentrated in the areas of pain relief and physical

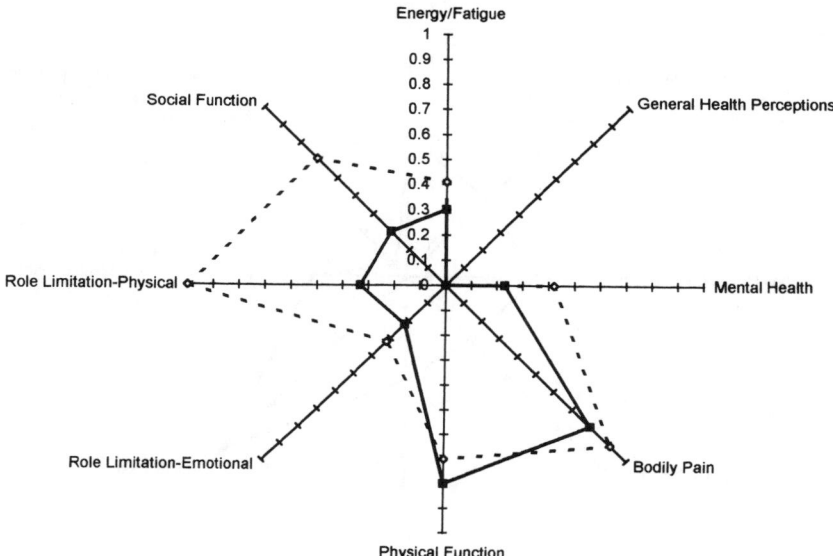

Figure 7. Outcomes profile for patients with lumbar impairments comparing one practice with all practices within the FOTO network. (---□--- = Practice X, —■— = FOTO network.)

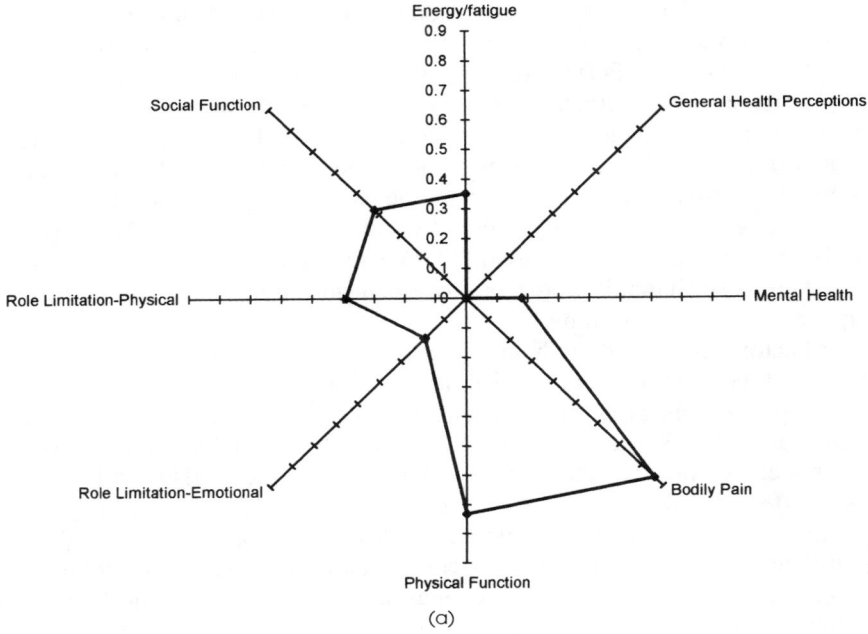

(a)

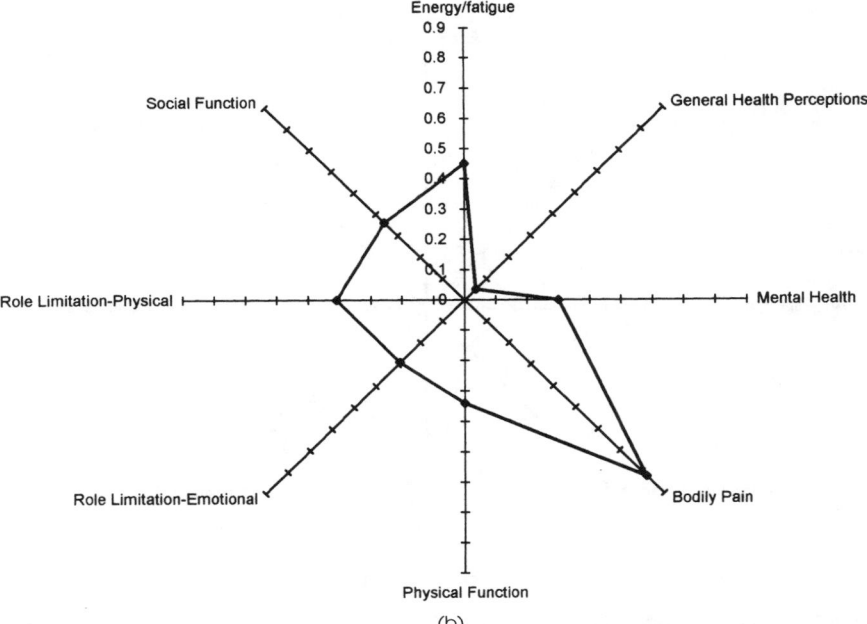

(b)

Figure 8. Patient outcomes profile: (a) with lumbar impairment and (b) with cervical impairment.

functioning. For patients with cervical impairment, reduction in pain and energy fatigue are the two areas of greatest improvement. A greater degree of change is seen for patients with a lumbar injury compared with those with a cervical injury.

Figure 9 demonstrates the different degrees of change in the FSQ dimensions associated with level of pulmonary disease severity as determined by pulmonary function testing. There appears to be little difference in health status between those with greater and lesser degrees of impairment. Figure 10 demonstrates the different degrees of change in the FSQ in these same patients following a course of rehabilitation. This figure suggests that those with greater impairment experience large changes in instrumental ADL compared with patients with lesser impairments.

CHALLENGES TO IMPLEMENTING HEALTH STATUS ASSESSMENT

There are several methodologic challenges to be faced in applying health status measurement in rehabilitation. These include the selection of appropriate health status instruments that are methodologically sound and have been psychometrically tested. Health status instruments must be shown to

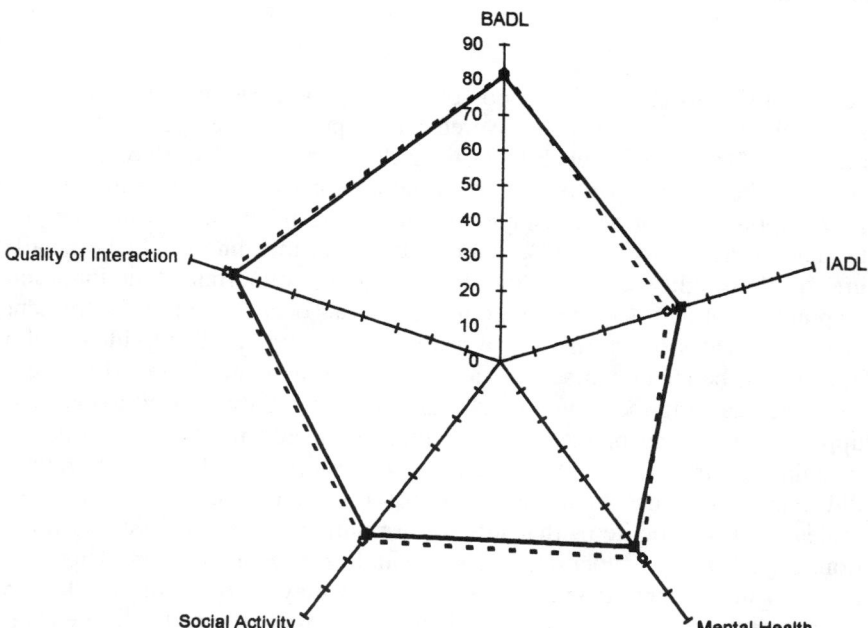

Figure 9. Admission profile for patients with pulmonary impairments according to disease severity. (BADL = Basic activities of daily living, IADL = Instrumental activities of daily living, ---□--- = FEV1 < 50% of predicted, —■— = FEV1 ≥ 50% of predicted.)

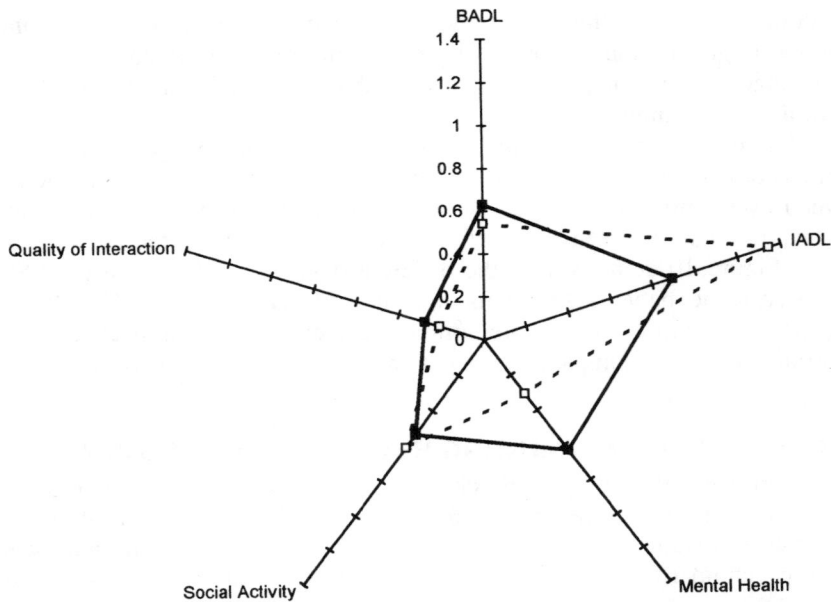

Figure 10. Outcomes profile for patients with pulmonary impairments according to disease severity. (BADL = Basic activities of daily living, IADL = Instrumental activities of daily living, ---□--- = FEV1 < 50% of predicted, —■— = FEV1 ≥ 50% of predicted.)

be responsive to change in groups of rehabilitation patients in which they are applied. The dimensions covered and depth of coverage must be appropriate for specific rehabilitation applications. Finally, they must be shown to be feasible for use in rehabilitation contexts. Potential limitations in the application of health status instruments to rehabilitation include potential ceiling or floor effects, inability to detect meaningful changes, failure to thoroughly evaluate the full range of important function, and respondent burden. Ceiling or floor effects can occur when an instrument or certain scales of an instrument are used for a group of individuals who have much better or worse function than the scales are designed to measure, thus causing the scores for the group to be highly skewed toward the upper or lower end of the scale. Such scales would not be able to detect meaningful differences in health among the group, even though differences did exist. For scales to be useful across different groups of individuals, scales must include items that solicit information about low levels of function, high levels of function, and the middle range of function. This may result in instruments that are so lengthy that they increase the burden on the respondent, thereby making the instrument less than practical. The challenge is finding instruments that are both practical and useful for application in the population of interest.

McHorney, Ware, Lu, and Sherbourne (1994) provided data concerning the distribution of scores of the SF-36 for patients seen in health providers' offices and addressed the extent of ceiling and floor effects in this group of subjects and in subsets of patients. For almost all subgroups of patients, ceiling and floor effects were substantial for the two role limitation scales. Ceiling effects were also notable for the social functioning scale. The presence of ceiling or floor effects suggests that the scales may not be graded finely enough and may not reflect important but subtle differences among individuals at the higher or lower levels of functioning. Addition of items within scales may reduce these problems; however, the advantage gained by adding items may be outweighed by the additional respondent burden attributed to a longer instrument.

Interpretation of scores is facilitated by published norms for particular health status instruments, as well as published scores for various groups of individuals with different health problems. Benchmarks for an instrument, denoting levels of function below which an individual is considered to have a significant problem, can assist in interpretation of scores. Interpretation also is improved when scales contain items that are hierarchical; in other words, items represent a continuum from severe deficit to high-level function and are spaced evenly along the continuum (Haley et al., 1994).

Beyond the outcomes research arena, another application is the use of health status instruments in clinical practice. Assuming that useful instruments that produce quality measurement are chosen, health status assessment meets several purposes and can be accomplished in most practice settings. Assessment of health status provides objective information about the presence and extent of disability, although interpretation requires comparative or normative data. This knowledge may add to the ability of a practitioner to determine effective treatment interventions or the need for referral. For example, practitioners might be able to objectively determine the need for the intervention of a social worker, psychologist, or homemaker based on levels of function as measured by scales for mental health, social interaction, or instrumental ADL. Furthermore, treatment effectiveness, at least for groups of patients, can be objectively determined based on patient-focused goals.

Many challenges exist in implementing health status assessment as a routine screening and monitoring mechanism for individuals seen in a rehabilitation setting. Because most of the health status instruments were designed for use in groups of individuals, the degree of error inherent with most instruments in the measurement of health status prohibits their use in monitoring individual change in health (Feinstein, 1992; Nelson & Berwick, 1989; Street, Gold, & McDowell, 1994). This limitation may deter practitioners from routinely using health status assessment for screening individual patients (Wasson et al., 1992).

There are instruments, such as the Chronic Respiratory Disease Questionnaire (Guyatt, Walter, & Norman, 1987), that have been developed specifically for use with individual patients. The reliability of instruments such as the Chronic Respiratory Disease Questionnaire is enhanced by individualizing the items and by making them specific to the symptoms of one type of condition. The SF-36 and FSQ, in contrast, were designed to measure health status in the general population or groups of patients, and, although generally sufficiently reliable for aggregate analysis, some of the subscales may not have sufficient reliability for monitoring the status of individual patients over time. McHorney, Kosinski, and Ware (1994), for example, reported that the reliability of the physical functioning scale of the SF-36 (> 0.9) is sufficient to allow for individual comparison. Other scales of the SF-36 instrument, however, may not be sufficiently reliable for such use.

Despite the limitations of using health status instruments such as the FSQ and SF-36 to monitor individual change in health status, use of health status assessment data may facilitate communication between patient and practitioner. In addition, patient satisfaction may increase when practitioners have useful information about a patient's daily functioning and overall abilities and can explicitly address these concerns with the patient. In a 1994 study, patients indicated a preference for physicians' addressing issues of physical functioning and role limitations, but the study found that these issues were not addressed (Street et al., 1994). Moreover, in this same group of patients, satisfaction with care was related to the perception that the physician asked about overall health status.

On a broader scale, information about the health status of patients in the rehabilitation setting can assist with planning for the personnel and financial resources needed to address the needs of the patients. Health status measures also can be used to assess the impact of changes in policy and procedure made in the process of total quality improvement (Lansky et al., 1992).

There is an additional challenge in determining linkages between health status and treatments best suited to effect change in health status. Many interventions are directed at limiting or reversing impairments in the biologic component with the belief that there is a direct relationship between organ system impairments and the physical function component, although this assumption may not hold true in many cases.

CONCLUSIONS

In spite of the challenges presented in this chapter, applying the SF-36 and FSQ instruments within separate rehabilitation studies illustrates their potential utility for rehabilitation outcomes research. In the majority of instances, they have been found to be practical and feasible to use in busy clinical settings. The data demonstrate that these instruments reflect different health profiles in different patient populations. Furthermore, they have demonstrated considerable responsiveness to change during the course of rehabilitation episodes of care. They should be further tested and examined within other rehabilitation patient groups and different treatment settings because they have the potential for becoming a valuable resource in rehabilitation outcomes research.

REFERENCES

Andrews, F., & Withey, S. (1976). *Social indicators of well-being: Americans' perceptions of life quality.* New York: Plenum.

Barnett, G.O. (1984). The application of computer-based medical record systems in ambulatory practice. *New England Journal of Medicine, 310,* 1643–1650.

Bergner, M.B., Bobbitt, R.A., Carter, W.B., & Gilson, B.S. (1981). The Sickness Impact Profile: Development and final revision of a health status measure. *Medical Care, 19,* 787–805.

Bousquet, J., Knani, J., Dhivert, H., Richard, A., Chicoye, A., Ware, J.E., Jr., & Michel, F. (1994). Quality of life in asthma: 1. Internal consistency and validity of the SF-36 questionnaire. *American Journal of Respiratory Critical Care Medicine, 149,* 371–375.

Chambers, L., Haight, M., Norman, G., & MacDonald, L. (1987). Sensitivity to change and the effect of mode of administration on health status measurement. *Medical Care, 25*(6), 470–480.

Chambers, L.W., MacDonald, L.A., Tugwell, P., Buchanan, W., & Kraag, G. (1982). The McMaster health index questionnaire as a measure of quality of life for patients with rheumatoid disease. *Journal of Rheumatology, 9,* 780–784.

Cleary, P., Greenfield, S., Mulley, A., Pauker, S., Schroeder, S., Wexter, L., & McNeil, B. (1991). Variations in length of stay and outcomes for six medical and surgical conditions in Massachusetts and California. *Journal of the American Medical Association, 266*(1), 73–79.

Cronbach, L.J. (1951). Coefficient alpha and the internal structure of test. *Psychometrika, 16,* 297–334.

Einarsson, G., & Grimby, G. (1990). Disability and handicap in late poliomyelitis. *Scandinavian Journal of Rehabilitation Medicine, 22,* 113–121.

Elinson, J., & Siegmann, A. (Eds.). (1979). *Socio-medical health indicators.* Farmingdale, NY: Baywood.

Ellwood, P. (1988). Outcomes management: A technology of patient experiences. *New England Journal of Medicine, 318,* 1549–1551.

Engel, G. (1980). The clinical application of the biopsychosocial model. *American Journal of Psychiatry, 137*(5), 535–544.

Epstein, A. (1990). The outcomes movement. Will it get us where we want to go? *New England Journal of Medicine, 323,* 266–270.

Fanshel, S., & Bush, J. W. (1970). A health-status index and its application to health-services outcomes. *Operations Research, 18,* 1021–1066.

Feinstein, A. (1992). Benefits and obstacles for development of health status assessment measures in clinical settings. *Medical Care, 30*(5), MS50–MS56.

Fuhrer, M.J. (Ed.). (1987). *Rehabilitation outcomes: Analysis and measurement.* Baltimore: Paul H. Brookes Publishing Co.

Ganiats, T., Palinkas, L., & Kaplan, R. (1992). Comparison of quality of well-being scale and Functional Status Questionnaire in patients with atrial fibrillation. *Medical Care, 30*(10), 958–964.

Garratt, A., Ruta, D., Abdalla, M., Buckingham, K., & Russell, I. (1993). The SF-36 health survey questionnaire: An outcome measure suitable for routine use within the NHS? *British Medical Journal, 306,* 1440–1444.

Granger, C., & Gresham, G. (Eds.). (1984). *Functional assessment in rehabilitation medicine.* Baltimore: Williams & Wilkins.

Guyatt, G., Walter, S., & Norman, G. (1987). Measuring change over time: Assessing the usefulness of evaluative instruments. *Journal of Chronic Disease, 40*(2), 171–178.

Haley, S., McHorney, C., & Ware, J. (1994). Evaluation of the MOS SF-36 physical functioning scale (PF-10): I. Unidimensionality and reproducibility of the Rasch item scale. *Journal of Clinical Epidemiology, 47*(6), 671–684.

Hunt, S., McEwen, J., & McKenna, S. (1985). Measuring health status: A new tool for clinicians and epidemiologists. *Journal of the Royal College of General Practice, 35,* 185–188.

Jenkinson, C. (1994). *Measuring health and medical outcomes.* London: UCL Press.

Jette, A.M. (1993). Using health-related quality of life measures in physical therapy outcomes research. *Physical Therapy, 73*(8), 528–535.

Jette, A.M., Davies, A.R., Cleary, P.D., Calkins, D., Rubenstein, L., Fink, A., Kosecoff, J., Young, R., Brook, R., & Delbanco, T. (1986). The Functional Status Questionnaire: Reliability and validity when used in primary care. *Journal of General and Internal Medicine, 1*(3), 143–149.

Jette, D.U., & Jette, A.M. (1996). Physical therapy and health outcomes in patients with knee impairments. *Physical Therapy, 76*(9), 930–941.

Jette, D.U., & Jette, A.M. (in press). Physical therapy and health outcomes in patients with spinal impairments. *Physical Therapy.*

Jette, D.U., Manago, D., Medved, E., Nickerson, A., Warzycha, T., Bourgeois, M.C., & Zadai, C.C. (1996). *The disablement process in patients with pulmonary disease.* Manuscript submitted for publication.

Katz, J., Larson, M., Phillips, C., Fossel, A., & Liang, M. (1992). Comparative measurement sensitivity of short and longer health status instruments. *Medical Care, 30*(10), 917–925.

Kazis, L., Anderson, J., & Meanan, R. (1989). Effect sizes for interpreting changes in health status. *Medical Care, 27*(3), 5178–5189.

Keith, R.A. (1994). Functional status and health status. *Archives of Physical Medicine and Rehabilitation, 75*(4), 478–483.

Kirshner, B., & Guyatt, G. (1985). A methodological framework for assessing health indices. *Journal of Chronic Disease, 38*(1), 40–66.

Lansky, D., Butler, B., & Waller, F. (1992). Using health status measures in the hospital setting: From acute care to "outcomes management." *Medical Care, 30*(5)(Suppl.), MS57–MS73.

McDowell, I., & Newell, C. (1996). *Measuring health: A guide to rating scales and questionnaires* (2nd ed.). New York: Oxford University Press.

McHorney, C., Kosinski, M., & Ware, J. (1994). Comparisons of the costs and quality of norms for the SF-36 health survey collected by mail versus telephone interview: Results from a national survey. *Medical Care, 32*(6), 551–567.

McHorney, C., Ware, J., Lu, R., & Sherbourne, C. (1994). The MOS 36-item short-form health survey (SF-36): III. Tests of data quality, scaling assumptions, and reliability across diverse patient groups. *Medical Care, 32*(1), 40–66.

McHorney, C., Ware, J., & Raczek, A. (1993). The MOS 36-Item Short Form Health Survey (SF-36): II. Psychometric and clinical tests of validity in measuring physical and mental health constructs. *Medical Care, 31*(3), 247–263.

Moriyama, I. (1968). Problems in the measurement of health status. In E.B. Sheldon & W. Moore (Eds.), *Indicators of social change: Concepts and measurements* (pp. 573–599). New York: Russell Sage.

Nelson, E., & Berwick, D. (1989). The measurement of health status in clinical practice. *Medical Care, 27*(3)(Suppl.), S77–S90.

Nelson, E., Wasson, J., & Kirk, J. (1987). Assessment of function in routine clinical practice: Description of the COOP Chart method and preliminary findings. *Journal of Chronic Disease, 40*(Suppl. 1), 55S–69S.

Parkerson, G.R., Gehlbach, S.H., Wagner, E.H., James, S., Clapp, N., & Muhbaier, L. (1981). The Duke–UNC Health Profile: An adult health status instrument for primary care. *Medical Care, 19*, 806–828.

Patrick, D., & Bergner, M. (1990). Measurement of health status in the 1990s. *Annual Review of Public Health, 11*, 165–183.

Patrick, D.L., & Erickson, P. (1993). *Health status and health policy.* New York: Oxford University Press.

Relman, A. (1988). Assessment and accountability: The third revolution in medical care. *New England Journal of Medicine, 319*, 1220–1222.

Reuben, D., Rubenstein, L., Hirsch, S., & Hays, R. (1992). Value of functional status as a predictor of mortality: Results of a prospective study. *American Journal of Medicine, 93*(6), 663–669.

Stevens, S. (1962). The surprising simplicity of sensory metrics. *American Journal of Psychology, 19*, 29–39.

Street, R., Gold, W., & McDowell, T. (1994). Using health status surveys in medical consultations. *Medical Care, 32*(7), 732–744.

Ware, J., Brook, R., Davies, A., & Lohr, K. (1981). Choosing measures of health status for individuals in general populations. *American Journal of Public Health, 71*, 620–625.

Ware, J., & Sherbourne, C. (1992). The MOS 36-Item Short-Form Health Survey (SF-36). *Medical Care, 30*(6), 473–483.

Wasson, J., Keller, A., Rubenstein, L., Hays, R., Nelson, E., & Johnson, D. (1992). Benefits and obstacles of health status assessment in ambulatory settings. *Medical Care, 30*(5), MS42–MS49.

Willer, B., Ottenbacher, K., & Coad, M. (1994). The community integration questionnaire. *American Journal of Physical Medicine and Rehabilitation, 73*(2), 103–111.

World Health Organization. (1958). *The first ten years of the World Health Organization.* Geneva, Switzerland: Author.

CHAPTER 9

Socioeconomic Approaches to Assessment

Pennifer Erickson

Socioeconomic analysis in general and cost–utility analysis in particular have much to contribute to the examination of health care issues and to the evaluation of medical treatments, surgical procedures, and rehabilitation practices. Socioeconomic evaluations have two conceptual and analytic features that distinguish them from other types of policy analyses: 1) they incorporate both health care costs and outcomes, and 2) they involve making choices under the assumption of scarcity of resources. The three most commonly used types of socioeconomic analysis are cost–benefit, cost-effectiveness, and cost–utility.

This chapter briefly reviews these three types of analysis within the context of medical rehabilitation, focusing on issues in the use of cost–utility analysis. Key features of health-related quality-of-life assessments are summarized and linked to cost–utility analysis. One use of cost–utility analysis is decision making across a range of treatment alternatives. The ranking of ratios of the added cost per additional year of life gained for various alternative health interventions, although mechanically straightforward, requires an understanding of the assumptions and methods used if this procedure is to provide a basis for allocating resources equitably and efficiently.

COST–BENEFIT, COST-EFFECTIVENESS, AND COST–UTILITY ANALYSES

The focus on linking health care costs to health outcomes is leading policy makers to consider using economic models that allow costs and outcomes to be considered simultaneously (Commonwealth of Australia, 1990; Office of Technology Assessment, 1981, 1990, 1992; Ontario Ministry of Health,

1991; Welch & Larson, 1988). In addition to using socioeconomic analysis for guiding policy concerning a wide array of health interventions and programs, these methods can be used at a micro level to evaluate benefits of diverse health interventions such as stroke rehabilitation, medical treatment for hypertension, and exercise to promote health (Dobkin, 1995; Hatziandru, Koplan, Weinstein, Caspersen, & Warner, 1988; Johannesson, 1994; Johnston & Keith, 1983).

Cost–benefit, cost-effectiveness, and cost–utility analyses have been developed to compare the relative impact of alternative health interventions (see Table 1). In each type of analysis, costs are expressed as the additional expenditures associated with a given intervention $(C_1 - C_2)$. Outcomes are measured as the gain in health that is attributed to the same intervention (either $B_1 - B_2$, $E_1 - E_2$, or $YHL_1 - YHL_2$). Each type of analysis evaluates change in benefit due to an intervention in relationship to the change in cost of the intervention.

Programs designed to improve health may yield four possible categories of results:

1. Increased costs and decreased benefits
2. Increased costs and increased benefits
3. Decreased costs and decreased benefits
4. Decreased costs and increased benefits

Ideally, health interventions increase the level of health at reduced costs; such relative efficiency has been demonstrated in screening programs such as those for phenylketonuria and for antepartum anti-D (Bush, Chen, & Patrick, 1973; Torrance & Zipursky, 1984). Interventions including some life-extending treatments, such as artificial respiration and nutritional support, that result in increased costs and decreased outcomes are to be avoided. Some health policies, such as explicit rationing and capping reimbursements, may encourage the use of interventions that decrease health expenditures and result in decreased health outcomes. Most health interventions, however, appear to result in increased outcomes with increased costs. It is with these programs that economic analyses can be a useful aid in allocating scarce health resources (Anderson, Bush, Chen, & Dolenc, 1986).

As suggested by the definitions in Table 1, the main difference between cost–benefit, cost-effectiveness, or cost–utility analysis is the outcomes measure that is used to determine the health effect gained from an intervention. In most cases, the availability of the outcomes data determines which type of analysis is used.

Cost–Benefit Analysis

In cost–benefit analysis, gains in health outcomes from implementing a health intervention, as well as costs, are expressed in dollars. The use of money as a measure of value reflects the origin of cost–benefit analysis as

Table 1. Comparison of three types of economic evaluations that consider health costs and outcomes simultaneously

Type of analysis	Measurement of costs	Identification of outcomes	Measurement of outcomes	Comparison of costs/outcomes
Cost-benefit	Dollars	Single or multiple outcomes that may be achieved by different degrees by the alternatives	Benefits in monetary terms (B)	$(C_1 - C_2) - (B_1 - B_2)$
Cost-effectiveness	Dollars	Single effect of interest that is common to both alternatives but achieved to different degrees	Effects expressed in natural units (e.g., life years, disability days saved) (E)	$(C_1 - C_2) \div (E_1 - E_2)$
Cost-utility	Dollars	Single or multiple outcomes that may be achieved by different degrees by the alternatives	Years of healthy life (YHL)	$(C_1 - C_2) \div (YHL_1 - YHL_2)$

Adapted from Drummond, Stoddart, and Torrance (1987).
1 = with intervention; 2 = without intervention.

a technique identified by Jules Dupuit in 1844 as a way of evaluating the social benefit of publicly supplied services and relating this benefit to the cost of providing the service (Blaug, 1983). In the middle of the 20th century, cost–benefit analysis was introduced as an aid to government decision making. One of the earliest applications was in the Flood Control Act of 1936 (Gramlich, 1981; Pearce, 1983; Warner & Luce, 1982). Subsequently, cost–benefit analysis was used for allocating resources to military spending, water resources, and agricultural programs. The use of cost–benefit analysis greatly expanded in the 1960s, especially with the federal government's adoption of the Program Planning Budgeting System.

In applying cost–benefit analysis to health programs, analysts encountered difficulties in translating health benefits into monetary units. Such a translation requires that a monetary value be assigned to an individual's life. Various methods including the human capital approach, willingness to pay, and revealed preference have been used for this purpose. With the human capital approach, health outcomes are associated with worker productivity and are valued in terms of earnings. Cooper and Rice (1976) used the human capital approach to assess the impact of various illnesses in terms of their economic costs to society. The total cost of illness was found to be $188 billion in 1972, with almost 20% of these costs being attributable to diseases of the circulatory system.

Willingness to pay attempts to value health outcomes in terms of the maximum cost that a person is willing to spend to purchase some level of health. In a 1973 study, Acton compared willingness to pay with the human capital approach to evaluate the social impact of selected heart diseases. Depending on the method used to value the health outcome, the discrepancy in the estimates of the societal impact of the diseases studied was significant, ranging from more than $46 billion when the human capital approach was used to $57 billion when the willingness-to-pay method was used. Thompson (1986) evaluated the use of willingness-to-pay methods in a sample of patients with rheumatoid arthritis who were participating in a pharmaceutical clinical trial. The percentage of income that these patients were willing to pay for improved functioning increased with level of dysfunction and with increased levels of pain.

With the revealed preference approach to valuing health, social decisions are used to estimate values placed on alternative health interventions and competing uses of resources. Court decisions for disability compensation may be one source of these values; administrative decision-making processes may be another source. Of the three methods for assigning a monetary value to human life, revealed preferences has received the least attention.

Although each of these methods has its proponents and has proved useful in selected studies, conceptual and practical concerns have prevented any single method from becoming widely accepted. For example, critics have argued that willingness-to-pay measures tend to allocate resources to the rich, who have more ability to pay for health interventions than the poor (Thompson, Read, & Liang, 1982). On a practical level, willingness-to-pay methods have been criticized for poor response rates and measurement biases in data acquisition efforts (O'Brien & Viramontes, 1994; Sirken, 1986).

Cost-Effectiveness Analysis

The difficulty in using monetary units to compare costs and outcomes was an important impetus for the development of cost-effectiveness analysis (Klarman, Francis, & Rosenthal, 1968). In cost-effectiveness analysis, outcomes are expressed in any one of a number of natural, or biologically meaningful, units, including years of life saved, number of disability days saved, number of cases averted, and number of cases treated. For example, Dasbach, Fryback, Newcomb, Klein, and Klein (1991) studied the cost-effectiveness of a health program designed to screen and treat patients with diabetic retinopathy. This analysis demonstrated that annual screening of people with early-onset diabetes and at least 5 years' duration of disease would result in a higher number of sight years gained than it would if the program were implemented among older people with non–insulin-dependent diabetes or late-onset diabetes.

In another example, Cameron, Lyle, and Quine (1994) evaluated the cost-effectiveness of an accelerated rehabilitation program compared with conventional care in a sample of 252 older adults with fractured femur. Effectiveness was measured in terms of ability to live independently as measured by a Barthel index (Mahoney & Barthel, 1965) score of 80 or higher 4 months after the fracture occurred. For accelerated rehabilitation, the cost per recovered patient was $21,240 compared with $31,190 for patients treated with conventional care. Weinberger, Smith, Katz, and Moore (1988) studied the impact of increased ambulatory care on hospital readmission rates. The overall cost reduction of $60 per patient suggests that increasing the intensity of ambulatory care after hospital discharge may result in lower readmission costs.

Because cost-effectiveness analysis measures health outcomes in different ways in different studies (e.g., sight years in one study, recovered patients in another), comparison of costs and outcomes across different health interventions may be meaningless. Thus, the lack of commensurate units of measurement limits the use of cost-effectiveness analysis in policy applications that cut across a large number of different health interventions or programs.

Cost–Utility Analysis

To overcome this limitation, cost–utility analysis emerged in the late 1960s as a form of economic evaluation that allows for the comparison of multiple health interventions without putting a monetary value on human life. Cost–utility analysis uses years of healthy life, or quality-adjusted life years, to measure health outcome. Broadly defined, a year of healthy life is the duration of life adjusted by some fraction between 0 and 1 that estimates quality of life during 1 year. For example, a person who is prevented from working for 1 year due to health problems may have a quality-of-life score of 0.75 or can be said to experience an average of three fourths of full function for the year. The concept of years of healthy life can be expanded to cover more than 1 year and more than one person. For example, if the duration of life is 10 years and the average quality of life associated with this interval is 0.75, then a person is said to have an average of 7.5 years of healthy life. Alternatively, 10 people living 1 year each with a quality of life of 0.75 also have an average of 7.5 years of healthy life in the aggregate. Through the mid-1990s, the majority of the applications of cost–utility analysis had compared medical or surgical treatment interventions.

As long as the methods for arriving at the quality-of-life component of the years of healthy life measure are the same across studies, results from various analyses are comparable. Years of healthy life have another advantage over other quality-of-life or health outcomes measures in that they are based on biologically meaningful units—namely, life years. Hence, measuring years of healthy life is more intuitively meaningful than measuring approaches based on arbitrary scoring systems. The next section details measuring quality of life and constructing a years-of-healthy-life measure and discusses its application in cost–utility analysis.

HEALTH CARE COSTS

In health care, as in other sectors of the economy, costs represent the inputs that are used in the production of a given output. Health care costs are usually categorized into three types of costs: 1) direct costs, 2) indirect costs, and 3) external costs (see Table 2). Although economists use the concept of opportunity cost (i.e., the value of alternative outputs foregone), in practice, this is rarely used, owing to difficulties of estimation (Warner & Luce, 1982). Most frequently, health services researchers rely on expenditures, prices, or charges when doing cost analyses.

Organizational and operating costs that are associated with developing and operating a specific health care program or providing a given intervention (Drummond, Stoddart, & Torrance, 1987; Eisenberg et al., 1988) are referred to as direct medical costs. Such costs include services of physicians, nurses, pharmacists, and other health care providers. Supplies and equipment (e.g., solutions, catheters, tubing costs) that are needed for making a diagnosis or providing treatment are also considered to be direct medical costs. Personal out-of-pocket expenditures that might be incurred

Table 2. Types of costs included in the economic evaluation of health interventions

- Direct costs
  Direct medical costs
    Physician and ancillary services
    Supplies, including devices and appliances, research and development, and
      diagnostic tests
    Overhead allocated to the technology, such as fixed costs of utilities, space,
      and storage
    Institutional inpatient care
    Institutional outpatient care
    Home health care
    Volunteers
    Prescription and nonprescription medications, such as drug costs, treating side
      effects or toxicity of medications
  Direct nonmedical costs
    Care provided by family and friends
    Transportation to and from medical services
    Child care and housekeeping
    Modification to home to accommodate patients
    Social services
- Indirect costs
  Time and productivity
      Change in productivity resulting from change in health status
      Lost productivity on the job
      Income lost by family members
      Foregone leisure time
- External costs
  Immunization programs
  Safety programs in occupational settings
  Laws mandating the use of seat belts

Adapted from Luce and Elixhauser (1990).

for medical devices and appliances, prescription medicines, and other medical supplies, for example, are also examples of direct medical costs (Luce & Elixhauser, 1990).

Direct costs that arise as a result of costs borne by patients and their families are referred to as direct nonmedical costs. These costs include modification of a home to accommodate health care needs of the patient, for example, to add access ramps to accommodate people in wheelchairs; care provided by relatives and friends; and transportation to obtain care (Eisenberg & Kitz, 1986; Eisenberg et al., 1988; Luce & Elixhauser, 1990).

In addition to direct costs of health care, patients and their families can incur indirect costs that are generally expressed as those that might be due to lost productivity (Luce & Elixhauser, 1990). In health care, such activities are usually described as changes in work schedules due to health problems. Indirect costs of morbidity include reduced levels of work output, time spent to obtain health care, loss of productivity that results from a change of employment caused by illness, and lost leisure time (Rice & Hodgson, 1981). Estimation of indirect costs requires that a monetary value be assigned to lost productivity through a method such as human capital or willingness to pay. The controversy associated with assigning a money value to human life is one explanation of why indirect costs are frequently excluded in cost–utility analysis. Another reason is to avoid double counting when quality of life is included in the denominator (Gold, Siegel, Russell, & Weinstein, 1996). In addition, lost earnings may be an inappropriate concept for evaluating rehabilitation programs that are designed to aid patients who are too dysfunctional to be able to return to work (Johnston, 1987).

Some analysts also consider external costs borne by consumers as another category of health care costs. A health intervention that generates external costs is designed to benefit other groups of individuals who may or may not be the direct beneficiaries of the output or intervention. For example, an immunization program benefits not only people who participate but also those who refuse to participate but benefit from the reduced probability of contracting the infectious disease due to others being vaccinated. As this example suggests, external costs are especially important to consider when evaluating health promotion activities. In considering rehabilitation programs, these costs may be more relevant to include when the goal is to prevent accidents and injuries that lead to the need for rehabilitation rather than when evaluating the effectiveness of alternative medical rehabilitation programs.

Any or all of these types of costs might be used to develop a cost estimate for use in socioeconomic evaluations. The particular components actually used depend on the purpose of analysis and the availability of data. In special studies, data on direct medical costs might be obtained by surveying medical providers (Thompson, Read, Hutchings, Paterson, & Harris, 1988; Weinstein & Stason, 1982). Although surveys can be designed to collect study-specific information on health care costs, the data generally are not comparable across studies, because different definitions and methods of collecting information are used. Whereas general population surveys, such as the National Medical Expenditure Survey, use standardized methods to collect information on all survey participants, cost data from large-scale sample surveys may give less precise estimates because they usually are based on respondents' self-report of information about their health care use and expenditures (Benson & Marano, 1994; Edwards & Berlin, 1989).

Generally, the costs associated with a health intervention occur over a relatively long time. Because money available in 1995 has a higher value than the same amount of money that will be available in the future, economists convert future dollars to present values through the process of discounting (Warner & Luce, 1982). Although economic theory provides a method for estimated net present value, the theory gives little guidance about which discount rate to use. When gains from an intervention extend into the future, as is the case with rehabilitation programs, the analyst may want to use a lower rather than higher discount rate. Because no single rate is recommended, the usual practice is to pick a range of rates to present an alternative understanding of the effect of discounting.

HEALTH OUTCOMES

Investigators have drawn on many concepts, including handicap, disability or dysfunction, and impairment, to include in a comprehensive definition of *health* (see Table 3). Each of these concepts has a number of domains that represent more specific levels of functioning. For example, the concept of *functional status* is usually described as having three domains: 1) social function, 2) psychological function, and 3) physical function. Each of these, in turn, has a set of subdomains. For example, physical function may be thought of as comprising two subdomains: activity restrictions and fitness. The right-hand column in this table presents a brief definition or an example of each subdomain. Although other authors have used slightly different ordering and terminology, general consensus exists among health status researchers that this table represents the range of concepts and domains to be included in a multidimensional definition of *health*.

The disability community, however, has adopted the World Health Organization's (WHO's; 1980) *International Classification of Impairments, Disabilities, and Handicaps* (ICIDH), which uses many of the same terms, some with different interpretation. Although impairment seems to be used in the same manner in both classification systems, the health services community tends to define *disability* more broadly by including social function and dysfunction, which are more closely represented in the definition *handicap* in the WHO classification. Opportunity for health and perceptions are two concepts that are not defined in the ICIDH.

In developing composite measures of health-related quality of life, whether generic or disease- or treatment-specific, investigators have adopted one of two approaches for modeling the interrelationship of multiple concepts. The first model views individual characteristics of the person and his or her disease as being at the core of a set of concentric circles. Moving out from the center, forces external to the individual have an increasing impact. The outer circle in this model is social and role functioning. At this level, the individual's social and cultural environment, including the possibility for treatment, shapes his or her reaction to illness (Ware, 1984). This general model offers researchers little guidance in specifying the relationships between different concepts of health. Measures based on this model include the Medical Outcomes Study Short Form (Stewart & Ware, 1992; Ware & Sherbourne, 1992), Functional Independence Measure (FIM)

Table 3. Core concepts and domains of health-related quality of life

Concepts and domains	Definitions/indicators
● **Handicap**	
Opportunity for health	
Social or cultural disadvantage	Disadvantage because of health, stigma, societal reaction
Resilience	Capacity for health, ability to withstand stress, physiologic reserves
Health perceptions	
General health perceptions	Self-rating of health, health concern or worry
Satisfaction with health	Satisfaction with physical, psychological, social function
● **Disability or dysfunction**	
Social function	
Limitations in usual roles	Acute or chronic limitations in usual social roles (major activities) of child, student, worker
Integration	Participation in the community
Contact	Interaction with others
Mental function	
Affective attitudes	Psychological attitudes and behaviors, including distress and well-being
Cognitive function	Alertness, disorientation, problems in reasoning
Physical function	
Activity restrictions	Acute or chronic reduction in physical activity, mobility, self-care, sleep, communication
Fitness	Performance of activity with vigor and without excessive fatigue
● **Impairment**	
Symptoms/subjective complaints	Reports of physical and psychological symptoms, sensations, pain, health problems, or feelings not directly observable
Signs	Physical examination: Observable evidence of defect or abnormality
Self-reported disease	Patient listing of medical conditions or impairments
Physiologic measures	Laboratory data, records, and their clinical interpretation
Tissue alterations	Pathologic evidence
Diagnoses	Clinical judgments after ``all the evidence''
● **Death and duration of life**	Mortality, survival, years of life lost

Source: Patrick and Erickson (1993).

(Granger, Hamilton, Linacre, Heinemann, & Wright, 1993; State University of New York at Buffalo, 1993), and the Craig Handicap Assessment and Reporting Technique (Whiteneck, Charlifue, Gerhart, Overholser, & Richardson, 1992).

The second model views health as a continuum that ranges from perfect health to death, with states representing intermediate levels of health ranked along this continuum (Fanshel & Bush, 1970). Relationships along this continuum are seen as a progression from positive health, including concepts such as health perceptions and resilience, to negative health, including activity restrictions and signs and symptoms of disease (Patrick & Bergner, 1990). Although issues of interrelationships between concepts have been addressed in this model, the linear progression is considered to be an oversimplification of the complex interactions that might occur between domains. Measures based on this model include the Health Utilities Index (Torrance, 1982), the Quality of Well-Being Scale (Kaplan & Bush, 1982), and the Q-TWiST (Goldhirsch & Gelber, 1986).

As suggested by this brief discussion of theoretical models underlying composite measures of health-related quality of life or measures of single concepts that have been used together to form batteries of measures, many questionnaires and rating scales are available for assessing medical rehabilitation outcomes. Of these, however, fewer than 20 measurement strategies have been developed using the continuum model and thus are available for estimating years of healthy life as required in a cost–utility analysis.

Among the earliest research aimed at measuring years of healthy life for use in cost–utility analysis was that of Fanshel and Bush (1970). These investigators specified that a years-of-healthy-life measure consists of three components:

1. A set of health state descriptors that comprises the concepts and domains of health-related quality of life included in the measure
2. A weighting scheme that represents preferences that individuals have for the concepts and domains in the classification system
3. A method for estimating years of healthy life by combining quantity and quality of life

Health State Descriptors

For developing an operational definition of *health-related quality of life,* the perfect health-to-death continuum is divided into a set of states defined in terms of concepts and domains. The states are specified by means of either holistic descriptors or a classification system. Although the holistic approach to formulating health state descriptors is intuitively appealing, health state classification systems are more commonly used because of ease of measurement and data collection (Patrick & Erickson, 1993; Torrance, 1982). A simple classification system that represents the concept of disability might comprise four states: dead, inpatient, outpatient, and nonpatient (Whitmore, 1973). An important feature is that states in the classification system are developed so that they are mutually exclusive in that a person cannot be both a nonpatient and an outpatient simultaneously.

Originally, investigators developed classification systems and questionnaires that were used with primary data collection. Erickson and colleagues (Erickson, Kendall, Anderson, & Kaplan, 1989; Erickson, Kendall, Odle, & Torrance, 1992) have shown that survey respondents can be assigned to a classification system without the use of a specific questionnaire. These constructed measures have been found to result in valid measures of population health status and have been shown to detect differences in health for people with various diagnoses, including hypertension, depression, and diabetes.

In adopting the continuum model of health-related quality of life, investigators accept that health states can be arrayed along the continuum according to the value that individuals place on them. Various assumptions and methods have been developed for measuring these values, which are also referred to as utilities or preferences.

Preferences for Health

In assigning preferences to health states, researchers use axioms of expected utility theory that were put forth by Von Neumann and Morgenstern (1953) to develop cardinal utilities under uncertainty. Thus, the meaning of the term *utility* as it is used in measuring health-related quality of life, and years of healthy life in particular, differs from that used by early economists such as Jeremy Bentham and John Stuart Mill, who thought that satisfaction for consumer bundles could be measured in terms of cardinal utility (Holcombe, 1990). Utilities based on the Von Neumann–Morgenstern (VN–M) axioms also differ from ordinal utility theory, which was developed during the early part of the 20th century. More appropriately, preferences that are based on expected utility theory should be referred to as VN–M utilities to avoid confusion (Torrance & Feeny, 1989). Although some researchers have criticized the normative basis of the expected utility model as not representative of individual behavior, the VN–M approach to utility estimation is the most widely used (Gafni, Birch, & Mehrez, 1993; Torrance & Feeny, 1989).

Information on preferences is usually collected by using one of three methods: 1) standard gamble, 2) time trade-off, and 3) category scaling. Each of these methods is briefly summarized in this section; for more detailed information about the methods and their application, see Torrance (1986). The standard gamble technique has been referred to as the gold standard or classical method of measuring preferences because it stems directly from the work of Von Neumann and Morgenstern (Gafni et al., 1993; Gyldmark & Morrison, 1993). Although the link between the standard gamble technique and expected utility theory makes it the method of choice from a theoretical perspective, investigators and respondents often indicate that the method is confusing. The findings of Wolfson, Sinclair, Bombardier, and McGeer (1982) are representative of the problems with using the standard gamble method. In a study of stroke patients, these investigators found that respondents had difficulties understanding what was expected of them and that respondents sometimes resisted the notion of gambling with one's health.

The time trade-off technique was developed as an easier-to-administer version of the standard gamble (Torrance, Thomas, & Sackett, 1972). Wolfson et al. (1982) found that preferences were generally higher when assessed by the standard gamble than by the time trade-off method. Gafni and colleagues (1993) suggested that because the time trade-off method is not directly related to a behavioral theory, it is impossible to interpret such discrepancies between preferences obtained by different methods.

The third method, category scaling, sometimes referred to as the rating scale approach, requires that a person rank states along a continuum with clearly specified end points, such as *most desirable* and *least desirable*. The feeling thermometer is a similar exercise; but instead of a sorting board, states are placed on a thermometer. Category scaling has been found to be acceptable to respondents (Carter, Bobbitt, Bergner, & Gelson, 1976; Patrick, Bush, & Chen, 1973; Torrance, 1982). In a comparison of rating scale and time trade-off techniques, O'Leary and colleagues (O'Leary, Fairclough, & Jankowski, 1995) found that the methods gave different results, suggesting that respondents perceived the experiments to be conceptually different.

When the data from one of these methods, either standard gamble, time trade-off, or category scaling, have been collected, they are converted to preferences, usually using a multiattribute utility theory to accommodate the large number of health states that can be formed from even a simple classification system. Multiattribute utility theory was developed by Keeney and Raiffa (1976) to extend expected utility theory to decisions involving multiple objectives (Torrance & Feeny, 1989). With this method, preferences can be assigned to all of the states in the classification system by collecting preference information on the individual domains, or attributes, and on a small number of holistic states (Torrance, 1982). Although the functional form for combining attributes can be additive, multiplicative, and multilinear, the multiplicative form has been found to be appropriate for developing multiattribute, utility-based measures of health (Drummond et al., 1987).

In collecting information on preferences, an investigator may ask respondents to rate health states while supplying information about their current health status; this approach is most frequently used with clinical studies. Alternatively, investigators can design a preference study in which data on the values that people place on health states would be collected independently of the survey in which health state information is collected. The independent approach has been used most frequently with classification systems created for use with policy analysis (Drummond et al., 1987; Fanshel & Bush, 1970; Ontario Ministry of Health, 1991).

One alternative to designing a special study is to use a set of preferences that have been collected for another purpose. Multiattribute measures of the health of the U.S. population have been developed using preferences associated with the Quality of Well-Being Scale and the Health Utilities Index (Erickson et al., 1989, 1992). Another alternative for arriving at a set of preferences might be based on the approach taken for developing a set of preferences for the Healthy People 2000 Years of Healthy Life measure (Torrance, Erickson, Patrick, & Feldman, 1995). These approaches might be used in other applications, as long as the results are interpreted cautiously.

Preferences based on different methods, for example, time trade-off, standard gamble, or category rating, may give different numerical values for the same health states. Also, different health state descriptors may be associated with different values or preferences. Thus, a measure of an individual's health-related quality of life is a function of the specific health state descriptors and preference elicitation methods used in the estimation procedure. Whichever descriptors or methods are used, this score can be used to adjust quantity of life to estimate years of healthy life.

Years of Healthy Life

One way of estimating years of healthy life is to follow an individual over time and observe changes in his or her health-related quality of life. Another, perhaps more commonly used, method of combining quality and quantity of life is to adjust life expectancy by a health-related quality-of-life score. The use of the life table for generating a measure of health that summarizes both mortality and morbidity experience was first suggested by Sanders (1965). In one of the earliest applications, Sullivan (1971a, 1971b) used disability data from the National Health Interview Survey (NHIS) and other national data sets to partition life expectancy into the proportion of the year that was lived with and without disability. In the early 1990s, this method was used to estimate Healthy Life Expectancy and Disability Adjusted Life Years (Robine, Michel, & Branch, 1992; Robine & Ritchie, 1991; World Bank, 1993). Although these measures combine morbidity and mortality, they are not years of healthy life, because they do not adjust quantity of life by assessing quality of life by including a measure that reflects preferences for health states.

The basic approach to estimating years of healthy life using the life table method is the same, regardless of the health state descriptors or the method used to obtain preferences. Two data sets are required. One is a life table that expresses the age-specific death rates in terms of a standard population and gives the number of people alive at the beginning of each age interval and the number alive in the interval. The other type of data needed is a set of age-specific, health-related, quality-of-life average scores for the population of interest. These scores are used to adjust the total person years in the interval, thus giving an estimate of the total quality-adjusted person years that are then used to calculate the years of healthy life remaining for each age group using the same methods as are used to calculate age-specific life expectancies (Erickson, Wilson, & Shannon, 1995). Comparing the life years and years of healthy life remaining indicates the impact of both mortality and health-related quality of life on a population and its subgroups.

RANKING OF COSTS AND OUTCOMES

Costs and outcomes comparisons using cost–utility analysis are shown in Table 4 for a selected set of interventions that have been evaluated using the Health Utilities Index. The ratios shown in this table have been devel-

Table 4. Estimated cost per year of healthy life gained using the Health Utilities Index

Intervention (reference)	Reported cost/YHL gained in U.S. dollars (year)	Adjusted cost/YHL* gained in U.S. dollars (1991)
Postpartum anti-D (Torrance & Zipursky, 1977)	<$0 (1977)	<$0
Antepartum treatment of primiparae and multiparae (average) (Torrance & Zipursky, 1984)	$1,223 (1983)	$ 2,150
Neonatal intensive care of low birth weight infants, 1,000 g–1,499 g (Boyle et al., 1983)	$2,800 (1978)	$ 8,000
Neonatal intensive care of very low birth weight infants, 500 g–999 g (Boyle et al., 1983)	$19,600 (1978)	$56,100
Continuous ambulatory peritoneal dialysis (Churchill, Morgan, & Torrance, 1984)	$35,100 (1980)	$82,900
Hospital hemodialysis (Churchill et al., 1984)	$40,200 (1980)	$94,000

Adapted from Patrick and Erickson (1993).

*Method of adjustment

$$C/YHL_{1991} = (MCPI_{1991}/MCPI_{py}) \times C/YHL_{py},$$

where

C/YHL_{1991} = adjusted cost/YHL gained in 1991,

$MCPI_{1991}$ = Medical Care Price Index for 1991,

$MCPI_{py}$ = Medical Care Price Index for previous year,

C/YHL_{py} = Cost/YHL gained for previous year.

For example, for antepartum treatment the adjusted ratio has been calculated as follows:

$$C/YHL_{1991} = MCPI_{1991}/MCPI_{1983} \times C/YHL_{1983} = 177/100.6 \times \$1,223 = \$2,152.$$

Note: MCPI data are from U.S. Bureau of the Census (1993).

oped by one team of investigators, thus enhancing their comparability. The use of a standard measure of years of healthy life as well as standard methods and assumptions for estimating costs resolves the problem of making comparisons between interventions when different indexes are used. Ratios of cost per year of healthy life have been ranked from low to high, indicating that postpartum anti-D screening is the most cost-effective and hospital hemodialysis is the least cost-effective of the interventions compared in this table. The data in this table illustrate the diverse types of health interventions to which cost–utility analysis has been applied.

Tables that summarize ratios of cost per year of healthy life for different health interventions are frequently referred to as "league" tables (Drummond, Torrance, & Mason, 1993; Mason, Drummond, & Torrance, 1993). Because not all league tables are based on a common methodology, Gerard and Mooney (1993) pointed out that care must be exercised in interpreting the information in league tables that rank interventions using different methods for estimating costs and outcomes. These differences mean that the ratios are not strictly comparable, even though they all reflect cost per year of healthy life gained.

Another problem with many compiled cost-per-year-of-healthy-life ratios is that they are based on average costs and outcomes that are appropriate for choosing among alternative interventions to fund. When the decision focuses on how much of an intervention to fund, as is most frequently encountered in health care, then marginal estimates of costs and outcomes, representing the additional costs and benefits gained from a unit of output, are more appropriate.

In a review of 21 interventions that had been evaluated using cost–utility analysis, Drummond, Torrance, and Mason (1993) found only 1 that was based on marginal analysis; 19 were based on average values; and, for 1, the information about how costs and outcomes were estimated was not ascertainable. Use of average rather than marginal estimates, especially for comparing interventions as is done in a league table, may mislead policy makers. In a classic example of the impact of using average rather than marginal data, Neuhauser and Lewicki (1975) showed that among the recommended six screening tests for colonic cancer, the marginal cost could be as much as 20,000 times higher than the average cost. Thus, decisions based on average, rather than marginal, values may underestimate the impact that implementation of an intervention may have on the overall cost.

League tables that show only the ratios for each intervention, as in Table 4, are also of limited use for policy making. In addition to the relative cost-effectiveness information conveyed by the ratios, policy makers also benefit from having information about the total amount of resources needed for and the total health benefit gained from each intervention. With aggregate costs, policy makers can evaluate the budgetary impact of interventions. By comparing the aggregate costs and benefits for competing interventions, policy makers should be able to develop a set of interventions that the community can afford (Gafni & Birch, 1993; Laupacis, Feeny, Detsky, & Tugwell, 1993).

The use of selected populations or treatment centers is another limitation of league tables. Selection may be defined in terms of the type of patient, such as *healthier, younger, better educated,* or *more compliant.* For example, if treatment comparisons in a clinical study are made on a relatively young and probably healthy subset of people who have a given condition, the findings will probably differ from those when the medicine becomes widely used in the general population. The selection also may be based on the application of a given intervention at a specialized treatment center, for example, the evaluation of neonatal intensive care units (see Table 4). Data from local areas that can be characterized by different practice patterns represent another type of selection that might introduce bias into league tables (Gerard & Mooney, 1993; Wennberg & Gittelsohn, 1973).

These criticisms of league tables suggest that if cost–utility analysis is to assist policy makers in containing costs while maintaining, or increasing, the level of health, then the same methods for assessing health care costs and outcomes need to be applied systematically to all interventions. Toward this end, researchers have called for the adoption of a set of standards that might include the following topics: methods for estimating direct and indirect health care costs, techniques for valuing health outcomes, and recommended ranges of discount rates (Drummond, Brandt, Luce, & Rovira, 1993; Gold et al., in press). Ideally, systematic analysis and implementation of standards will be applied on a common database such as the one developed for the Oregon Medicaid experiment (Office of Technology Assessment, 1992) or a general population survey such as the National Medical Expenditure Survey.

ETHICAL CONCERNS

Socioeconomic analysis—cost–utility analysis in particular—is frequently criticized as discriminating on the basis of age, functional status, and ability to benefit from treatment (Dougherty, 1995; LaPuma & Lawlor, 1990). These criticisms stem in part from the use of years of healthy life to measure treatment benefit. On the one hand, the use of life expectancy is erroneously considered to give an advantage to the young in the calculation of years of healthy life. On the other hand, the inclusion of explicitly measured preferences is considered to favor people without disability.

Years of healthy life, however, need not be any more discriminatory than any other type of health data used for decision making, a process that is inherently dependent on people's preferences. Thus, a major responsibility of both decision makers and decision stakeholders is to develop mechanisms suitable for including preference information in the decision process that reflects the concerns of all members of the society, and not just a select, possibly elite, few.

Perhaps the most equitable approach is through the use of large-scale general population surveys, such as the NHIS, to collect information on preferences for health states. The NHIS is being used to collect information about the prevalence of various types of disability in the United States, with a questionnaire that has been designed with input from people with disabilities. Although the model for questionnaire design and data collection developed for the NHIS disability supplement would need to be expanded, the collection of preference information in such a survey setting is not beyond the state of knowledge about how to collect this information. A major advantage of the use of a national survey is the potential for representativeness of all people living in the community. Thus, a national survey helps ensure that all people have direct input into the decision-making process.

CONCLUSIONS

Overall, socioeconomic analysis and cost–utility analysis in particular are important methods for understanding the relationships between health care costs and outcomes associated with alternative treatment interventions, whether these are rehabilitation programs or medical or surgical treatments. In developing the components to be used in these analyses, careful attention is needed in deciding on which operational definitions of costs and outcomes to use and the methods adopted to measure them. With a thoughtful approach to the assessment of both costs and outcomes, socioeconomic analysis is a powerful tool to guide policy makers in allocating resources so that costs are contained and a high level of health-related quality of life is maintained.

REFERENCES

Acton, J.P. (1973). *Evaluating public health programs to save lives: The case of heart attacks* (Rand Report R-950-RC). Santa Monica, CA: Rand Corp.

Anderson, J.P., Bush, J.W., Chen, M., & Dolenc, D. (1986). Policy space areas and properties of benefit-cost/utility analysis. *Journal of the American Medical Association, 255*(6), 794–795.

Benson, V., & Marano, M.A. (1994). Current estimates from the National Health Interview Survey, 1993. *Vital and Health Statistics* (Series 10, No. 190).

Blaug, M. (1983). *Economic theory in retrospect* (3rd ed., pp. 337–339). Cambridge, England: Cambridge University Press.

Boyle, M.H., Torrance, G.W., Sinclair, J.C., & Horwood, S.P. (1983). Economic evaluation of neonatal intensive care of very-low-birth-weight infants. *New England Journal of Medicine, 308*(22), 1330–1337.

Bush, J.W., Chen, M.M., & Patrick, D.L. (1973). Health status index in cost-effectiveness: Analysis of PKU program. In R. Berg (Ed.), *Health status indexes* (pp. 172–208). Chicago: Hospital Research and Educational Trust.

Cameron, I.D., Lyle, D.M., & Quine, S. (1994). Cost-effectiveness of accelerated rehabilitation after proximal femoral fracture. *Journal of Clinical Epidemiology, 47*(11), 1307–1313.

Carter, W.B., Bobbitt, R.A., Bergner, M., & Gelson, B.S. (1976). Validation of an interval scaling: The Sickness Impact Profile. *Health Services Research, 11*(4), 516–528.

Churchill, D.N., Morgan, J., & Torrance, G.W. (1984, January–March). Quality of life in end-stage renal disease. *Peritoneal Dialysis Bulletin,* 20–23.

Commonwealth of Australia. (1990). *Guidelines for the pharmaceutical industry on preparation of submissions to the pharmaceutical benefits advisory committee: Including submissions involving economic analyses.* Woden (ACT): Canberra, Australia: Department of Health, Housing and Community Services.

Cooper, B.S., & Rice, D.P. (1976). The economic cost of illness revisited. *Social Security Bulletin, 39*(2), 21–36.

Dasbach, E.J., Fryback, D.G., Newcomb, P.A., Klein, R., & Klein, B.E. (1991). Cost-effectiveness of strategies for detecting diabetic retinopathy. *Medical Care, 29*(1), 20–39.

Dobkin, B. (1995). The economic impact of stroke. *Neurology, 45*(Suppl. 1), S6–S9.

Dougherty, C.J. (1995). Quality-adjusted life years and the ethical values of health care. *American Journal of Physical Medicine and Rehabilitation, 73*(Suppl. 1), S29–S33.

Drummond, M., Brandt, A., Luce, B., & Rovira, J. (1993). Standardizing methodologies for economic evaluation in health care: Practice, problems, and potential. *International Journal of Technology Assessment in Health Care, 9*(1), 26–36.

Drummond, M.F., Stoddart, G.L., & Torrance, G.W. (1987). *Methods for the economic evaluation of health care programmes.* Oxford, England: Oxford University Press.

Drummond, M., Torrance, G., & Mason, J. (1993). Cost-effectiveness league tables: More harm than good? *Social Science and Medicine, 37*(1), 33–40.

Edwards, W.S., & Berlin, M. (1989). *National Medical Expenditure Survey: Questionnaires and data collection methods for the household survey and the survey of American Indians and Alaska Natives, methods 2.* Rockville, MD: Department of Health and Human Services, Public Health Service, National Center for Health Services Research and Health Care Technology Assessment. (DHHS Publication No. [PHS] 89-3450).

Eisenberg, J.M., et al. (1988). Measuring the economic impact of perioperative total parenteral nutrition: Principles and design. *American Journal of Clinical Nutrition, 47,* 382–391.

Eisenberg, J.M., & Kitz, D.S. (1986). Savings from outpatient antibiotic therapy for osteomyelitis: Economic analysis of a therapeutic strategy. *Journal of the American Medical Association, 255*(12), 1584–1588.

Erickson, P., Kendall, E.A., Anderson, J.P., & Kaplan, R.M. (1989). Using composite health status measures to assess the nation's health. *Medical Care, 27*(Suppl. 3), S66–S77.

Erickson, P., Kendall, E.A., Odle, M.P., & Torrance, G.W. (1992). *Assessing health-related quality of life in the National Health and Nutrition Examination Survey.* Hyattsville, MD: National Center for Health Statistics.

Erickson, P., Wilson, R.W., & Shannon, I. (1995). *Years of healthy life. Statistical Note Number 7.* Hyattsville, MD: National Center for Health Statistics.

Fanshel, S., & Bush, J.W. (1970). A health status index and its application to health services outcomes. *Operations Research, 18*(6), 1021–1066.

Gafni, A., & Birch, S. (1993). Guidelines for the adoption of new technologies: A prescription for uncontrolled growth in expenditures and how to avoid the problem. *Canadian Medical Association Journal, 148*(6), 913–917.

Gafni, A., Birch, S., & Mehrez, A. (1993). Economics, health and health economics: HYEs versus QALYs. *Journal of Health Economics, 11,* 325–339.

Gerard, K., & Mooney, G. (1993). QALY league tables: Handle with care. *Health Economics, 2,* 59–64.

Gold, M., Siegel, J., Russell, L.B., & Weinstein, M.C. (1996). *Cost-effectiveness in health and medicine.* New York: Oxford University Press.

Goldhirsch, A., & Gelber, R.D. (1986). A new endpoint for the assessment of adjuvant therapy in postmenopausal women with inoperable breast cancer. *Journal of Clinical Oncology, 4,* 1772–1779.

Gramlich, E.M. (1981). *Benefit-cost analysis of government programs.* Englewood Cliffs, NJ: Prentice Hall.

Granger, C.V., Hamilton, B.B., Linacre, J.M., Heinemann, A.W., & Wright, B.D. (1993). Performance profiles of the Functional Independence Measure. *Journal of Physical Medicine and Rehabilitation, 72,* 84–89.

Gyldmark, M., & Morrison, G.C. (1993). Re-appraising the use of contingent valuation: A reply. *Health Economics, 2,* 363–365.

Hatziandru, E.I., Koplan, J.P., Weinstein, M.C., Caspersen, C.J., & Warner, K.E. (1988). A cost-effectiveness analysis of exercise as a health promotion activity. *American Journal of Public Health, 78*(11), 1417–1421.

Holcombe, R.G. (1990). Social welfare. In J. Creedy (Ed.), *Foundations of economic thought* (pp. 159–185). Cambridge, MA: Basil Blackwell.

Johannesson, M. (1994). The impact of age on the cost-effectiveness of hypertension treatment: An analysis of randomized drug trials. *Medical Decision Making, 14*(3), 236–245.

Johnston, M.V. (1987). Cost–benefit methodologies in rehabilitation. In M.J. Fuhrer (Ed.), *Rehabilitation outcomes: Analysis and measurement* (pp. 99–113). Baltimore: Paul H. Brookes Publishing Co.

Johnston, M.V., & Keith, R.A. (1983). Cost–benefits of medical rehabilitation: Review and critique. *Archives of Physical Medicine and Rehabilitation, 64*(4), 147–154.

Kaplan, R.M., & Bush, J.W. (1982). Health-related quality of life measurement for evaluation research and policy analysis. *Health Psychology, 1,* 61–80.

Keeney, R.L., & Raiffa, H. (1976). *Decisions with multiple objectives: Preferences and value tradeoffs.* New York: John Wiley & Sons.

Klarman, H.E., Francis, J.O'S., & Rosenthal, G.D. (1968). Cost-effectiveness analysis applied to the treatment of chronic renal disease. *Medical Care, 6*(1), 48–54.

LaPuma, J., & Lawlor, E.F. (1990). Quality-adjusted life years: Ethical implications for physicians and policymakers. *Journal of the American Medical Association, 263*(21), 2917–2921.

Laupacis, A., Feeny, D., Detsky, A., & Tugwell, P.X. (1993). Tentative guidelines for using clinical and economic evaluations revisited. *Canadian Medical Association Journal, 148*(6), 927–929.

Luce, B.R., & Elixhauser, A. (1990). *Standards for socioeconomic evaluation of health care products and services.* New York: Springer-Verlag.

Mahoney, F.I., & Barthel, D.W. (1965). Functional evaluation: The Barthel Index. *Maryland State Medical Journal, 14,* 61–65.

Mason, J., Drummond, M., & Torrance, G. (1993). Some guidelines on the use of cost-effectiveness league tables. *British Medical Journal, 306*(6877), 570–572.

Neuhauser, D., & Lewicki, A.M. (1975). What do we gain from the sixth stool guaiac? *New England Journal of Medicine, 293*(5), 226–228.

O'Brien, B., & Viramontes, J.L. (1994). Willingness to pay: A valid and reliable measure of health state preference? *Medical Decision Making, 14*(3), 289–297.

Office of Technology Assessment. (1981). *Cost-effectiveness of influenza vaccination.* Washington, DC: U.S. Government Printing Office.

Office of Technology Assessment. (1990). *Costs and effectiveness of colorectal cancer screening in the elderly.* Washington, DC: U.S. Government Printing Office. (OTA-BP-H-74)

Office of Technology Assessment. (1992). *Evaluation of the Oregon Medicaid proposal.* Washington, DC: U.S. Government Printing Office. (OTA-H-531)

O'Leary, J.F., Fairclough, D.L., & Jankowski, M.K. (1995). Comparison of time-tradeoff utilities and rating scale values of cancer patients and their relatives: Evidence for a possible plateau relationship. *Medical Decision Making, 15*(2), 132–137.

Ontario Ministry of Health. (1991). *Guidelines for preparation of economic analysis to be included in submission to Drug Programs Branch for listing in the Ontario drug benefit formulary/comparative drug index.* Toronto, Ontario, Canada: Author.

Patrick, D.L., & Bergner, M. (1990). Measurement of health status in the 1990s. *Annual Review of Public Health, 11,* 165–183.

Patrick, D.L., Bush, J.W., & Chen, M.M. (1973). Towards an operational definition of health. *Journal of Health and Social Behavior, 14*(1), 6–23.

Patrick, D.L., & Erickson, P. (1993). *Health status and health policy: Quality of life in health care evaluation and resource allocation.* New York: Oxford University Press.

Pearce, D.W. (1983). *Cost-benefit analysis* (2nd ed., pp. 14–24). New York: St. Martin's Press.

Rice, D.P., & Hodgson, T.A. (1981). Social and economic implications of cancer in the United States. *Vital and Health Statistics.* Hyattsville, MD: National Center for Health Statistics.

Robine, J.M., Michel, J.P., & Branch, L.G. (1992). Measurement and utilization of healthy life expectancy: Conceptual issues. *Bulletin of the World Health Organization, 70*(6), 791–800.

Robine, J.M., & Ritchie, K. (1991). Healthy life expectancy: Evaluation of global indicator of change in population health. *British Medical Journal, 302*(6774), 457–460.

Sanders, B. (1965). Measuring community health levels. *American Journal of Public Health, 54*(7), 1063–1070.

Sirken, M.G. (1986). Error effects of survey questionnaires on the public's assessments of health risks. *American Journal of Public Health, 76*(4), 367–368.

State University of New York at Buffalo. (1993). *Guide for the Uniform Data Set for Medical Rehabilitation (Adult FIM), version 4.0.* Buffalo, NY: Author.

Stewart, A.L., & Ware, J.E. (1992). *Measuring functioning and well-being: The Medical Outcomes Study approach.* Durham, NC: Duke University Press.

Sullivan, D.F. (1971a). A single index of morbidity and mortality. *HSMHA Health Reports, 86*(4), 347–355.

Sullivan, D.F. (1971b). Disability components for an index of health. *Vital and Health Statistics* (Series 2, No. 42). Hyattsville, MD: National Center for Health Statistics.

Thompson, M.S. (1986). Willingness to pay and accept risks to cure chronic disease. *American Journal of Public Health, 76*(4), 392–396.

Thompson, M.S., Read, J.L., Hutchings, H.C., Paterson, M., & Harris, E.D., Jr. (1988). The cost-effectiveness of auranofin: Results of a randomized clinical trial. *Journal of Rheumatology, 15*(1), 35–42.

Thompson, M.S., Read, J.L., & Liang, M. (1982). Willingness-to-pay concepts for societal decisions in health. In R.L. Kane & R.A. Kane (Eds.), *Values and long-term care* (pp. 103–125). Lexington, MA: Lexington Books.

Torrance, G.W. (1982). Multiattribute utility theory as a method of measuring social preferences for health states in long-term care. In R.L. Kane & R.A. Kane (Eds.), *Values and long-term care* (pp. 127–156). Lexington, MA: Lexington Books.

Torrance, G.W. (1986). Measurement of health state utilities for economic appraisal: A review. *Journal of Health Economics, 5*(1), 1–30.

Torrance, G.W., Erickson, P., Patrick, D.L., & Feldman, J.J. (1995). Technical notes. In P. Erickson, R. Wilson, & I. Shannon, *Years of healthy life, Statistical Note 7.* Hyattsville, MD: National Center for Health Statistics.

Torrance, G.W., & Feeny, D. (1989). Utilities and quality-adjusted life years. *International Journal of Technology Assessment in Health Care, 5,* 559–575.

Torrance, G.W., Thomas, W.H., & Sackett, D.L. (1972). A utility maximization model for evaluation of health care programs. *Health Services Research, 7*(2), 118–133.

Torrance, G.W., & Zipursky, A. (1977). *Cost-effectiveness of treatment with anti-D.* Rh Prevention Conference, McMaster University, Hamilton, Ontario, Canada.

Torrance, G.W., & Zipursky, A. (1984). Cost-effectiveness of antepartum prevention of Rh immunization. *Clinics in Perinatology, 11*(2), 267–281.

U.S. Bureau of the Census. (1993). *Statistical abstract of the United States: 1992* (112th ed.). Washington, DC: U.S. Government Printing Office.

Von Neumann, J., & Morgenstern, O. (1953). *Theory of games and economic behavior.* Princeton, NJ: Princeton University Press.

Ware, J.E. (1984). Conceptualizing disease impact and treatment outcomes. *Cancer, 53*(Suppl.), 2316–2323.

Ware, J.E., & Sherbourne, C.D. (1992). The MOS 36-Item Short Form Health Survey (SF-36): I. Conceptual framework and item selection. *Medical Care, 30*(6), 473–483.

Warner, K.E., & Luce, B.R. (1982). *Cost–benefit and cost-effectiveness analysis in health care: Principles, practice, and potential.* Ann Arbor, MI: Health Administration Press.

Weinberger, M., Smith, D.M., Katz, B.P., & Moore, P.S. (1988). The cost-effectiveness of intensive postdischarge care: A randomized trial. *Medical Care, 26*(11), 1092–1102.

Weinstein, M.C., & Stason, W.B. (1982). Cost-effectiveness of coronary artery bypass surgery. *Circulation, 66*(Suppl. 3), 56–66.

Welch, H.G., & Larson, E.B. (1988). Dealing with limited resources: The Oregon decision to curtail funding for organ transplantation. *New England Journal of Medicine, 319*(3), 171–173.

Wennberg, J., & Gittelsohn, A. (1973). Small area variations in health care delivery. *Science, 182,* 1102–1108.

Whiteneck, G.G., Charlifue, S.W., Gerhart, K.A., Overholser, J., & Richardson, G. (1992). Quantifying handicap: A new measure of long-term rehabilitation outcomes. *Archives of Physical Medicine and Rehabilitation, 73*(6), 519–526.

Whitmore, G.A. (1973). Health state preferences and the social choice. In R.L. Berg (Ed.), *Health status indexes* (pp. 135–145). Chicago: Hospital Research and Educational Trust.

Wolfson, A.D., Sinclair, A.J., Bombardier, C., & McGeer, A. (1982). Preference measurements for functional status in stroke patients: Interrater and intertechnique comparisons. In R.L. Kane & R.A. Kane (Eds.). *Values and long-term care* (pp. 127–156). Lexington, MA: Lexington Books.

World Bank. (1993). *World development report 1993: Investing in health.* New York: Oxford University Press.

World Health Organization (WHO). (1980). *International classification of impairments, disabilities, and handicaps.* Geneva, Switzerland: Author.

CHAPTER 10

Designing and Interpreting Clinical Studies

Kenneth J. Ottenbacher

In discussing priorities in rehabilitation research, Kirby (1994) noted, "Because it can be argued that we are doing a fairly good job in patient care and teaching, and because there is evidence . . . that in research we are not, I submit that research is the major priority in rehabilitation today" (p. 56). According to Kirby (1994) and others (Fuhrer, 1987), the goal of rehabilitation outcomes research is to improve the services provided to people with a disability. This might sound like a rather straightforward undertaking. If a working knowledge of the scientific method is acquired and the knowledge is applied systematically to the problems of disability and handicap, we should be able to achieve the goal. As it turns out, however, few undertakings are quite as ambitious as the scientific study of therapeutic outcomes. There is little scientific evidence of what distinguishes effective from ineffective treatment in many areas of medical rehabilitation (Bach, Findley, & Klecz, 1993; Kirby, 1994). The question of what constitutes good, valid, and useful scientific evidence of effectiveness is not a trivial one. Without a good understanding of what composes useful scientific evidence, that is, evidence that can withstand the test of time, today's rehabilitation science may be tomorrow's therapeutic alchemy.

The purpose of this chapter is to discuss issues of design, analysis, and interpretation of rehabilitation outcomes studies. A primary goal of this discussion is to assist rehabilitation investigators in the production of research that will positively affect the lives of people with a disability and their families. The chapter addresses three major issues affecting outcomes research in clinical environments. The first issue relates to the selection of

This chapter was completed while the author was a faculty member in the Department of Rehabilitation Medicine, and Associate Director of the Center for Functional Assessment Research, State University of New York at Buffalo.

designs appropriate for examining rehabilitation outcomes. The second issue is differentiating between outcomes that are clinically significant and those that are statistically significant. The third issue is the importance of replication in establishing a body of knowledge that will help refine and guide the development of effective rehabilitation services. These three issues are part of the empirical matrix that forms the foundation for planning and implementing medical rehabilitation outcomes research.

DESIGN OF OUTCOMES RESEARCH

Definitions and Terms

Outcomes research is an attempt to describe and explain systematic covariations between events. In discussing outcomes research in medical rehabilitation Johnston and Granger (1994) stated, "Outcomes research measures the impact of medical interventions experienced by patients," and "intervention-oriented or clinical outcomes research is essential in understanding the effectiveness of medical and rehabilitation intervention and answering the questions that confront clinical professionals and case managers" (p. 297).

Common to all clinical outcomes studies is the act of comparison. Clinical experiments involve a comparison of dependent (i.e., outcomes) variable values in the presence of different values of the independent (i.e., treatment) variable. In extreme form, the independent (i.e., manipulated) variable may take on dichotomous values, usually present versus absent, that is, treatment versus no treatment. The basic question, of course, is whether different values of the dependent (i.e., outcomes) variables are associated with different values of the independent (i.e., treatment) variable. This comparison is usually accomplished by one of two basic strategies: within-subject designs and between-subjects designs.

Within-Subject Designs

As the term implies, in *within-subject designs,* the comparison is made within the same subjects across time. That is, the dependent variable is measured after the introduction of the independent variable and perhaps before and during intervention. Guyatt and colleagues (Guyatt, Heyting, Jaeschke, Keller, Adachi, & Roberts, 1990; Guyatt, Sackett, Taylor, Chung, Roberts, & Pugsley, 1986) have discussed and demonstrated the use of within-subject designs using small numbers of subjects in clinical medicine. They refer to these designs as randomized trials involving individual patients, or $N = 1$ randomized trials. Variations of these same designs are more commonly referred to as interrupted time-series designs (Cook & Campbell, 1979). The essence of the interrupted time-series design is the presence of repeated measurements and the introduction into the measurement process of an intervention (i.e., experimental change) (Cook & Campbell, 1979). The ability to apply these designs to individual patients has been identified as a major advantage in rehabilitation environments (Gonnella, 1989; Ottenbacher, 1993).

A schema for the simplest form of interrupted time-series design is 0 0 0 0 0 X 0 0 0 0 0, where 0 represents observations or measurements both before and after the introduction of treatment (X) (Campbell & Stanley, 1966). When applied to a single individual or a small series of individuals, these designs are referred to by a variety of terms including single-subject, single-case experimental designs, single-system designs, or $N = 1$ clinical or randomized trials (Barlow & Hersen, 1984; Bloom, Fisher, & Orme, 1995; Kazdin, 1982; Ottenbacher, 1986).

An excellent example of an interrupted time-series design was reported in the rehabilitation research literature by Carey, Matyas, and Oke (1993). They examined the effectiveness of an intervention program designed to improve the tactile and proprioceptive discrimination of people who have had a stroke. The time-series trial involved four AB designs and four multiple baseline experiments. An adaptation of the AB design for Patient 1 from the Carey et al. (1993) investigation is presented in Figure 1. This design illustrates the basic characteristics of the simplest form of interrupted time-series design applied to a single patient. These characteristics include the repeated collection of data and the comparison of within-subject performance on the dependent variable.

The example illustrates a within-subject (i.e., interrupted time series) design where the unit of analysis was a single subject or series of subjects. Interrupted time-series designs can also be used with groups in which the comparison is within or across the same subjects over time. For example, Meythalre and colleagues (1992) examined the effect of intrathecal administration of baclofen in reducing muscle tone in 10 patients with spinal cord spasticity using an interrupted time-series design.

As noted earlier, the distinguishing characteristic of interrupted time-series designs is the presence of repeated measurements. A single application of the treatment (X), however, is not sufficient to establish a cause-and-effect association in an interrupted time-series design, regardless of how many measurements (0's) are taken prior to or following the intervention. To establish confidence in the cause-and-effect connection between the independent and dependent variable using an interrupted time-series design, the researcher must provide sequential applications. An illustration of this concept is presented in Figure 2, where data are repeatedly collected during a baseline phase and following introduction of the treatment for three different subjects. Inspection of the figure reveals that the introduction of the treatment is staggered across each subject. This interrupted time-series design is referred to as a multiple baseline design

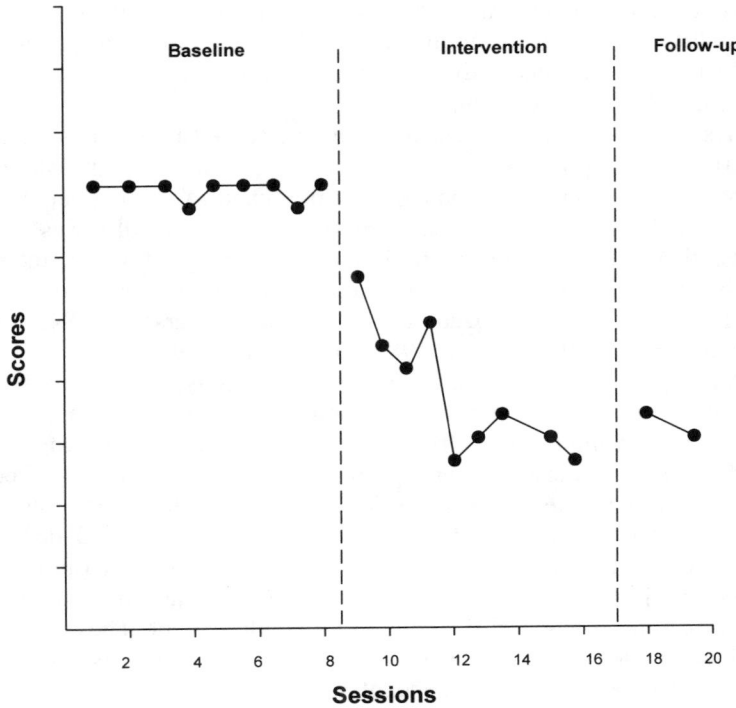

Figure 1. Performance of one subject on a tactile discrimination task displayed across three phases: Baseline, intervention, and follow-up. (Adapted from Carey, Matyas, & Oke (1993).)

across subjects (Ottenbacher, 1986) and provides convincing evidence of an intervention effect, assuming, of course, that there is consistent observable change each time the treatment is introduced (see Figure 2).

The analysis of interrupted time-series designs ranges from simple to quantitatively complex. At the simple end of the analysis continuum, the investigator plots the data using an $x-y$ chart (see Figure 1) and visually examines the results to determine whether a clinically important change in performance has occurred over the phases. At the complex end of the analysis continuum are autoregressive integrated moving average (ARIMA) models (McCleary, Hay, Medinger, & Powell, 1980). Between these two extremes, a large number of statistical procedures and supplements to visual inspection are available for analysis of interrupted time-series data. A substantial debate has developed since the mid-1980s regarding the relative merits (and demerits) of both visual and statistical analysis of interrupted time-series data (Ottenbacher, 1992, 1993). A researcher interested in using interrupted time-series designs to examine rehabilitation outcomes must

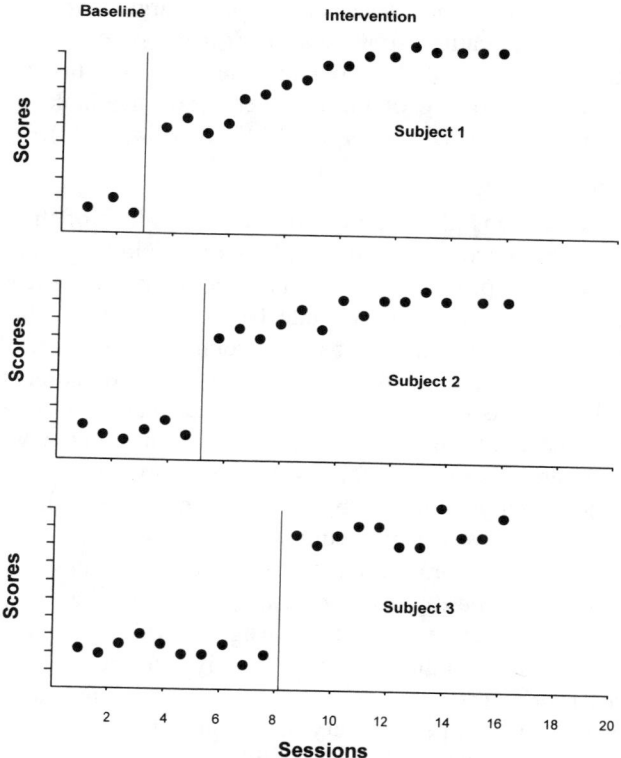

Figure 2. Interrupted time-series design (multiple baseline) across subjects. All subjects begin the study at the same time, but the intervention is introduced at different times for each subject.

make a decision regarding the most appropriate method of analysis based on the research question, the nature of the data collected, and the type of within-subject design used.

There are many variations of within-subject designs. Some of these designs provide powerful methods of examining outcomes, particularly outcomes for individual patients. These include reversal designs and versions of the multiple baseline design (see Figure 2). Bloom and associates (1995) provided an excellent discussion and description of many interrupted time-series designs, and their text should be a valuable resource to clinicians and researchers planning rehabilitation outcomes investigations using a within-subject approach.

One limitation of interrupted time-series designs applied to a small series of subjects is the inability to generalize the findings using a statistical model. The findings from within-subject designs based on a small N can be generalized, but the strategy for generalization is based on replication, not on the random selection of subjects from a target population. Information regarding replication strategies and other issues associated with interrupted time-series research is beyond the scope of this chapter, and the reader is referred to one of the excellent texts available in this area (Barlow & Hersen, 1984; Bloom et al., 1995; Kazdin, 1982).

Between-Subjects Designs

Between-subject designs also attempt to compare values of the dependent variables in the presence of different values of the independent variable. In these designs, the primary strategy is to look at differences *between* people. Ideally, the comparison is made between subjects who have not been exposed to the treatment (i.e., independent variable) and those who have received the treatment. Historically, most between-subjects designs have involved comparisons between groups rather than between individual subjects; thus, the between-subjects design is often equated with group-comparison research. Between-subjects designs, particularly those associated with random assignment of subjects to groups, have traditionally been defined as the most powerful procedures to establish cause-and-effect relationships. In the behavioral and social sciences, these designs are commonly referred to as *true experiments* (Campbell & Stanley, 1966). In the biomedical sciences, between-subjects designs involving random assignment of participants to conditions are frequently referred to as *randomized clinical trials, randomized controlled trials,* or *RCTs*. This category of between-subjects designs is held in very high regard because of its ability to control for multiple threats to internal validity. The internal validity of an investigation refers to the degree of confidence the investigator (and reader) can have that any change in observed outcome is a function of the independent variable and not a function of some extraneous or uncontrolled factor.

In discussing various research approaches available to rehabilitation researchers, Reilly and Findley (1989) noted that "true random experiments are the best way to establish causation" (p. 197). The true experimental design involves a comparison in which participants are randomly assigned to groups or conditions (Reilly & Findley, 1989). This random assignment provides an equality between groups based on probability. That is, the probability is high that the two groups are equal on the outcomes measure of interest. The subjects in one group are exposed to the independent (i.e., treatment) variable, and the performance of both groups is measured on some operationally defined dependent (i.e., outcomes) variable. Based on the obtained results, a null hypothesis, which generally states that there is no difference between the performance of the two groups, is evaluated. If the results are found to be statistically significant at a predetermined probability level, then the null hypothesis is rejected. The alternative hypothesis, that the two groups differ on the dependent variable, is supported. Properly implemented, the RCT provides a high degree of confidence regarding cause-and-effect relationships between independent and dependent variables. This confidence is based on the fact that the RCT controls for many of the threats to internal validity originally identified by Campbell and Stanley (1966).

The disadvantage of the true experimental configuration is that it is often difficult or impossible to implement in a clinical setting. The limitations of RCTs were described by Kramer and Shapiro (1984), who noted that "despite the obvious advantages and impressive track record of RCT's, clinical investigators have become increasingly aware of certain difficulties in the interpretation, feasibility and ethics" (p. 2739). The primary difficulties involved in conducting RCTs in clinical environments are small sample size, lack of homogeneity in people with disabling conditions, inability to withhold or delay intervention for people in comparison or control groups, difficulty in establishing a standard intervention protocol appropriate for all patients, and the inability to collect information on functional outcomes measures that can be blindly recorded (Andrews, 1991; Gladman, 1991; Kramer & Shapiro, 1984).

In discussing this issue in rehabilitation research, Johnston and Granger (1994) made an important distinction between effectiveness research and efficacy investigations:

> Randomized clinical trials (RCT's) . . . are frequently limited in their generalizability. RCT's are typically efficacy studies involving distinctly selected patient subgroups at university medical facilities. In contrast, outcomes research studies effectiveness in facilities with a staff of average competency, practical levels of funding and the normal range of variation in patients served. (p. 298)

They also noted that the distinction between ideal efficacy and real-world clinical effectiveness is particularly important in rehabilitation, where large variations exist across patients, treatments, and facilities.

The difficulty in meeting the requirements of RCTs in clinical environments has led investigators to use modified versions of classic experimental (i.e., between-subjects) designs. Variations of true experimental designs are referred to as quasi-experiments. They do not provide the same degree of methodologic control over threats to internal validity as do true experiments. For example, many quasi-experimental designs do not include random assignment of subjects to treatment and control groups.

The use of quasi-experimental designs in clinical fields has led to criticism of the research literature. Detractors frequently argue that the reported studies are methodologically weak and scientifically uninterpretable (Pollock, Freemantle, Seldon, Song, & Mason, 1993). Researchers proposing or reporting outcomes investigations not using RCTs or other randomized experimental designs frequently find that their proposals are not funded or their papers are not published (Andrews, 1991). Some rehabilitation investigators have suggested that a restrictive conceptualization of acceptable research design has reduced our ability to conduct and collect outcomes research on the effectiveness of rehabilitation practice (Andrews, 1991; Gladman, 1991; Spencer, 1993).

The design, whether within-subject or between-subjects, provides a framework for manipulating variables and collecting data. A primary function of any design is to ensure that information is collected in a way that will maximize interpretation and explanation. The ultimate goal of any experimental study is to help understand the phenomenon being investigated. There is an interaction between the design and level of empirical explanation that is attained.

EXPLICATION AND EXPERIMENTATION

Research design, broadly conceived, refers to the methods of arranging observations so that principles and relationships can be identified. Campbell and Stanley (1966) originally divided research strategies into three categories: pre-experimental, quasi-experimental, and true experimental. Within this framework, research designs are viewed along a continuum of control. Pre-experimental designs are considered weak because these designs demonstrate little control over various threats to internal validity. In contrast, true experimental designs are considered more powerful and provide maximum control in minimizing threats to internal validity, which Campbell and Stanley (1966) identified as the sine qua non of experimental research.

The design framework proposed by Campbell and Stanley (1966) is well established and widely taught in the behavioral, social, and biomedical sciences. The ability to infer causal relationships from true experimental designs is undisputed. Several authorities have argued, however, that the view of research design along a continuum of control reflects a narrow operationalism that limits applied research (Barlow, Hayes, & Nelson, 1984; Cronbach, 1983). A more flexible approach to research design in which relevance is considered as important as internal validity is emerging. Cronbach (1983) suggested that outcomes studies should be guided by attempts to construct designs that meet situational needs, rather than focusing strictly on the requirements of an idealized true experiment. Creating the best research design, in this view, involves multiple considerations, including the purpose of the investigation, the specific setting, and the available resources. Cronbach (1983) argued that there is no single ideal standard for designs in clinical or applied environments. Any design is an interplay of resources, possibilities, creativity, and personal judgments.

The way research design is usually taught to students and portrayed in the professional journals implies that the design is an open window through which the phenomenon of interest can be studied in an unobstructed manner. The stronger the design in terms of control, as defined by Campbell and Stanley (1966), the sharper the view of the outside world. This window analogy suggests that the design allows researchers to uncover a phenomenon, but that the design does not directly contribute to the results. Evidence now exists that this assumption is false (Colditz, Miller, & Mosteller, 1986; Gehan, 1984; Grice & Hunter, 1964; Ottenbacher, 1992). The findings of a clinical trial, no matter how well it is designed, do not provide a picture of the world independently of the methods used to collect the information. Therefore, no investigation can isolate a relationship between independent and dependent variables outside the context of the design.

Numerous articles and tutorials have been published providing guidelines regarding the design attributes and statistical criteria a clinical outcomes trial should include (Rieglman & Hirsch, 1989; Sackett, 1986). These design checklists educate readers about various components of the research process as they relate to conducting and interpreting a single clinical trial. They are less informative, however, when the question turns from interpreting a single investigation to synthesizing the results of multiple clinical trials. When the task shifts to interpreting a series of clinical trials rather than a single investigation, the idealized design approach can be misleading. Using preselected design criteria to interpret a series of therapeutic trials may lead to a form of methodologic myopia. Research suggests that judgments regarding how design quality variables interact with clinical outcomes should be an empirical question, not an a priori assumption derived from a pre-established design hierarchy (Ottenbacher, 1992).

The assumption exists on the part of journal editors and grant reviewers that clinical trials not meeting some predetermined design criterion (such as random assignment) are biased in favor of the independent variable and produce spurious positive results (Pollock et al., 1993). This assumption was operationalized by Sackett (1986) and by others (Rieglman & Hirsch, 1989) in various strategies to interpret and integrate multiple studies. Sackett's (1986) model provides a framework based on design characteristics that translates to five levels of evidence. The levels of evidence model assumes that trials of poor design quality are more likely to produce positive (i.e., statistically significant) results.

The issue of how design attributes interact with clinical outcomes was addressed by Williamson, Goldschmidt, and Colton (1986). In their comprehensive methodologic review, Williamson and colleagues (1986) found eight articles in which the authors compared research findings for a given topic with the quality of the research design. In analyzing these methodologically adequate reviews, Williamson and colleagues found that 305 investigations were judged methodologically adequate. Of these 305 trials, approximately 25% reported statistically significant findings. Conversely, approximately 80% of those clinical trials judged to be methodologically inadequate ($N = 449$) reported statistically positive findings. The clear implication from this analysis is that trials of poor methodologic quality are biased and more likely to produce (spurious) positive results in favor of the independent variable. An alternative explanation for the findings reported in the Williamson et al. (1986) investigation is that those studies judged to be methodologically adequate—that is, affiliated with rigorous designs—were also associated with smaller sample sizes. In addition, the smaller sample sizes contributed to low statistical power and therefore produced fewer statistically significant results. The influence of statistical power is discussed in more detail in the next section.

The findings of meta-analytic reviews specifically examining design as a moderator variable indicate that the assumption underlying the levels of evidence model is not universally warranted. This is particularly true when statistical results are translated to measures of effect size, such as weighted d-indexes, that are not sample-size-sensitive (Cooper & Hedges, 1994; Wortman, 1994). In fact, the opposite argument (assumption) regarding outcomes in therapeutic clinical trials has been made (Weiss & Weiss, 1990). That is, trials with poor designs allow the introduction of random variation or error and make it more difficult to uncover a treatment effect when one is present. Thus, clinical trials with poor (i.e., weak) designs are more likely to contain large error variance and produce negative (i.e., nonsignificant) results. Conversely, a well-controlled trial eliminates or reduces random variability or noise and therefore increases between-groups variability.

Examples exist in the biomedical and behavioral science literature of specific research areas in which design characteristics are associated with positive outcomes, negative outcomes, or show no relationship to outcomes (Colditz et al., 1986; Gehan, 1984; Shapiro & Shapiro, 1982). For example, Ottenbacher (1992) examined the covariation between design characteristics and trial outcomes in 60 articles published in two premier medical journals, the *Journal of the American Medical Association* and the *New England Journal of Medicine*. The design characteristics of each study were coded and analyzed in relation to the study outcome. All trials examined the effectiveness of some therapeutic intervention. The findings revealed that statistically significant results were more frequently reported for designs where random assignment of subjects was not used. However, when the statistical results were transformed to effect sizes (d-indexes) and examined by type of assignment, there was no significant difference in effect size between trials using random assignment and those not using random assignment. The effect size values were weighted to account for sample size differences. Sample size is a factor that is known to influence the results of statistical significance testing.

The results of these studies suggest that design attributes should be considered as potential moderator variables and the relationship of design to trial outcome investigated. If covariation is found between a design attribute and a statistical result in a series of trials, then this characteristic must be considered as a moderator variable in the evaluation and interpretation of trial results and in the planning of future investigations. For example, if clinical trials that use random assignment to conditions are associated with results more (or less) favorable than trials that do not include this design characteristic, then the design attribute must be considered in any attempt to evaluate and synthesize related trials. If, however, no relationship exists between a particular design characteristic and trial outcome, then studies with and without the design feature should not be treated differently when examining a series of clinical trials. This empirical judgment can be made by considering research design as a moderator variable and determining its contribution to aggregated research outcomes as we would any other important moderator variable.

The preceding discussion should not be interpreted as an argument against the use of randomized clinical trials or against the consideration of design quality factors in the evaluation and synthesis of clinical research. On the contrary, design attributes are of the utmost importance. In fact, design considerations are too important to be conceptualized as predetermined categories that capture empirical quality. Design characteristics should be examined in relation to specific research outcomes whenever any attempt is made to integrate and interpret multiple clinical trials. If investigators adopt such a practice, we will avoid the rigidity that sometimes allows empirical habit to overpower scientific originality and subordinates research problems to methodology.

STATISTICAL VERSUS CLINICAL SIGNIFICANCE

One area of well-established empirical habit is the interpretation of statistical significance. Rehabilitation researchers and clinicians often operationalize clinical significance by equating it with statistical significance. This is a practice that has caused considerable confusion in the research literature on rehabilitation outcomes. Positive results from these investigations are usually interpreted as those associated with statistically significant outcomes (Anscombe, 1990). Statistical significance is a function of several factors. One of the most important contributors to statistical significance is sample size (Anscombe, 1990; Gore, 1981).

The tendency of some clinical researchers to treat the $p < .05$ alpha level as a probability cliff where a result associated with a p-value of .04

is treated as clinically important and a result with a p-value of .06 is judged as clinically nonsignificant represents an unfortunate misinterpretation of significance testing. As a result of this misinterpretation, research results supporting the null hypothesis are treated as if they were qualitatively different from research reports failing to support the null hypothesis.

Statistical significance depends on several factors unrelated to the magnitude of any real-world experimental effect. First, whether a finding is statistically significant depends on the alpha level that the investigator selects, which, by convention, is set at .05 or .01. The statistical significance of a finding is also a function of sample size, although the relationship of significance level to sample size is nonlinear, being generally a function of $\sqrt{N}$. Consequently, studies with large numbers of subjects tend to yield smaller p-values, all other factors being equal.

Statistical significance also depends, in part, on the power of the statistical evaluation, and the precision with which the experiment is carried out. According to Cohen (1977), "the power of a statistical test of a null hypothesis is the probability that it will lead to the rejection of the null hypothesis, i.e., the probability that it will result in the conclusion that the phenomenon exists" (p. 4). Power is typically defined as 1-beta. Beta is the probability of making a Type 2 error. A Type 2 error occurs when a researcher, mistakenly, supports the null hypothesis when it should have been rejected.

When all other factors are kept constant, the larger the effect size, the smaller the p-value will be. The relation, however, between effect size and statistical significance is nonlinear, and drawing inferences about the magnitude of a treatment effect from the statistical significance associated with it is not warranted. Rosenthal (1991) provided an excellent example of how confusion associated with traditional statistical significance testing can lead to spurious conclusions regarding treatment effectiveness. Suppose a rehabilitation researcher, "White," conducts a between-subjects study using a true experimental design with treatment and control groups. The statistical results of White's study are $F = 4.88$ ($df = 1, 78; p < .05$). Based on this statistically significant result, White rejects the null hypothesis. A second rehabilitation investigator, "Black," performs a replication experiment using the same design and variables as White, but Black reports a statistically nonsignificant result ($F = 1.12$ ($df = 1, 18; p < .30$). The statistical findings of the two studies conflict. The second trial by Black is considered a failure to replicate, and the effectiveness of the treatment is called into question. The results appear to be black (i.e., nonsignificant) and white (i.e., significant). But are they?

Calculation of effect sizes for the two studies reveals that both the White and Black studies produced the same d-index ($d = 2\sqrt{F} \div \sqrt{df} = .50$). This finding suggests that the standardized mean difference (i.e., presumed treatment effect) is the same in both investigations, yet one trial reported a statistically significant result and the other reported a nonsignificant statistical outcome. Further analysis reveals that the statistical power of White's study is approximately 0.80, and the power of Black's study is less than 0.30. In this example, the effect of the independent variable (i.e., treatment) is equal in both investigations (i.e., $d = 0.50$), in spite of the difference in statistical outcomes. The discrepancy is due to the difference in sample size. White used a larger sample ($N = 80$) that resulted in adequate power to test the hypothesis and relatively low probability of a Type 2 error. Black, with a smaller sample ($N = 20$) and low power, did not report a statistically significant result, despite the fact that the effect size was the same in both trials. The low power in Black's trial indicates the high probability ($> 70\%$) of a Type 2 error (supporting a false null hypothesis).

Research on the statistical power of published rehabilitation research suggests that many clinically based studies have potentially high rates of Type 2 errors (Ottenbacher, 1995; Ottenbacher & Barrett, 1989, 1990). These errors produce statistical confusion in attempting to establish a research literature on treatment effectiveness in rehabilitation.

The limitations of significance testing have been well documented, and numerous supplements or alternatives have been proposed (Cohen, 1988; Lipsey, 1990; Oakes, 1987; Pocock, 1983). At one extreme, several authors have argued that researchers should abandon statistical significance testing and apply other methods of evaluating outcomes (Carver, 1993; Salsburg, 1992). The reality is, however, that significance testing is an established component of the research process, and there are few indications that rehabilitation researchers will stop using p-levels (Anscombe, 1990). Assuming that significance testing remains an integral part of the way in which clinical researchers evaluate hypotheses, there are procedures that can be used to help ensure the integrity of the inferences that are made and reduce the incidence of Type 2 errors. One frequently advocated supplement to statistical significance testing is the calculation of effect size measures. Cohen (1977, 1988) proposed various measures of effect size appropriate for a wide range of designs and statistical procedures. For example, the d-index, described earlier, measures the difference between two means in terms of their common standard deviation units. If $d = .20$, then a .2 standard deviation separates the average subject in one group from the average subject in the control or comparison group.

Several researchers in the biomedical and rehabilitation sciences have proposed that investigators routinely report effect sizes as an indicator of how much of a treatment effect is present (Ottenbacher, 1992, 1995). The emphasis on reporting effect size measures is particularly strong in clinical fields, where the distinction between effect sizes of clinical significance and effect sizes of statistical significance are not easily made. For example, the editor of the *Journal of Gerontology* has stated:

> We are increasingly insistent that authors address the issue of effect magnitude, both in terms of the statistics reported and the discussion of the implications of the research. Any effect can be shown to be significant given sufficiently large sample sizes. The real question is whether or not the effect is important; measures of effect size help the researcher answer this question. (Storandt, 1983, p. 2)

Another frequently suggested supplement to significance testing is the use of confidence intervals. Gardner and Altman (1989) argued that the use of confidence intervals would produce a move away from a single-value estimate (*p*-value) to a range of values considered plausible for the population. The width of a confidence interval based on a sample statistic depends partly on its standard error; thus, both the standard deviation and sample size are included in the computation. If the scores from the hypothetical White and Black trials described earlier are assumed to be normally distributed and the population variances are assumed to be approximately equal, then the computation of confidence intervals would have revealed that the confidence intervals for the Black study did not include 0. This finding suggests that supporting the null hypothesis was not an appropriate inference in the Black trial, despite the fact that the result was not statistically significant. The concept of confidence intervals is widely understood, if not widely used, in rehabilitation research. Many examples and illustrations of confidence intervals exist in the clinical research literature (Anscombe, 1990).

THE IMPORTANCE OF REPLICATION

In their classic article on the law of small numbers, published in 1971, Tversky and Kahneman observed that "the emphasis on significance levels tends to obscure a fundamental distinction between the size of an effect and its statistical significance. Regardless of sample size, the size of an effect in one study is a reasonable estimate of the size of an effect in replication" (p. 110), and concluded that "unrealistic expectations concerning the replicability of significance levels may be corrected if the distinction between sample size and significance is clarified, and if the computed size of observed effects is routinely reported" (p. 110). Along similar lines, Hedges (1987) observed, "A fundamental question for any scientific research program is, How cumulative should we expect empirical results to be? That is, how much consistency should we expect of the results of replicated experiments?" (p. 453).

Standard Model of Replication

Hedges (1987) defined *scientific consensus* as the "degree of agreement among replicated experiments, or the degree to which related experimental results fit into a simple pattern that makes conceptual sense" (p. 443). The development of a *body of knowledge* in rehabilitation research implies a series of trials examining a particular research question. To establish a body of knowledge examining medical rehabilitation outcomes requires replication research (Lindsay & Ehrenberg, 1993; Mulkay & Gilbert, 1986). Successful replication is generally taken to mean that a null hypothesis that has been rejected in the original experimental trial will be rejected in a second or subsequent investigation. This model of replication, based on the results of traditional statistical significance testing, was discussed in detail by Rosenthal (1991) and is presented in Figure 3. The logic associated with the model in Figure 3 was described by Goodman (1992). He states that "in practice, if a *p*-value is low enough to be considered significant, the observed effect is often claimed to be 'real,' with the subsequent thought that a replication of the experiment should, with high probability, produce a similar statistical verdict" (Goodman, 1992, pp. 875–876).

The assumption made in using this model is that, if a real treatment effect exists in the population, it should produce statistically significant results (i.e., reject the null hypothesis) in the initial experimental trial and when the investigation is repeated. If the null hypothesis is rejected in follow-up studies, researchers can conclude that a successful replication has been achieved and that the theory tested or the intervention under investigation is supported. Conversely, if the first study produces statistically significant results and the second investigation produces statistically nonsignificant results, then the frequent conclusion is that the results of the two studies conflict. There is a lack of consensus, that is, a failure to replicate. (See the hypothetical White and Black example in the previous section.)

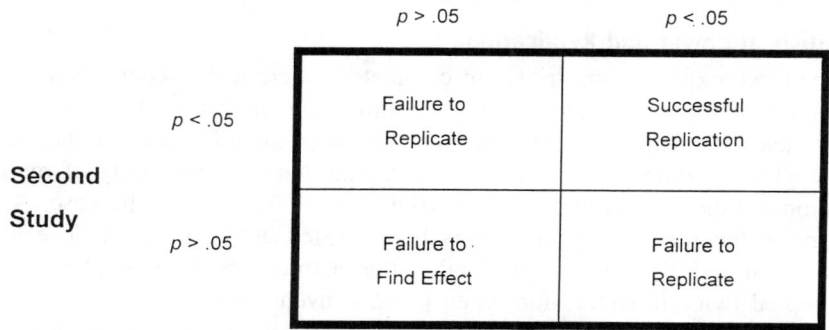

Figure 3. Standard model of replication based on statistical significance testing.

Reliance on the results of statistical significance testing to confirm or refute empirical consensus has a long history in the social and behavioral sciences (Freeman, 1993; Johnstone, 1986; Lykken, 1968; Oakes, 1987; Tversky & Kahneman, 1971). Light and Smith (1971) referred to the practice of using the results of tests of statistical significance to confirm the success of replication efforts as the *vote-counting method*. Hedges and Olkin (1985) noted that "conventional vote counting or box score methodology uses the outcome of the tests of significance in a series of replicated studies to draw conclusions about the magnitude of the treatment effects" (p. 48). Using the vote-counting method, the investigator identifies replicated studies and counts the number with statistically significant results and compares this number to the number of studies with nonsignificant results.

Vote counting fits the model of replication presented in Figure 3. Its main attractions are simplicity and the ability to quickly confirm consistent findings. Despite its apparent simplicity, vote counting can lead to serious errors in the attempt to develop consensus from the statistical results of replicated clinical trials. For instance, assume that 7 of 10 replicated studies reported statistically nonsignificant results. The conclusion based on the vote-counting method (see Figure 3) would be that the seven statistically nonsignificant studies reflect a failure to replicate. If the program is genuinely ineffective, only about 5% of the experimental trials should report statistically significant outcomes due to chance alone (assuming a $p < .05$ probability of Type 1 error). Yet 30% of the studies in the example produced statistically significant results. This large number of statistically significant effects does not reflect random variation around a null hypothesis.

A second and perhaps more important problem with vote counting and the logic of replication presented in Figure 3 is that it ignores statistical power. When sample size and effect size are small, a simple vote count often fails to identify a significant overall treatment effect and leads to the conclusion that a failure to replicate has occurred.

Statistical Power and Replication

When two experimental trials are conducted wherein the second is a replication of the first, what is the probability that both investigations will produce statistically significant results? Based on the information contained in Figure 3, some investigators may imagine that the probability of replication for the second experimental trial is 95%. This is not the case. Assuming that the null hypothesis is being tested at the $p < .05$ level of statistical significance, the probability that a true hypothesis (H_0) will be accepted twice in succession when using conventional statistical methods is $.95^2$, or .9025. In contrast, the probability that it will be falsely rejected twice is $.05^2$, or .025. Thus, the overall probability of replication is $.9025 + .025$, or approximately .93 when H_0 is true.

In general, if a replication study uses the same sample size and thus has the same power as the original study, then the probability of a replication is $p^2 + (1 + p)^2$. The value of .93 for the preceding example is an approximation that does not take into consideration the influence of statistical power. If the investigator conducting a replication study is examining a genuine effect (the true research [alternative] hypothesis, H_a), then power becomes a critical factor in determining the success of any replication effort.

The impact of low statistical power on successful replication is easily illustrated with an example. Assume that a researcher has conducted a series of appropriately designed replication studies with a mean power of .40, the probability of replication p(replication) $= .40^2 + (1 - .40)^2$ is .52. This value is even less encouraging if it is considered that, because of the low power, the majority of the replications in this example represent confirmations of a false impression. In fact, $(1 - .40)^2 + [.40^2 + (1 - .40)^2 = .88$, or 88% of the replications' strength, a false impression (a Type 2 error).

The overall probability of replication in a given field further depends on the proportion of times the researcher has selected a true null or non-null hypothesis, that is, on the a priori probability of the research hypothesis (H_a) being true. If it is assumed that $p(H_a) = .30$, $\alpha = .05$, and a power of .40 to detect a medium effect size ($d = .50$), then the overall probability of replication is p(replication) $= .7[.05^2 + (1 - .05)^2] + .3[.40^2 + (1 - .40)^2] = .79$.

Of course, it is preferable to imagine that theories, observations, and prior studies in medical rehabilitation are valuable guides to future research, so that investigators are led to conduct research where the population effect does exist more often than 30% of the time. If the preceding example is reversed, so that $p(H_a) = .70$ and $p(H_0) = .30$, the result is p(replication) $= .63$, a lower value. The paradoxical conclusion is that the more often the researcher is well guided by theory and prior observation but conducts a *low-power study,* the more the probability of replication is decreased! Of course, if theories and prior observations lead researchers to test what are true null hypotheses, the practice of setting α at $p < .05$ will allow a high probability of replication. It thus appears that the best chance of replication under current practice occurs when no effect is discovered, that is, when a true null hypothesis is examined.

IMPLICATIONS

At the beginning of this chapter, it was noted that three methodologic factors can be identified that interfere with establishing a useful knowledge base regarding rehabilitation outcomes. The first is a narrow conceptualization of research design in which clinical trials that do not meet certain predetermined criteria are considered scientifically unacceptable. The second is confusion regarding statistical significance testing and the tendency of researchers to misinterpret clinical and statistical significance. The third factor is failure to appreciate the negative impact that low statistical power and Type 2 errors have on the ability to establish a consensus regarding what is effective intervention, that is, to produce a body of knowledge on rehabilitation effectiveness.

These three factors are not mutually exclusive. The factors interact in a complex manner to potentially obscure the interpretation of rehabilitation effectiveness. The first factor limits the number of investigations that researchers are willing to seriously consider in developing an empirical knowledge base regarding rehabilitation outcomes. The second and third factors reduce researchers' ability to accurately interpret the results of individual clinical trials, and, perhaps more important, they prevent researchers from synthesizing existing investigations to determine whether a consensus exists regarding the effectiveness of various rehabilitation interventions.

An illustration of the problems caused by these three factors can be found by examining the research literature on the effectiveness of stroke rehabilitation. Lind (1982) reviewed the findings of what he identified as the eight best clinical trials investigating stroke rehabilitation. The trials were examined according to type of research design and statistical analysis, with particular attention being paid to threats to internal validity. Lind (1982) concluded his review by stating that the "results of these studies conflict and the conclusions vary widely" (p. 149). This conclusion was based on the fact that some trials reported statistically significant results, whereas others produced statistically nonsignificant results. Lind's (1982) interpretation relied on the model of replication presented in Figure 3. Some of the stroke rehabilitation trials he examined rejected the null hypothesis ($p < .05$), and other trials that he examined did not reject the null hypothesis ($p > .05$). A meta-analysis of 36 experimental and quasi-experimental trials examining the effectiveness of stroke rehabilitation revealed a mean effect size (d-index) of .40 ($SD = .33$) (Ottenbacher & Jannell, 1993). This effect size would be considered small according to Cohen's (1988) criteria. In a related analysis, Matyas and Ottenbacher (1993) demonstrated that the mean power values required to determine population effect sizes in the ranges Cohen defines as small, medium, and large were 0.12, 0.41, and 0.67, respectively. These power values correspond to Type 2 error rates ranging from .88 to .33.

The stroke rehabilitation d-index of .40, though moderate, may have important practical, clinical, or cost-effectiveness implications. The probability of this effect being identified as statistically significant through replication research appears quite low, given the power of stroke rehabilitation clinical trials. The conclusion by Lind (1982) that the results of stroke rehabilitation trials "conflict and the conclusions vary widely" (p. 133) is understandable when the low statistical power and high probability of a Type 2 error in the individual clinical trials are recognized. Lind's conclusion, however, may reflect confusion regarding the interpretation of the statistical results as opposed to the actual impact of the treatment. As Lipsey, Crosse, Pankle, Pollard, and Stobart (1985) accurately noted, "research with low statistical power has the potential for falsely branding a program as a failure when, in fact, the problem is the inability of the research to detect an effect, not the inability of the program to produce one" (p. 26).

CONCLUSIONS

The debate and discussion regarding the advantages and strengths of various research strategies for outcomes research have the potential to infuse clinical investigation in rehabilitation with flexibility and relevance (Wortman, 1994). Many investigators (this author included) have displayed a tendency to be overzealous in their use and promotion of traditional experimental methods and associated statistical procedures, much like the young child who, when first given a hammer, finds that everything he encounters needs pounding. Not all rehabilitation research questions need to be hammered with the RCT and statistical null hypothesis testing. The evolving discussion concerning the merits of various research strategies makes it clear that traditional experimental designs are a valuable and viable empirical option, but that they are not the absolute ideal in every situation (Whyte, 1995). The debate regarding strategies to assess effectiveness will help legitimize and increase the acceptance of qualitative, idiographic, and other alternative research approaches. The continuing discussion will force investigators to focus not only on outcomes as traditionally defined but also on rehabilitation process and the ecology of disability.

These topics have not been afforded a high priority in the traditional experimental paradigm (Spencer, 1993; Whiteneck, 1994). To develop a useful body of knowledge, researchers must become proficient in a variety of empirical strategies so that they can explore research problems without quantitative or qualitative parochialism. Rehabilitation researchers must strive to learn new ways of combining methods and reconciling discrepant findings without arbitrarily rejecting one set of procedures in favor of another. Investigators should be modest in their claims regarding specific designs and realize that, in clinical settings, all designs and statistical procedures are fallible. The discovery of a bias or weakness in a research strategy is not necessarily a reason to reject the method but is instead a challenge to improve it, just as we strive to improve or to refine a theory in the face of disconfirming data.

In reporting and interpreting the results of outcomes trials, particularly those that use statistical tests to assist in data analysis, rehabilitation researchers must realize that the ultimate judgment regarding the clinical importance of a finding cannot be a statistical one. Judgments regarding the clinical importance of rehabilitation outcomes trials can be improved if investigators consistently report descriptive statistics and present statistical significance in the appropriate context. In most cases, this will involve supplementing the results of statistical significance testing with a measure of effect size or confidence levels. If the results of a statistical significance test are negative, then the researcher should report the power of the test and the corresponding probability of a Type 2 error. The probability of a Type 1 error (usually $p < .05$) is always known and is essential in interpreting the results of statistical tests where the null hypothesis is rejected, that is, where the results are statistically significant. When the results are not statistically significant, researchers rarely provide any information regarding the probability that they made the correct decision. Lipsey (1990) argued that the failure to report information on Type 2 errors and statistical power "degrades our ability to learn from research, to differentiate successful treatments from unsuccessful ones and find the keys to making the successful ones work even better" (p. 26). Information on statistical power is essential in planning and interpreting rehabilitation outcomes research trials where null hypothesis testing is used.

Replication research is required to develop a body of knowledge on the effectiveness of rehabilitation interventions. Ideally, the results of accumulated clinical investigations provide consensus on the research question of interest. The development of empirical consensus is an important aspect of establishing the effectiveness of rehabilitation interventions, regardless of the research approach used to conduct the individual investigations. The reporting of effect size values and developments in meta-analysis has direct implications for how we conduct and report replication studies. These implications suggest that the model of replication based on statistical significance testing as depicted in Figure 3 should be abandoned and replaced with a model that emphasizes consistency of effect size values across studies examining similar hypotheses. Rosenthal (1990) and Hedges (1987) argued that the traditional view of replication success, defined by dichotomous significance testing decisions, should be replaced by a new view of replication success defined by degree of agreement of effect sizes obtained across replicated investigations.

The philosopher of science, John Ziman, has stated that the "goal of science is a consensus of rational opinion over the widest possible field"

(Ziman, 1978, p. 3). This consensus is achieved through the replication of previous research. Ziman (1978) notes that "the results of repetitions of the same experiments are fundamental to the creation of any body of knowledge" (p. 56). Replication research should be promoted in the field of rehabilitation by professional organizations, funding agencies, and individual investigators. The effectiveness of rehabilitation interventions will be convincingly established only through the development of empirical consensus. This consensus must be based on clinical research that is appropriately designed, accurately analyzed, and clearly interpreted.

REFERENCES

Andrews, K. (1991). The limitations of randomized controlled trials in rehabilitation research. *Clinical Rehabilitation, 5,* 5–8.

Anscombe, F.J. (1990). The summarizing of clinical experiments by significance levels. *Statistics in Medicine, 9,* 703–708.

Bach, J.R., Findley, T.W., & Klecz, R. (1993). Physical medicine and rehabilitation: Trends in academic productivity. *American Journal of Physical Medicine and Rehabilitation, 72,* 62–66.

Barlow, D.H., Hayes, S., & Nelson, R.O. (1984). *The scientist practitioner: Research and accountability in clinical and educational settings.* New York: Pergamon.

Barlow, D.H., & Hersen, M. (1984). *Single case experimental designs* (2nd ed.). New York: Pergamon.

Bloom, M., Fisher, S., & Orme, J.G. (1995). *Evaluating practice: Guidelines for the accountable professional* (2nd ed.). Boston: Allyn & Bacon.

Campbell, P.T., & Stanley, J.C. (1966). *Experimental and quasi-experimental designs for research.* Chicago: Rand McNally.

Carey, L.M., Matyas, T.A., & Oke, L.E. (1993). Sensory loss in stroke patients: effective training of tactile and proprioceptive discrimination. *Archives of Physical Medicine and Rehabilitation, 74,* 602–611.

Carver, R.P. (1993). The case against statistical significance testing. Revised. *Journal of Experimental Education, 61,* 287–292.

Cohen, J. (1977). *Statistical power analysis for the behavioral sciences* (Rev. ed.). New York: Academic press.

Cohen, J. (1988). *Statistical power analysis for the behavioral sciences* (2nd ed.). Hillsdale, NJ: Lawrence Erlbaum Associates.

Colditz, G.A., Miller, J., & Mosteller, F. (1989). How study design affects outcome in comparison therapy: I. Medical. *Statistics in Medicine, 8,* 441–454.

Cook, T.P., & Campbell, P.T. (1979). *Quasi-experimentation: Design and analysis issues in field settings.* Chicago: Rand McNally.

Cooper, H., & Hedges, L.V. (Eds.). (1994). *The handbook of research synthesis.* New York: Russell Sage.

Cronbach, L.J. (1983). *Designing evaluations of educational and social programs.* San Francisco: Jossey-Bass.

Freeman, P.R. (1993). The role of *P*-values in analyzing trial results. *Statistics in Medicine, 12,* 1443–1452.

Fuhrer, M.J. (Ed.). (1987). *Rehabilitation outcomes: Analysis and measurement.* Baltimore: Paul H. Brookes Publishing Co.

Gardner, M.J., & Altman, D.G. (Eds.). (1989). *Statistics with confidence.* London: British Medical Journal Publication.

Gehan, E.A. (1984). Progress in therapy in acute leukemia 1948–1981: Randomized versus non-randomized trials. *Controlled Clinical Trials, 3,* 199–208.

Gladman, J.R.F. (1991). Some solutions to problems of the randomized controlled trial in rehabilitation research. *Clinical Trials, 5,* 9–13.

Gonnella, C. (1989). Single subject experimental paradigm as clinical decision tool. *Physical Therapy, 69,* 286–292.

Goodman, S.N. (1992). A comment on replication *P*-values and evidence. *Statistics in Medicine, 11,* 875–879.

Gore, S.M. (1981). Assessing methods: Art of significance testing. *British Medical Journal, 283,* 600–602.

Grice, C., & Hunter, J. (1964). Stimulus intensity effects depend upon the type of experimental design. *Psychological Review, 71,* 247–256.

Guyatt, G., Heyting, A., Jaeschke, R., Keller, J., Adachi, J.D., & Roberts, R. (1990). *N* of 1 randomized trials for investigating new drugs. *Controlled Clinical Trials, 11,* 88–100.

Guyatt, G., Sackett, D., Taylor, W., Chung, J., Roberts, R., & Pugsley, S. (1986). Determining optimal therapy randomized trials in individual patients. *New England Journal of Medicine, 314,* 889–892.

Hedges, L.V. (1987). How hard is hard science; how soft is soft science? *American Psychologist, 42,* 443–455.

Hedges, L.V., & Olkin, I. (1985). *Statistical methods for meta-analysis.* New York: Academic Press.

Johnston, M.V., & Granger, C.V. (1994). Outcomes research in medical rehabilitation: A primer and introduction to a series. *American Journal of Physical Medicine and Rehabilitation, 73,* 296–303.

Johnstone, D.J. (1986). Test of significance in theory and practice. *Statistician, 35,* 491–498.

Kazdin, A.E. (1982). *Single-case research designs: Methods for clinical and applied settings.* New York: Oxford University Press.

Kirby, R.H. (1994). Priorities and rehabilitation research. *American Journal of Physical Medicine and Rehabilitation, 73,* 56–57.

Kramer, M.S., & Shapiro, S.H. (1984). Scientific challenges in the application of randomized trials. *Journal of the American Medical Association, 252,* 2739–2745.

Light, R.J., & Smith, P.V. (1971). Accumulating evidence: Procedures for resolving contradictions among different studies. *Harvard Educational Review, 41,* 429–476.

Lind, K. (1982). A synthesis of studies on stroke rehabilitation. *Journal of Chronic Disease, 35,* 133–149.

Lindsay, R.M., & Ehrenberg, A.S. (1993). The design of replicated studies. *American Statistician, 47,* 217–228.

Lipsey, M.W. (1990). *Design sensitivity: Statistical power for experimental research.* Newbury Park, CA: Sage Publications.

Lipsey, M.W., Crosse, S., Pankle, J., Pollard, T., & Stobart, G. (1985). Evaluation: The state of the art and the sorry state of the science. In D. Cordary (Ed.), *Utilizing prior research in evaluation planning: New directions for program evaluation* (Vol. 27, pp. 7–27). San Francisco: Jossey-Bass.

Lykken, D.T. (1968). Statistical significance in psychological research. *Psychological Bulletin, 70,* 151–159.

Matyas, T.A., & Ottenbacher, K.J. (1993). Confounds of insensitivity and blind luck: Statistical conclusion validity in stroke clinical trials. *Archives of Physical Medicine and Rehabilitation, 74,* 559–565.

McCleary, R., Hay, R.A., Medinger, E., & Powell, C.D. (1980). *Applied time-series analysis for the social sciences.* Beverly Hills, CA: Sage Publications.

Meythalre, J.M., Steers, W.P., Tuel, S.M., Cross, L.L., & Haworth, L.S. (1992). Continuous intrathecal baclofen in spinal cord spasticity. *American Journal of Physical Medicine and Rehabilitation, 71,* 321–327.

Mulkay, M., & Gilbert, G.N. (1986). Replication and more replication. *Philosophy of the Social Sciences, 16,* 21–37.

Oakes, M. (1987). *Statistical inference: A commentary for the social and behavioral sciences.* New York: John Wiley & Sons.

Ottenbacher, K.J. (1986). *Evaluating clinical change: Strategies for occupational and physical therapists.* Baltimore: Williams & Wilkins.

Ottenbacher, K.J. (1992). The impact of random assignment on study outcome: An empirical examination. *Controlled Clinical Trials, 13,* 50–61.

Ottenbacher, K.J. (1993). Clinically relevant designs for rehabilitation research: The idiographic model. *American Journal of Physical Medicine and Rehabilitation, 72,* 144–150.

Ottenbacher, K.J. (1995). Why rehabilitation research does not work (as well as we think it should). *Archives of Physical Medicine and Rehabilitation, 76,* 123–129.

Ottenbacher, K.J., & Barrett, K. (1989). Measures of effect size in the reporting of rehabilitation research. *American Journal of Physical Medicine and Rehabilitation, 68,* 52–58.

Ottenbacher, K.J., & Barrett, K. (1990). Statistical conclusion validity of rehabilitation research: A quantitative review. *American Journal of Physical Medicine and Rehabilitation, 69,* 102–107.

Ottenbacher, K.J., & Jannell, S. (1993). The results of clinical trials in stroke rehabilitation research. *Archives of Neurology, 50,* 37–44.

Phelps, C.E. (1993). The methodologic foundation of studies of the appropriateness of medical care. *New England Journal of Medicine, 329,* 1202–1204.

Pocock, S.J. (1983). *Clinical trials: A practical approach.* New York: John Wiley & Sons.

Pollock, C., Freemantle, N., Seldon, T., Song, F., & Mason, J. (1993). Methodological difficulties in rehabilitation research. *Clinical Rehabilitation, 7,* 63–72.

Reilly, R.P., & Findley, T.W. (1989). Research in physical medicine and rehabilitation: IV. Some practical designs in applied research. *American Journal of Physical Medicine and Rehabilitation, 68,* 196–201.

Rieglman, R.K., & Hirsch, R. (1989). *Studying a study and testing a test: How to read the medical literature* (2nd ed.). Boston: Little, Brown.

Rosenthal, R. (1991). Replication in behavior research. In J.W. Neulieup (Ed.), *Handbook of replication research in the behavioral and social sciences* (pp. 1–30). Newbury Park, CA: Sage.

Sackett, D. (1986). Rules of evidence and clinical recommendations on the use of antithrombotic agents. *Chest, 89,* 25–35.

Salsburg, D. (1992). The use of statistical methods in the analysis of clinical studies. *Journal of Clinical Epidemiology, 46,* 17–27.

Shapiro, D.A., & Shapiro, D. (1982). Meta-analysis of comparative therapy outcome studies: A replication and refinement. *Psychological Bulletin, 92,* 581–604.

Spencer, J.C. (1993). The usefulness of qualitative methods in rehabilitation: Issues of meaning, of context and of change. *Archives of Physical Medicine and Rehabilitation. 74,* 119–126.

Storandt, M. (1983). Significance does not equal importance [Editorial]. *Journal of Gerontology, 38,* 2.

Tversky, A., & Kahneman, D. (1971). Belief in the law of small numbers. *Psychological Bulletin, 76,* 105–110.

Weiss, B., & Weiss, J.R. (1990). The impact of methodological factors on child psychotherapy outcome research: A meta-analysis for researchers. *Journal of Abnormal Child Psychology, 18,* 639–670.

Whiteneck, G.G. (1994). Measuring what matters: Key rehabilitation outcomes. *Archives of Physical Medicine and Rehabilitation, 75,* 1072–1076.

Whyte, J. (1995). Toward a methodology for rehabilitation research. *American Journal of Physical Medicine and Rehabilitation, 74,* 428–425.

Williamson, J.W., Goldschmidt, P.C., & Colton, T. (1986). The quality of medical literature: An analysis of validation assessments. In J.C. Blair & F. Mostellar (Eds.), *Medical uses of statistics* (pp. 370–391). Waltham, MA: NEJM Books.

Wortman, P.M. (1994). Judging research quality. In H. Cooper & L.V. Hedges (Eds.), *Handbook of research synthesis* (pp. 97–110). New York: Russell Sage.

Ziman, J. (1978). *Reliable knowledge: An exploration of the grounds for belief in science.* Cambridge, England: Cambridge University Press.

CHAPTER 11

The Role of Treatment Theory

Robert Allen Keith

Although health care providers and their patients have always been concerned about treatment results, it is doubtful that so much energy would be devoted to the search for outcomes information without the financial incentives present in the mid-1990s. The funders of health care are not only looking for the most effective procedures; they also want such procedures to be moderate in cost. Consequently, the cost-effectiveness of treatment has been thrust into the spotlight. Large-scale reviews of the scientific literature have found, however, that a high proportion of published studies do not provide answers on effectiveness, either because they do not address the issue or because research designs are too weak to demonstrate the value of interventions (Maklan, Greene, & Cummings, 1994). Because the subject of costs has been of interest to clinical investigators only since the early 1990s, the amount of research combining effectiveness and costs has been small.

Medical rehabilitation, as part of health care, is the target of considerable skepticism about its effectiveness and is a candidate for potentially far-reaching changes. The response to this has been an effort to provide evidence of the effectiveness of orthodox treatment. The Medical Rehabilitation Education Foundation, for example, a group whose aim is to further the interests of rehabilitation, has been combing the scientific literature for proof of effectiveness. Thus far, the results have been very modest. One of the few reviews of the costs and benefits and cost-effectiveness of rehabilitation was published in 1983 by Johnston and Keith. As of 1995, there had been no attempt to update that review, partially because of the limited research on the topic.

If support for the effectiveness of treatment in rehabilitation is insufficient, then a long-range strategy is needed to improve the body of information available. Medical rehabilitation is a small field in health care; resources available for research also have been small. It is important, then, to make the best use of funding and research personnel.

The premise of this chapter is that improving research is a matter of not only technical and methodologic advances but also an understanding of rehabilitation treatment and how it produces patient changes. Such understanding requires a coherent conceptual scheme into which research findings can be placed: the role of treatment theory. With this knowledge, the field can be more efficient in addressing key issues about the way treatment is related to outcomes and how treatment can be improved.

There are three goals in this chapter. The first is to demonstrate the importance of theory and theory building in the quest for more efficient and effective treatment. The second is to examine the paradigms of rehabilitation and how treatment theory might be developed in the unique context of rehabilitation. Third, there are a number of key questions to consider that furnish the direction for theory-driven research.

EFFECTIVENESS RESEARCH AND TREATMENT THEORY

The importance of theory in the determination of treatment effects can be seen in program evaluation. This field began during the 1960s stemming from concern about whether newly initiated social programs had any impact. New ways of looking at research were required. Investigators in evaluation research evolved an increasingly sophisticated array of analytic tools. Because of their ability to probe for answers about effectiveness, the demand for program evaluation grew.

Since the mid-1980s, however, dissatisfaction with the field has become evident. Too much of the intervention research failed to show that programs had the expected results, often in spite of the convictions of providers and others that there were positive effects. There also have been complaints of intellectual sterility and of evaluations conducted piecemeal without integrating evaluation results into a coherent body of knowledge (Finney & Moos, 1989). Dissatisfaction with "black box" formulations, that is, establishing relationships while ignoring causal processes, has become widespread.

As a remedy, Chen and Rossi (1980, 1983, 1987) advocated theory-driven evaluation, using explicit theorizing or modeling of program processes to account for outcomes. In a series of papers, these authors laid out evaluation strategies that require formulations about the nature of the assumptions made in treatment intervention. Chen (1989) advanced two subtheories of program theory, which is the usually implicit assumptions that are made about how a program works. First, there is normative theory, which provides the rationale and justification for program structure. This component furnishes the direction for program planning and implementation. It is usually assumed to be understood, with little systematic or explicit examination. The second subtheory is causal theory, which specifies how the program works and under what conditions. The emphasis here is on the worth of the program and how it might be improved. Both of these formulations are important in improving program outcomes.

Because of the difficulty of constructing comprehensive theories, Lipsey (1990) advocated the use of what he calls small theory, in which careful specification at each stage of research provides the conceptual building blocks. In this scheme, there are four major components to treatment theory:

1. A problem definition that specifies what conditions are treatable and under what circumstances
2. Specification of the critical inputs necessary to effect change
3. The important links in treatment transformation
4. Specification of expected outputs or outcomes

Although there may not be complete fulfillment of each step—it is difficult, for example, to specify linkages for what causes change—the closer an investigator is able to describe these components, the more explicit theoretical relations become.

Lipsey's (1990) small theory notions are grounded in the experimental method. Detailed specification at each stage of inquiry is in the best scientific tradition, but even careful investigators have difficulty fulfilling such requirements. Theory does not automatically spring from the results of such research. It is still necessary to examine the resulting relations and impose some conceptual order on them. This approach does maximize the potential for understanding the treatment process and the imposition of some theoretical structure.

In the search for sources of treatment theory, program evaluation specialists have begun to examine program theory, the assumptions about how a program works. There are three major avenues (Lipsey & Pollard, 1989). Existing theory is an obvious place to begin. In rehabilitation, there are relatively few explicit treatment theories. The use of learning theory in the treatment of chronic pain is one example (Fordyce, Roberts, & Sternbach, 1985) in which a theory that originated in a different field has been successfully applied to rehabilitation. A second source of program theory is in exploratory research, where promising relationships have been found but there is not a sufficient body of research from which to draw definitive conclusions. An example is the use of life table analysis for studying both the natural history and the effect of treatment with patients with stroke (Reding & Potes, 1988). The authors found differences in the probability of reaching independence in ambulation and self-care based on differences in deficit levels. The interval after stroke required to reach the plateau phase of recovery also was significant among subgroups. Both sensory and motor deficits and phase of recovery can then be used in the strategic application of treatment. A third source of program theory is the implicit assumptions held by those who design and apply treatment. They have some idea of the rationale of various procedures, and there are methods for formalizing such cognitive schemas. Clinical experience, although not as organized as formal research, should provide a beginning knowledge of how and perhaps why certain treatments work.

Even though program evaluation is required for accreditation from CARF . . . The Rehabilitation Accreditation Commission, this activity has not had much direct effect on the body of scientific evidence about rehabilitation. The management-oriented evaluation systems ordinarily in use do not employ research designs powerful enough to establish the validity of results, although the emphasis on better measurement and better data has had a propitious effect on the field.

Rehabilitation is a particularly challenging circumstance in which to establish treatment proof. The problems are well known. Links between pathology or impairment and the patient's functional performance are often poorly understood. Likewise, the relationship between patient performance in clinical as opposed to home and community settings has not been well established. The time spans necessary to establish long-term effects are a problem. Research designs that will separate therapeutic effects from natural recovery and a host of factors outside of treatment must be ingenious and are often outside the capability and resources of many investigators. The temptation is to address the technical design problems and not worry about theory. If the experience of evaluators in program evaluation is to be taken seriously, however, neglect of theory would be a mistake. Research has to be more than a series of isolated studies. Otherwise, a coherent body of knowledge will not be built, and new directions for research will continue to stem from trial-and-error methods.

TREATMENT PARADIGMS IN REHABILITATION

Treatment paradigms are a set of blueprints for how treatment should be conducted. They represent a distillation of wisdom from clinical experience, research, and training. The assumptions under which treatment paradigms operate are often unexamined, particularly if they have been in place for a long time or if there has been no reason to challenge them. Treatment paradigms change when assumptions upon which they are based are altered, when delivery system capabilities or characteristics change, or with fluctuations in external circumstance such as funding. When health care comes under pressure, such as in the mid-1990s, treatment paradigms become the subject of renewed interest. The development of clinical practice guidelines, now underway for a number of major diseases, is a way of reducing variability in procedures and, presumably, increasing quality of care.

Although existing practices are an obvious place in which to begin identifying treatment theory, treatment paradigms and treatment theories are not synonymous. Treatment paradigms are models of existing practice, but they may have little explanatory power. The most prominent paradigm in rehabilitation, although not the only one, is the use of the comprehensive team to deliver services. The rationale for its use is that individuals with severe disease or injury have an array of physical, cognitive, emotional, and social problems whose remediation requires equal therapeutic skills distributed among a number of professionals. There are many commentaries on this form of treatment delivery in rehabilitation, its origins (Gritzer & Arluke, 1985), its multidisciplinary nature (Melvin, 1989), and its effectiveness (Keith, 1991). Thus, the team is not discussed in detail in this chapter. Even though the comprehensive team is the system of choice, there has been relatively little research on its effectiveness as a method of treatment delivery (Keith, 1991).

There are a number of threats to the comprehensive team remaining the paradigm of choice. The deployment of a number of professionals, each with a fairly narrowly defined range of treatment responsibility, is very expensive. Arguments have been advanced that, even though it is costly in the short run, the benefits accumulated over several years more than balance treatment costs, a classic cost-effectiveness problem. Unfortunately, cost-effectiveness and cost–benefit studies have been in short supply in rehabilitation (Johnston & Keith, 1983); thus, research justifying orthodox treatment is lacking. The sponsors of health care have begun to select treatment on a pragmatic basis, looking for the most inexpensive way to accomplish acceptable outcomes. Alternate forms of treatment, such as subacute rehabilitation (nursing facility–based services) or rehabilitation in the home with small teams of therapists, have become popular. Their worth will be established more on the basis of clinical and fiscal experience than on formal research.

The second threat to traditional treatment will come with the advent of practice guidelines, the codification of appropriate practices by systematically examining how health care is conducted. Guidelines have been advanced as the panacea for most of health care's woes, particularly cost containment. A more realistic appraisal is that their principal function is in improving quality of care, with some cost savings from the reduction of inappropriate or unnecessary care (Field & Lohr, 1992). The impetus for establishing guidelines came from the pioneering work of Wennberg and Gittelsohn (1973, 1982), which demonstrated wide variations in clinical procedures within a local area. Variations in treatment, in which there is presumed common understanding of what is appropriate, imply that there is either poor consensus on the procedures or a number of factors contribute to the inability to implement care as formulated. Clinical guidelines for rehabilitation, such as earlier formulations for Professional Service Review Organizations, have come primarily from a pooling of clinical experience and research. They have not come from surveys of clinical practice. There is remarkably little systematic description of usual clinical practices in rehabilitation.

Changes to rehabilitation from either economic strictures or an examination of current practice represent threats to the orthodox model. What happens when clinicians and the public begin to lose confidence in a treatment paradigm? The field of mental health furnishes an example that might be useful to rehabilitation. Colby began a 1964 review of psychotherapy practices with the sentence "Chaos prevails" (p. 347). He found there to be no single paradigm on which there was consensus. Although there had been increasing signs of crisis in psychotherapy, it was not until there was public acknowledgment of the limitations of therapy that the crisis became acute. A major factor in producing this was the use of tape recordings for training and research. According to Colby, as long as what went on in therapy sessions remained secret, it was not difficult to perpetuate the myth that there was consensus about the therapeutic model. When tapes were listened to, it became apparent that there was great diversity in treatment and profound differences in perspectives among therapists. There was no agreement about what the treatment model should be.

Thus far, rehabilitation has been spared the equivalent of tape recordings for psychotherapy. As a result, it is claimed that there is a high degree of consensus about what should and does occur. However, it is not really known whether there is consensus or how it is manifested in treatment procedures. If research on practice variations in other fields is any indication, then it should be expected that there are significant variations in rehabilitation as well. The potential for variation may be even higher because of the number of individuals on the comprehensive team. Maintaining the current model may be difficult in the face of significant differences in practice.

Restructuring of treatment is underway in rehabilitation. Although team care is still the belief system under which rehabilitation operates, it is imperative to find a better understanding of what goes on in treatment and what it is that produces change. Understanding will come only with the integration of patient and treatment information into a coherent explanatory framework: the role of theory.

TREATMENT THEORY AND REHABILITATION

Theory building has never had a high priority in rehabilitation; there are only a few systems with any visibility. The practical problems of restoring functions, increasing strength and endurance, and reintegrating individuals into familiar surroundings have consumed the energies of clinicians. Much of the research has been directed toward fairly specific clinical problems. Foundations of treatment have often come from basic research in other fields, such as electrophysiology, kinesiology, and neurology. The span of phenomena is so wide, from physiologic processes to social roles, that it discourages construction of conceptual frameworks. Rehabilitation has not been entirely devoid of underlying concepts, however. There is a rich substratum of assumptions on which to base theory.

Functional Perspective

The functional orientation is basic to an understanding of the aims, processes, and outcomes of rehabilitation. Its emphasis is a defining characteristic of the field. Restoration of function has been contrasted with the medical model, which has the aim of alleviating disease and injury (Granger, 1984). Even though *function* is a fundamental concept in rehabilitation, it is a remarkably elusive term. When referring to physical, emotional, or social functioning, it includes most of life's activities. A better understanding of the concept of *function* requires some historical background.

Functionalism is a viewpoint found in biologic and social sciences and has its origins in the evolutionary adaptation of Charles Darwin. In biology, study of the isolated structure of organisms gave way to a holistic orientation in which it was recognized that structures are interrelated; a change in any part affects the whole. Organisms had to be examined as integrated systems. Changes in structure also affect functions, again in a holistic manner. Biologic systems also regulate themselves in such a way that they produce equilibrium or homeostasis.

Psychology took the idea behind biologic adaptation of a species and transferred it to the psychologic adjustment of the individual, a debatable jump in logic (Kendler, 1987). However, the notion of adaptation or adjustment has become a fundamental tenet in psychology. Even though functionalism in psychology has never had an integrated group of concepts or been a clearly defined school of thought, it has had considerable influence on the field. Gestalt psychology, in which the whole is seen as more than the sum of its parts, is one example of the impact of the functionalist orientation. Systems theory, particularly in the study of organizations, is another.

Although most American sociologists would not consider themselves strict functionalists, this perspective has had a strong impact on theory. Functionalist theory in sociology is concerned primarily with the concept of a system and the analysis of social patterns as parts of larger systems of behavior and belief (Gouldner, 1959). The interdependence of system parts and their tendency to maintain equilibrium in their relationships is of major interest. According to Patrick and Erickson (1993), the principal theoretical bases for defining health and quality of life come from functionalist theory in sociology, particularly from the work of Talcott Parsons. Parsons viewed illness as a deviation from the social expectations that go with social role performance, a temporary exemption from usual duties. Descriptions of role functions have been developed in terms of performance and capacity and form the basis for health and functional status indicators. They are an operationalization of society's ideas of health in productive roles, including work, school, housework, and independent care for one's own personal needs. Impairment, disability, and handicap in the World Health Organization (WHO; 1980) scheme incorporate the idea of disablement that comes from deficits in expected performance or from societal norms.

In rehabilitation, the concept of *function* is used constantly, although its most prominent place is in functional assessment. Halpern and Fuhrer (1984) defined *functional assessment* as "the measurement of purposeful behavior in interaction with the environment, which is interpreted according to the assessment's intended uses" (p. 3). *Purposeful behavior* was defined as activity that has some goal or objective. Granger (1984) had a broader definition:

> Functional assessment is the tool that allows one to (a) secure a comprehensive view of pathology and impairment, disability and handicap, (b) identify discordances between diagnoses, performance (behaviors), and social role, (c) identify apparent discrepancies through analyses of functional limitations as they interfere with fulfillment of social roles, and (d) plan appropriate interventions and mobilization of resources to address the various needs—medical, restorative, psychosocial, environmental, and supportive. (p. 21)

According to these definitions, *function* refers to task-oriented behavior in which performance adequacy is judged by comparison with social expectations or norms. Measurement of progress and outcomes goes beyond the realm of medicine into the social sciences, but the conceptual basis of such measures merits more attention (Keith, 1995).

Classification of Disablement

The most prominent theories in rehabilitation address ways to categorize the consequences of disease and injury that lead to disablement. The most well known is the *International Classification of Impairments, Disabilities, and Handicaps* (ICIDH) of the WHO (1980), designed as a supplement to the *International Classification of Diseases*. Although its authors recognize the limitations of the medical model, its major purpose is to aid in the planning of health care services. The ICIDH has proved very useful in separating the levels of function in disablement and the appropriate assessment and treatment procedures. There have been many commentaries on the ICIDH, including those of Granger (1984), Frey (1984), and Pope and Tarlov (1991).

The system of Nagi (1976), a medical sociologist, was used as a tool for epidemiologic analysis in a survey of disability in Columbus, Ohio. Its terminology of pathology, impairment, functional limitation, and disability parallels the WHO system but attaches different meanings to some of the terms. In a 1991 statement, Nagi clarified his scheme and compared it to the WHO publication, reaching the conclusion that his terminology is more precise.

A third conceptual framework comes from a committee on disability prevention sponsored by the Institute of Medicine (IOM) of the National Academy of Sciences (Pope & Tarlov, 1991). The request for this effort came from the Centers for Disease Control (CDC). The IOM formulations use the Nagi terminology but extend them to include risk factors causally associated with health-related conditions and quality of life. *Disability in America* represents a rare attempt at policy formation for disability, using the prevention orientation that is part of the CDC mission. The most promising aspect of this effort is the potential for the development of ways to keep track of populations with disability, a public health function.

All of these classification systems have the goal of conceptualizing the process and consequences of disease and injury, an important task for rehabilitation. They were not meant to be a theory of treatment, however. Whyte (1994) provided a useful theoretical framework that relates levels of intervention and their corresponding levels of outcomes assessment using the WHO scheme. It demonstrates that conceptualization of treatment in rehabilitation must take into account the level of disablement.

Learning Theory

Learning plays a central role in the conduct of therapy in rehabilitation. The physical therapist, for example, spends a high proportion of time instructing the patient in ways to improve motor skills. Even exercises designed for strength and endurance rather than skill acquisition require instruction. The patient's job is to observe or to listen to such instruction and then to practice. Much of the progress of patients comes as the result of learning or relearning. Although clinicians may unwittingly apply learning principles in their work, most of what they do comes from their experience or from procedures in which they have been trained, which may or may not incorporate learning theory. Most clinicians understand intuitively that reward, in the form of praise or encouragement, is an important motivator for patients. But should they receive praise every time? Should reward be used in the face of poor performance? Operant conditioning principles would say no. Is it more efficient to treat patients in a short, intensive course of treatment, or is it better to space sessions over a longer period? There is a body of work in learning on spaced versus massed practice that might be relevant (Underwood, 1961).

Despite the voluminous literature in psychology and education on learning principles, most of these principles have not been adopted by rehabilitation clinicians. Mosey (1986) pointed out that therapists want to be seen, not as teachers, but as members of a medical team. Aside from questions of occupational status, however, it is partially a question of professionals not venturing outside their own field when they read. Poole (1991) noted that, even though occupational therapists are constantly involved in motor learning tasks with their patients, most occupational therapy texts devote little space to motor learning and teaching. Motor learning principles are advocated in a few accounts of functional retraining for physical therapists, but they are not widespread (Carr & Shepherd, 1987).

Behavior Modification   The most visible use of learning principles in rehabilitation has been with behavior modification methods, pioneered in chronic pain programs by Fordyce and others (Fordyce, Fowler, Lehmann, & DeLateur, 1968). Using the principles of operant conditioning established by the behavioral psychologist B.F. Skinner, this treatment modality identifies the desired behavior, plots baselines and daily progress, and provides rewards only when the desired behavior is forthcoming. Strict attention is paid to the patient's environment and to sources of reinforcement. Because of the emphasis on environmental management, all members of the treatment team must be versed in behavioral methods. Even though the method has enjoyed success, particularly with patients who have chronic pain or brain injury, its requirement of a staff dedicated to a learning orientation has limited its use. Although the record keeping can be burdensome, behavior modification provides better insights into the mechanisms of change than many other treatment regimens.

Motor Learning   Occupational therapists have been particularly active in selecting principles from the motor learning literature. Mathiowetz and Haugen (1994) reviewed some of the work on motor learning behavior that might be relevant to therapy. Research in this area uses concepts and methods that help to define the problems in applying motor learning. One such issue is the best way to structure practice. Mere repetition is often not the best way to optimize skill acquisition. The role of feedback, whether it is intrinsic (proprioceptive or sensory information) or extrinsic (an external source, such as performance graphs or digital displays), is an important accompaniment to learning. Transfer of training, a traditional learning topic, is particularly relevant for therapy. If the patient is unable to perform the tasks learned in a clinical setting in other settings, the value of therapy is lost. Poole (1991) and Jarus (1994) provided discussions of the application of such principles in therapy. Motor learning is a particularly fertile source of conceptual and theoretical work for rehabilitation.

This short journey through existing theory in rehabilitation illustrates that thoughtful attempts at theory building are in short supply. An exposition of theories and concepts by Patrick and Erickson (1993) in the wider realm of health-related quality of life provides interesting background on health and functional status (see also Chapter 7 of this book for a detailed discussion of quality of life). The next section of this chapter turns to the more specific question of treatment theory for rehabilitation.

BUILDING TREATMENT THEORY

If Lipsey's (1990) advice on starting with small theory is taken, then detailed specifications of the components, processes, and outcomes of care are needed. Some of these details are known, but many are relatively unexplored. In looking at the common input, process, outcome model (taken here from Keith & Lipsey, 1993), inputs can be thought of as patient characteristics, organizational factors in the facility, and external factors from the health care and community environments. Patient characteristics, such as impairments, demographics, severity, stage of recovery, and comorbidities, have undergone the most research and are the easiest to specify. The influences on treatment of staff qualifications, their kinds and number, and how they are organized are virtually unknown in any systematic way. The exceptions are a few comparisons of freestanding and hospital units with case mix and length of stay (Hosek et al., 1986; Mullner, Nuzum, & Matthews, 1983). The effects of family or community support, health care funding, or health care regulations on treatment are also poorly researched.

Processes are the treatment procedures in rehabilitation, which are discussed in the next section. Focus on outcomes has become widespread; thus, a list of commonly used indicators, such as functional status level, discharge destination, or amount of assistance required, is not difficult to compile. However, conceptualization of the basis for such measures is still in an early stage (Keith, 1995). The utility of outcomes also would be enhanced with more research on their validity.

Treatment Components

The most strategic place to amplify details is in treatment itself. Before this can be done, however, there are some conceptual problems to be solved. How can various aspects of rehabilitation treatment be characterized? There are no formal classifications of treatment type. The most obvious first cut is by discipline (e.g., physical therapy, occupational therapy) although there are some overlaps in what these professional groups do. It is also probable that there are idiosyncratic applications of skills in various facilities. Nevertheless, a specification of number of hours of treatment by discipline would be of value. Whether treatment is administered to individual patients or groups is also relevant. In trying to group procedures in a logical fashion, such as building strength and endurance, increasing gross and fine motor skills, or cognitive retraining, the problems of complexity appear. What is required is a compilation of treatment activities that can then be grouped in an empirical or rational manner.

Strength of Treatment

One promising area for describing treatment is in establishing the strength of the interventions. For example, for a group of patients with stroke who require maximum assistance for ambulation, how many hours per day and for how long do they require physical therapy to become independent? There also are other issues involved, such as the severity of physical and cognitive impairments or medical complications; but ways are needed to quantify treatment to find out how well it works. Scott and Sechrest (1989), writing from the evaluation perspective, used concepts from medicine and pharmacology to quantify treatment elements.

Purity Purity is the extent to which treatment follows the intended protocol. There are many procedures for which there is reasonable agreement about how they should be administered. Significant deviations from standard methods may result in degradation of the effects of the therapy. The patient doing resistive exercises to strengthen an upper extremity may receive no benefit if the apparatus is set for zero resistance. Purity depends greatly on a common understanding of practices and on implementation of them.

Specificity The extent to which treatment is tailored to the characteristics of the patient is a measure of specificity. Some routines are designed to be of general benefit, such as a calisthenics class for a group of ambulatory patients. Also, there are procedures that are done fairly automatically that may not be of uniform value but, in the interest of efficiency, are given to everyone. Specialty units that treat only one impairment, such as strokes or brain injury, presumably plan treatment around the problems of particular impairments. An interesting question is the extent to which efficiency of treatment and billing arrangements blur specificity so that patients receive some treatment because it is expedient to give it to everyone or it is tied to revenue enhancement.

Dose The concept of *dose* is basic to medicine but has been used little in rehabilitation, aside from medical management. In rehabilitation, *dose* refers to type of treatment and amount, usually expressed in time units. Engaging in a particular activity for a specified time interval, then, is the metric of treatment. The accumulation of hours of treatment presumably leads to therapeutic improvement. This variable offers a fertile field for understanding treatment mechanisms.

Intensity In its simplest form, intensity is the amount of treatment per unit of time, such as the number of hours per day. Most billing systems can retrieve such information, so intensity should be one treatment quantity that is readily available. Despite its basic nature, few studies provide data on treatment intensity. In a comparison of acute versus subacute rehabilitation for stroke (Keith, Wilson, & Gutierrez, 1995), it was found that the acute (hospital-based) rehabilitation program provided an average of 4.92 therapy hours per day and the subacute program provided 2.62 therapy hours per day, a substantial difference. The differential resulted in greater Functional Independence Measure (FIM) gain (30.41 versus 20.56), but not much difference in the proportion discharged to a residential setting (71% versus 67%).

Duration This is the length of time of treatment. For inpatient programs, it is synonymous with length of stay. Duration is important for outpatient treatment as well; it is often translated into time in service or some other terminology. There are two concepts incorporated into treatment duration: the span of time during which treatment goes on and total treatment exposure. Length of stay has been used for years as a rough proxy for the amount of treatment, with the assumption being that there is reasonable uniformity in intensity from one program to the next. Because there has been little research on detailed treatment variables among facilities, it is not known if the assumption is correct.

Drastically shortened lengths of service and compressed treatment regimens have foreclosed the question of whether patients profit more from programs of longer or shorter length. Length of stay statistics need to be augmented by some index of total treatment exposure or intensity. In the acute–subacute rehabilitation comparison (Keith et al., 1995), patients with stroke received a total of 114 hours of therapy in 28.6 days in the acute facility, and 51 hours of therapy in 24.2 days in the subacute facility. Because these were billed hours, they did not include nursing time.

The Caregiver The characteristics of the person or people who deliver treatment would seem important: their discipline, gender, level of training, experience, personal competence, and motivation. Some of these, such as training and experience, can be quantified, but personal attributes defy easy indexing. A significant research problem with team configurations is how to identify the effects of individual treaters on outcomes. Although there is a division of labor in treatment tasks, it is difficult to find a one-to-one correspondence between treatment activity and patient performance. The physical therapist may be responsible for ambulation training, and ambulation skill can be measured; but cognitive factors may play a role. Also, the patient ambulates in many settings other than physical therapy.

The effect of treater discipline was addressed in a multifacility study coordinated at the Rehabilitation Institute of Chicago (Heinemann, Hamilton, Linacre, Wright, & Granger, 1995). Eight hospitals cooperated in producing treatment and outcomes data on patients with traumatic brain injury and spinal cord injury (SCI). Therapy hours were retrieved from billing information and categorized by individual and group services and by type of service (cognitive retraining, occupational therapy, physical therapy, speech therapy, psychology services, social services, patient education, therapeutic recreation, and vocational rehabilitation services). The FIM was used for functional assessment. Occupational, physical, and speech therapy intensities were not related to any outcome for patients with traumatic brain injury. The single exception was psychological service intensity, which was found to be related to greater cognitive function at discharge. For patients with SCI, occupational, physical, speech, and psychology therapy intensities were not related to outcomes. Psychology intensity was related to cognitive outcomes for these patients, but in a reverse direction: Patients with SCI who received *less* intense psychology services had *greater* cognitive gains.

These findings are certainly unexpected and also disconcerting. Heinemann et al. (1995) explored several possible explanations but did not find an adequate one. Functional status changes have been assumed to be related to the amount of treatment given by the various modalities. Most studies find gains between admission and discharge, but it is difficult to attribute all such improvement to spontaneous recovery or some other nontherapeutic influence. Additional research needs to be done on this topic.

Timing

The strategy with which therapies are applied over the course of treatment is the timing dimension. It refers both to the application of treatment in relation to phase of recovery and to phase of treatment during a stay. There is considerable research showing that the most significant improvement after stroke comes during the first 3 months of recovery (Andrews, Brocklehurst, Richards, & Laycock, 1981; Kelly-Hayes et al., 1989; Kotila, Waltimo, Niemi, Laaksonen, & Lempinen, 1984). It seems likely that rehabilitation, to be most effective, needs to occur within that time. Knowledge of the natural history of recovery is useful to maximize the effects of therapy for any impairment, but such information is not systematically gathered. A data system that tracked one individual through various treatment services, such as that advocated by Johnston and Hall (1994), would be an essential component in tracking recovery and establishing recovery curves.

As patients change during their stay, therapy is modified, but there has been little systematic work on phases of treatment. With physical recovery, both the amount and frequency of treatment should change. In a study at Casa Colina Hospital, Horowitz (1990) looked at the daily treatment hours for 210 patients with traumatic brain injury or stroke who had a length of stay between 28 and 32 days. His assumptions were that patients should gain in stamina and that treatment intensity should increase during the hospital stay. An analysis of intensity by week did show such a trend. The general pattern across all disciplines was for an increase in amount of treatment. In this case, research simply confirmed what is assumed to be the usual transition in treatment; but there are many other treatment strategies that need to be examined.

Building treatment theory in rehabilitation has to start at the basic level of many scientific enterprises—compiling and classifying. Counting and categorizing the many treatment procedures may seem tedious, but these procedures are needed to know what treatment patients receive. Without this knowledge, it is not possible to understand the nature of treatment intervention. With a treatment taxonomy in hand, it is then possible to turn to the delivery questions entailed in quantifying the strength of treatment, purity, specificity, dose, and so forth. Research that includes the content of the treatment and a quantification of its components can then be applied to a range of patient problems and characteristics. This will facilitate better understanding of the causal links between treatment and its effects and building of a treatment theory.

CONCLUSIONS

It is easy to advocate ambitious research programs as a way to improve treatment effectiveness, and indeed programmatic research is important, but there are more modest ways to further the cause. Most of them depend on more careful specification of the variables of investigation, particularly treatment. Every research report of outcomes, for example, should include a description of the treatment that was actually delivered, including hours of service by discipline, treatment intensity, and total treatment exposure. A general description of how treatment was intended to be delivered is not sufficient; there are always significant variations in delivery. The efforts of physicians and nurses also should be included, because they often are not in current billing practices. The interaction of patient characteristics with variations in treatment delivery is an important relationship often masked by analyses that use only measures of central tendency.

Controlled clinical trials, the most powerful research design in establishing efficacy of treatment, have been used relatively little in rehabilitation. Many such investigations have compared care in specialized units, such as stroke care, with care in general medical settings. The rationale for such comparisons is usually not explicitly stated beyond the general characteristics of both programs. Usually, there is insufficient documentation of treatment delivery to establish what it was that caused differential outcomes, if they exist. Such trials demonstrate only that there is a difference; the opportunity to examine why is usually not exploited. An exception is the controlled trial for stroke treatment reported by Smith et al. (1981). The authors reported hours of treatment by discipline with group and individual treatment, along with details of changes in patients over time. Intensity of treatment appeared to be an important difference between regimens.

With the demand for more economical courses of treatment, there is a pressing need to establish what is the minimum team configuration that will produce desired outcomes. Although it usually is not possible to manipulate team membership, changes in funding are producing a natural experiment in which it is possible to compare various patterns of minimal care with more elaborate schedules. If such differential effects can be isolated, they can contribute to building a theory of treatment.

Treatment theory is essential to the strategic use of research resources. It furnishes a systematic and rational direction of inquiry. Rehabilitation already has a number of underlying concepts that could contribute to theory if they were elaborated on and made more explicit. At the same time, careful specification of the characteristics of patients and of the various elements of treatment would lead to a better understanding of the rehabilitation process and would provide an avenue to treatment theory.

REFERENCES

Andrews, J., Brocklehurst, J.C., Richards, B., & Laycock, P.J. (1981). The rate of recovery from stroke—and its measurement. *International Rehabilitation Medicine, 3,* 155–161.

Carr, J.H., & Shepherd, R.B. (1987). A motor learning model for rehabilitation. In J.H. Carr, R.B. Shepherd, J. Gordon, A.M. Gentile, & J.M. Held (Eds.), *Movement science: Foundations for physical therapy in rehabilitation* (pp. 31–91). Rockville, MD: Aspen Publishers.

Chen, H. (1989). The conceptual framework of the theory-driven perspective. *Evaluation and Program Planning, 12,* 391–396.

Chen, H., & Rossi, P.H. (1980). The multi-goal, theory-driven approach to evaluation: A model linking basic and applied social science. *Social Forces, 59,* 106–122.

Chen, H., & Rossi, P.H. (1983). Evaluating with sense: The theory-driven approach. *Evaluation Review, 7,* 283–302.

Chen, H.T., & Rossi, P.H. (1987). The theory-driven approach to validity. *Evaluation and Program Planning, 10,* 95–103.

Colby, K.M. (1964). Psychotherapeutic processes. *Annual Review of Psychology, 15,* 347–370.

Field, M.J., & Lohr, K.N. (Eds.). (1992). *Guidelines for clinical practice: From development to use.* Washington, DC: National Academy Press.

Finney, J.W., & Moos, R.H. (1989). Theory and method in treatment evaluation. *Evaluation and Program Planning, 12,* 307–316.

Fordyce, W.E., Fowler, R.S., Jr., Lehmann, J.F., & DeLateur, B.J. (1968). Some implications of learning in problems of chronic pain. *Journal of Chronic Diseases, 21,* 179–190.

Fordyce, W.E., Roberts, A.H., & Sternbach, R.A. (1985). The behavioral management of chronic pain: A response to critics. *Pain, 22,* 113–125.

Frey, W. (1984). Functional assessment in the '80s: A conceptual enigma, a technical challenge. In A.S. Halpern & M.J. Fuhrer (Eds.), *Functional assessment in rehabilitation* (pp. 11–43). Baltimore: Paul H. Brookes Publishing Co.

Gouldner, A.W. (1959). Reciprocity and autonomy in functional theory. In L. Gross (Ed.), *Symposium on sociological theory* (pp. 241–270). New York: Harper & Row.

Granger, C.V. (1984). A conceptual model for functional assessment. In C.V. Granger & G.E. Gresham (Eds.), *Functional assessment in rehabilitation medicine* (pp. 14–25). Baltimore: Williams & Wilkins.

Gritzer, G., & Arluke, A. (1985). *The making of rehabilitation.* Berkeley: University of California Press.

Halpern, A.S., & Fuhrer, M.J. (1984). Introduction. In A.S. Halpern & M.J. Fuhrer (Eds.), *Functional assessment in rehabilitation* (pp. 1–9). Baltimore: Paul H. Brookes Publishing Co.

Heinemann, A.W., Hamilton, B.B., Linacre, J.M., Wright, B.D., & Granger, C.V. (1995). Functional status and therapeutic intensity during inpatient rehabilitation. *American Journal of Physical Medicine and Rehabilitation, 74,* 315–326.

Horowitz, J. (1990). *Treatment variations in acute inpatient medical rehabilitation.* Unpublished manuscript.

Hosek, S., Kane, R., Carney, M., Hartman, J., Reboussin, D., Serrato, C., & Melvin, J. (1986). *Charges and outcomes for rehabilitative care.* Santa Monica, CA: Rand Corp.

Jarus, T. (1994). Motor learning and occupational therapy: The organization of practice. *American Journal of Occupational Therapy, 48,* 810–816.

Johnston, M.V., & Hall, K.M. (1994). Outcomes evaluation in traumatic brain injury rehabilitation. Part I: Overview and system principles. *Archives of Physical Medicine and Rehabilitation, 75*(Suppl.), SC2-9.

Johnston, M.V., & Keith, R.A. (1983). Cost–benefits of medical rehabilitation: Review and critique. *Archives of Physical Medicine and Rehabilitation, 64,* 147–154.

Keith, R.A. (1991). The comprehensive treatment team in rehabilitation. *Archives of Physical Medicine and Rehabilitation, 72,* 269–274.

Keith, R.A. (1995). The conceptual basis of outcome measures. *American Journal of Physical Medicine and Rehabilitation, 74,* 73–80.

Keith, R.A., & Lipsey, M.W. (1993). The role of theory in rehabilitation assessment, treatment and outcomes. In R.L. Glueckauf, L.B. Sechrest, G.R. Bond, & E.C. McDonel (Eds.), *Improving rehabilitation assessment practices: Issues and new directions* (pp. 33–58). Beverly Hills, CA: Sage Publications.

Keith, R.A., Wilson, D.B., & Gutierrez, P. (1995). Acute and subacute rehabilitation for stroke: A comparison. *Archives of Physical Medicine and Rehabilitation, 76,* 495–500.

Kelly-Hayes, M., Wolf, P.A., Kase, C.S., Gresham, G.E., Kannel, W.B., & D'Agostino, R.B. (1989). Time-course of functional recovery after stroke: The Framingham Study. *Journal of Neurological Rehabilitation, 3,* 65–70.

Kendler, H.H. (1987). *Historical foundations of modern psychology.* Philadelphia: Temple University Press.

Kotila, M., Waltimo, O., Niemi, M.L., Laaksonen, R., & Lempinen, M. (1984). The profile of recovery from stroke and factors that influence outcomes. *Stroke, 15,* 1039–1044.

Lipsey, M.W. (1990). Theory as method: Small theories of treatment. In L. Sechrest, E. Perrin, & J. Bunker (Eds.), *Research methodology: Strengthening causal interpretations of nonexperimental data* (pp. 33–51). Washington, DC: Agency for Health Care Policy and Research, Public Health Service, U.S. Department of Health and Human Services.

Lipsey, M.W., & Pollard, J.A. (1989). Driving toward theory in program evaluation: More models to choose from. *Evaluation and Program Planning, 12,* 317–328.

Maklan, C.W., Greene, R., & Cummings, M.A. (1994). Methodological challenges and innovations in patient outcomes research. *Medical Care, 32*(Suppl.), JS13–JS21.

Mathiowetz, V., & Haugen, J.B. (1994). Motor behavior research: Implications for therapeutic approaches to central nervous system dysfunction. *American Journal of Occupational Therapy, 48,* 733–745.

Melvin, J.L. (1989). Status report on interdisciplinary medical rehabilitation. *Archives of Physical Medicine and Rehabilitation, 70,* 273–276.

Mosey, A.C. (1986). *Psychosocial components of occupational therapy.* New York: Raven Press.

Mullner, R., Nuzum, F.J., & Matthews, D. (1983). Inpatient medical rehabilitation: Results of the 1981 survey of hospitals and units. *Archives of Physical Medicine and Rehabilitation, 64,* 354–358.

Nagi, S.Z. (1976). An epidemiology of disability among adults in the United States. *Milbank Memorial Fund Quarterly: Health and Society, 54,* 439–467.

Nagi, S.Z. (1991). Disability concepts revisited: Implications for prevention. In A.M. Pope & A.R. Tarlov (Eds.), *Disability in America: Toward a national agenda for prevention* (pp. 309–327). Washington, DC: National Academy Press.

Patrick, D.L., & Erickson, P. (1993). *Health status and health policy.* New York: Oxford University Press.

Poole, J.L. (1991). Application of motor learning principles in occupational therapy. *American Journal of Occupational Therapy, 45,* 531–537.

Pope, A.M., & Tarlov, A.R. (Eds.). (1991). *Disability in America: Toward a national agenda for prevention.* Washington, DC: National Academy Press.

Reding, M.J., & Potes, E. (1988). Rehabilitation outcome following initial unilateral hemispheric stroke. *Stroke, 19,* 1354–1358.

Scott, A.G., & Sechrest, L. (1989). Strength of theory and theory of strength. *Evaluation and Program Planning, 12,* 329–336.

Smith, D.S., Goldenberg, E., Ashburn, A., Kinsella, G., Sheikh, K., Brennan, P.J., Meade, T.W., Zutshi, D.W., Perry, J.D., & Reeback, J.S. (1981). Remedial therapy after stroke: A randomised controlled trial. *British Medical Journal, 282,* 517–520.

Underwood, B.J. (1961). Ten years of massed practice on distributed practice. *Psychological Review, 68,* 229–247.

Wennberg, J., & Gittelsohn, A. (1973). Small area variations in health care delivery. *Science, 142,* 1102–1108.

Wennberg, J., & Gittelsohn, A. (1982). Variations in medical care among small areas. *Scientific American, 246,* 120–134.

Whyte, J. (1994). Toward a methodology for rehabilitation research. *American Journal of Physical Medicine and Rehabilitation, 73,* 428–435.

World Health Organization. (1980). *International classification of impairments, disabilities and handicaps.* Geneva, Switzerland: Author.

CHAPTER 12

Clinical Program Monitoring Systems

Current Capability and Future Directions

Deborah L. Wilkerson and Mark V. Johnston

A new health care order is emerging in which outcomes and cost-effectiveness are essential parts of the knowledge base for providers and purchasers of services. Clinical programs are encouraged, if not impelled, to conduct outcomes research to contribute to the knowledge base of rehabilitation and to ensure their own quality and cost-effectiveness.

As the health care industry in the United States attempts to rein in its costs, concern about maintaining quality has grown. Attention to outcomes and outcomes research has gone beyond the immediate efficacy of a specific intervention for a carefully controlled set of subjects to extend to entire health care systems, disciplines, and populations of consumers (Ellwood, 1988; Wennberg, 1990a). During the 1980s and 1990s, the availability and capabilities of clinical and administration information systems have grown astronomically, with greatly enhanced capabilities in recording, storing, and analyzing clinical service and outcomes data on an ongoing basis. Increasing resources are therefore potentially available for outcomes research.

CLINICAL PROGRAM MONITORING SYSTEMS

Clinical program monitoring systems refer to those clinical information systems developed for the purposes of outcomes management (Ellwood,

Preparation of this chapter was supported in part by grants H133 B4 0025 (Medical Rehabilitation Services and Health Policy) and H133B30041 (Functional Assessment and Evaluation of Rehabilitation Outcomes) from the National Institute on Disability and Rehabilitation Research, and Grant GR108 from the Henry Kessler Foundation.

1988), program evaluation (CARF . . . The Rehabilitation Accreditation Commission [CARF], 1995; Johnston, Wilkerson, & Maney, 1993), quality improvement (Batalden, Nelson, & Roberts, 1994), or clinical record keeping (DesHarnais, Marshall, & Dulski, 1994; Glaser, 1994). Clinical databases begin with the medical or clinical records of patients. Methods for capturing data range from retrospective abstracting from narrative records on paper to highly automated systems in which electronic records are created directly by clinicians (DesHarnais et al., 1994; Iezzoni, 1994).

Contemporary program monitoring information systems include computerized databases. Large databases have been created in acute medical care, for example, for trauma care (Gennarelli, Champion, Copes, & Sacco, 1994). Pooled, multi-institutional databases also have been created for rehabilitation programs and disciplines. Large numbers of cases can also accumulate from the databases of single facilities.

This chapter presents the case for use of clinical program monitoring databases in rehabilitation outcomes research. Many conditions must be met to ensure scientific integrity of the findings. Program monitoring systems can contribute to the development of better rehabilitation practice by identifying variation and areas for more detailed research. For many questions of the outcomes and cost-effectiveness of rehabilitation programs, only large program monitoring systems can provide answers. Efficacy, the capability of a treatment to produce a safe, positive outcome under controlled conditions, must be distinguished from effectiveness, the actual outcomes typically achieved under real-world circumstances (Iezzoni, 1994; Johnston & Granger, 1994). The results of efficacy research in artificial or limited circumstances must be linked to effective outcomes observed in practice, or such research risks isolation in an ivory tower. Real-world databases are essential to test whether rehabilitation interventions are effective in the real world by comparing outcomes for similar patients in different programs.

The Right Outcomes

Central to the utility of a database for outcomes research is the outcomes measure itself. Traditional outcomes measures in acute medicine are mortality or survival rate, length of stay (LOS), and cost, although these measures are being broadened to include functional status and quality-of-life indexes (Stewart & Ware, 1992). In rehabilitation, mortality is infrequently an issue, and functional status, quality of life, and community reintegration become the focus (Fuhrer, 1987; Wagner, 1987). In rehabilitation outcomes research, LOS and cost represent inputs to the treatment system. Since the 1960s, medical rehabilitation has been developing, refining, and using functional outcomes measures (Forer, 1987; Fuhrer, 1987; Granger & Gresham, 1984; Johnston, Keith, & Hinderer, 1992; Wade, 1992) and thus in some ways is more advanced than acute care disciplines. Nonetheless, the identification of the "right outcomes" is still a major issue in rehabilitation.

Since the early 1980s, substantial and growing attention has been given to the World Health Organization's (1980) *International Classification of Impairments, Disabilities, and Handicaps* as a conceptual framework, if not a coding system, for the consequences of disease. However, there is controversy over the language of the classification (Pope & Tarlov, 1991), especially the use of the term *handicap* to refer to the societal-level disadvantage of having a disability or impairment when the physical or social environment is not accommodating. *Handicap* should not be used in describing individuals, but rather the negative circumstances created by the environment. Ignoring this debate for the moment and simply adopting the term *handicap* to refer to societal or environmental disadvantage, there is a fundamental issue of where the rehabilitation program's responsibility for outcomes lies.

Some argue that the ultimate rehabilitation outcomes goal, and hence the desired measure for research on long-term outcomes, is the elimination or reduction of handicapping situations (DeJong, 1979; Johnston & Wilkerson, 1992; Johnston et al., 1993; Whiteneck, 1994; Whyte, 1994). Yet rehabilitation programs, especially inpatient or residential programs, have little or no control over social and environmental determinants of handicap, such as attitudinal barriers, lack of funding of or access to community-based support and programs, and the values and role choices of the individual. It is expected that inpatient or residential medical rehabilitation programs would affect physical independence, but it is not clear whether other dimensions can be affected. Generally, the use of ultimate outcomes measures, such as measures of handicap or quality of life, could commit programs to outcomes they cannot control. Glueckauf (1990) argued that the most common error in program evaluation is assuming overgenerality of the effects of treatment.

Rather than rehabilitation programs giving up on reducing handicap or measuring it routinely, more needs to be known about the relationship between measures of proximal treatment effects, such as increased functional independence in the clinic, and sustained improvement in real-world outcomes, such as reduced handicap. Program monitoring systems that measure all three domains—impairment, disability, and handicap—are fertile ground for the growth of such knowledge.

A complementary way of conceiving rehabilitation outcomes is in terms of a hierarchy or levels of functions (Wilkerson, 1992)—micro, meso, and macro—in which the basic building block functions must be assembled to achieve higher-order function. Micro-level functions (e.g., endurance, range of motion, strength) are packaged into meso-level functions (e.g., dressing, communicating, ambulation), and those in turn into macro-level functions (e.g., homemaking, working, leisure activity) (see Table 1). Understanding the relationship among the levels of function is crucial to justifying the continued need for an individual's rehabilitation services. More needs to be known about how rehabilitation interventions focusing at the micro- and meso-levels of function can affect the macro-level outcomes most often of interest to patients and to the payers of their care.

USING CLINICAL PROGRAM MONITORING DATABASES FOR OUTCOMES RESEARCH

Outcomes Research in Acute Medical Care

Outcomes researchers have found large variations in treatment intensity, type, and patient outcomes in different areas of the United States. In now-classic studies, Wennberg (1990b), for instance, found that children were almost 10 times more likely to have their tonsils removed if living in one area of Vermont than in another. Similarly, women were three and one half times as likely to undergo hysterectomies if living in certain areas (Wennberg & Gittelsohn, 1982). No differences in health or disease rates could be found to account for these differences in practice. In other well-known studies, Wennberg and colleagues found that inpatient care expenditures

Table 1. Levels of function

Micro
* Range of motion
* Memory
* Cognition
* Strength
* Endurance

Meso
* Activities of daily living
* Walking
* Wheelchair propulsion
* Talking, operating equipment
* Interacting with people

Macro
* Working
* Parenting
* Recreation
* Homemaking
* Social life
* Community participation
* Creating

From Wilkerson, D. (1996). *Level of function as an organizing framework for functional assessment applications.* Manuscript submitted for publication.

per resident of Boston were virtually twice that of New Haven, Connecticut (Wennberg, 1987; Wennberg, Freeman, & Culp, 1987; Wennberg, Freeman, Shelton, & Bubolz, 1989).

Wide variations in intensity of medical treatment have been found for prostatectomy, back surgery, and many other medical procedures in different areas of the United States, with strikingly poor or absent correlations with population morbidity or mortality (Wennberg, 1990b). Variations in intensity of treatment do, however, correlate with the availability of hospital beds, trained specialists, and other treatment resources (Phelps, 1993; Wennberg, 1990a, 1990b).

The notion of outcomes management has begun to affect the organization of American health care. Outcomes management, "a technology of patient experience" (Ellwood, 1988, p. 1551), is based on improvements in health status measurement and increasing expectations regarding the effectiveness and scientific basis of medicine. Outcomes management involves the application of knowledge of the efficacy of treatment and effectiveness in practice to improve the real-world outcomes and cost-effectiveness of health care (Ellwood, 1988). Understanding how outcomes can be improved, while controlling costs, requires the use of large clinical outcomes monitoring systems. Ellwood pointed out that, in rehabilitation and in other fields, databases, even with their imperfections, can and should be used immediately to enhance this understanding.

An example of outcomes management and quality improvement using a clinical database is provided by Horn (1993) from the Intermountain Health Care system. Using the system's clinical information system, the lowest rates of postsurgical infection were found to be related to early administration of prophylactic antibiotics. Hospital practice standards were set to require 2-hour preoperative administration of prophylactic antibiotics, and infection rates and hospital costs subsequently dropped precipitously (Horn, 1993).

Several principles in the use of clinical program monitoring (CPM) databases for outcomes research can be identified. First, key data elements for study—the right outcomes, resources used, and some information about treatment process—must be routinely and uniformly collected. Second, outcomes measures need to be chosen that reflect health-related quality of life, function (disability), or handicap (disadvantage). It is possible to do valuable outcomes research using generic indicators of health (Ware & Sherbourne, 1992), functional activities, or handicap (e.g., institutionalization, return to work). Third, it is important to include disease-specific measures to understand medical outcomes. The Horn Computerized Severity Index, for instance, containing approximately 32 disease-specific variables per case, is of use in assessing case-mix severity in acute hospitals (Horn & Horn, 1986). The Medical Outcomes Study, although most famous for development of a generic health outcome measure, the SF-36 (Ware & Sherbourne, 1992), used a health status questionnaire with many condition-specific items (Stewart & Ware, 1992; Ware & Sherbourne, 1992). A number of condition-specific indicators have been developed to supplement the SF-36 (e.g., for pain, cf. Krousel-Wood, McCune, Abdoh, & Re, 1994).

Fourth, and perhaps most important, changing clinical practice based on CPM systems requires a three-step process. In Step 1, outcomes variation patterns and their correlates are analyzed using the CPM database. If the right data elements are available, there is substantial ability to understand variations and probable processes at this point. However, Step 2, which involves the gathering of additional data, is typically necessary to understand likely causal processes. Step 2 usually involves the gathering and analysis of more detailed information on interventions and processes involved in producing the observed outcomes. Step 3 involves communicating or changing practice standards (a sort of experimental intervention) and continued monitoring to determine the effect, if any, on patient outcomes. Examples of such effects include the drop in postsurgical infection rates and costs documented by Horn (1993) or the decrease in surgical rates documented by Wennberg (Wennberg, 1990a; Wennberg & Gittelsohn, 1982). It is changes such as these that are the intended end point of real quality improvement efforts based on outcomes management systems.

HISTORY AND CRITIQUE OF REHABILITATION CPM DATABASES

Origins and Purposes of Existing Databases

Medical rehabilitation has an extensive history of CPM systems. CARF has, since the 1990s, required accredited organizations to have ongoing program evaluation systems, encouraging providers to collect data on patient outcomes (CARF, 1995). The Joint Commission on Accreditation of Healthcare Organizations (JCAHO; 1995), as of 1995, requires an information management plan that includes the use of aggregate and comparative information in clinical management.

CPM databases for rehabilitation have many common elements, whether they are large shared systems or facility-specific ones. A smaller number of more technologically and conceptually advanced databases, usually organization specific or government funded, include data elements that add analytic power for study of cost-effectiveness, risk adjustment, or outcomes prediction. Table 2 shows examples of both basic data elements, commonly found in CPM data systems in rehabilitation, and more advanced elements.

Three types of CPM databases will be discussed: 1) those developed by facilities or organizations for their own internal use; 2) shared systems, which are multifacility but for the private use of system subscribers; and 3) those developed with public funding, usually for research purposes.

Table 2. Data elements in typical and advanced rehabilitation program monitoring databases

Domain or type of data	Availability	
	Typical of databases in medical rehabilitation	Also available in more fully developed databases
Impairment	Diagnoses, impairments	Severity of impairments and comorbidities; common complications
Disability	Rated independence in a minimum set of physical activities of daily living and cognitive or communicative function at discharge	Assessment of much wider range of abilities, including abilities specific to different conditions or patient needs
Handicap	Home vs. institutional discharge Return to work	Fuller assessment of independent living, social integration, productive activities, and personal well-being 3–12 months postdischarge
Demographics	Age, race, gender, marital status, living arrangement, residence location, referral source	Same as typical, but with more informaton on education, employment, family, resources
Consumer satisfaction	Simple satisfaction with services, staff, service environment	Satisfaction with outcomes, team, participation in plan, input on content of program
Process and interventions	Program name, general type, length of stay	Units of service, types of services, charges, costs and cost ratios, team clinician traits

Facility-Specific Databases

Many rehabilitation providers have developed CPM databases for their own use in program evaluation and outcomes management, often in preparation for CARF accreditation. Most early systems used "homegrown" measures and data elements. Some of these systems have developed into well-validated systems that have contributed to the development of shared systems.

Patient Evaluation and Conference System The Patient Evaluation and Conference System (PECS) developed by Marianjoy Rehabilitation Hospital (Harvey & Jellinek, 1981, 1983; Marianjoy, 1992) was designed for internal use by the hospital's programs. Used to guide periodic review of patient function and progress by the interdisciplinary team, the PECS system has evolved since the early 1980s into a substantial research vehicle.

The PECS now includes 93 items, which comprise validated subscales of impairment severity, applied self-care, motoric competence, and cognition (Harvey et al., 1992; Kilgore, Fisher, Silverstein, Harley, & Harvey,

1993; Marianjoy, 1993; Silverstein, Fisher, Kilgore, Harley, & Harvey, 1992; Silverstein, Kilgore, Fisher, Harley, & Harvey, 1991). Each inpatient is scored just before each team conference, and these data are entered into a computer using the PECS software and displayed for team review and communication to external sponsors. Marianjoy also uses the PECS for outcomes measurement in outpatient clinics and subacute rehabilitation settings. The PECS instrument and the accompanying software are sold for use by other organizations, although no pooled database is created (Marianjoy, 1992).

Rehabilitation Institute of Chicago Functional Assessment Scale (RIC-FAS) The RIC-FAS includes 70 items across the spectrum of rehabilitation disciplines that assess impairment, disability, and, to a limited degree, handicap. The Functional Independence Measure (FIM) (Hamilton, Granger, Sherwin, Zielzny, & Tashman, 1987; State University of New York at Buffalo, 1993) is embedded within the 70 items. (See the discussion of the FIM under shared systems on p. 283.) Two types of rating scales are used: 1) The independence scale rates the degree of assistance needed from another person to accomplish the activity, and 2) the problem scale rates the degree to which the individual has a problem accomplishing the activity. Each item is scored from 1 (complete dependence or severe problem) to 7 (independence or no problem).

The interrater reliability of the RIC-FAS has been assessed, unlike many such tools. Correlation coefficients for RIC-FAS items varied from .36 to 1.0, with the majority achieving coefficients above .80 (RIC, 1989). The RIC-FAS is made available for cost to other providers who wish to use it (RIC, 1989, 1996).

Other Data Sets There are many other organization-specific data sets that have not been as widely publicized but that could be the basis of valuable outcomes research. Typically, these data sets as well as their descriptors are proprietary and unavailable to investigators not employed by the organization.

Private Shared Data Systems

Private shared data systems feature defined data sets, formal training and/or credentialing opportunities, and pooled databases. They are private in that users must pay for participation in the systems, which are run by commercial enterprises. A key advantage of shared systems is the availability of normative information that allows subscribers to compare their average outcomes to other similar facilities. It should be noted that new private shared data system companies are entering this arena as the need for and interest in outcomes management increases. Those described below were well established by the early 1990s.

Uniform Data System for Medical Rehabilitation The Uniform Data System for Medical Rehabilitation (UDSMR) was developed in the mid-1980s as an effort of a joint task force of rehabilitation disciplines and organizations, with funding from the National Institute on Disability and Rehabilitation Research (NIDRR) (Hamilton et al., 1987; State University of New York at Buffalo, 1993). The UDSMR is the largest data system in medical rehabilitation, currently serving more than 800 rehabilitation facilities. Participating facilities must demonstrate conformance with rater credentialing and data quality standards. The UDS primarily contains descriptive and functional status data at admission and discharge, although many providers also obtain data on patient functioning 90 days after discharge.

The FIM is the core functional status and outcomes measure in the UDS. The FIM is an 18-item scale measuring disability in terms of assistance needed to accomplish certain basic physical activities of daily living (ADL) and mobility, plus cognitive and communicative activities. Its reliability is high, and motor and cognitive subscales have been identified (Granger, Hamilton, Linacre, Heinemann, & Wright, 1993; Heinemann, Linacre, Wright, Hamilton, & Granger, 1993). Other variables in the data set include patient demographic characteristics, diagnoses, impairment group, time from onset to rehabilitation, discharge setting, payer, LOS, and hospital charges.

Subscribers to the UDSMR Data Management Service receive quarterly reports summarizing their own data, along with regional and national averages for elements of the data set, and summary measures of the FIM. The service is the most common basis for program evaluation and outcomes management for a large number of rehabilitation organizations.

Formations in Healthcare Formations in Healthcare, Inc., a Medirisk Company, is another company that provides pooled data management services to subscribing rehabilitation providers. Formations maintains databases for inpatient medical rehabilitation, subacute inpatient rehabilitation, outpatient rehabilitation, and industrial rehabilitation (Formations, 1993). Formations began by using the Level of Rehabilitation Scale (LORS) (Carey & Posavac, 1978, 1982) but now also offers data processing for organizations using the FIM. RESTORE, the Formations system for outpatient programs, uses as a part of its data set the SF-36 measure of health status (Ware & Sherbourne, 1992). This measure, developed to assess outcomes in general ambulatory medicine, contains subscales for general health, mental health, and physical functioning. Subscribers to Formations receive periodic reports summarizing their own data and normative comparisons to other subscribers (Formations, 1993).

Focus on Therapeutic Outcomes (FOTO) The FOTO organization specializes in outpatient rehabilitation, primarily freestanding outpatient physical therapy practices dealing with back, knee, and neck impairments. FOTO now uses a derivative of the SF-36, the SF-12, plus other demographic, impairment-related, and service process-related items (FOTO, 1996). FOTO was developed with funding from six national provider organizations. The database is under contract to New England Research Institute. The FOTO data set is brief but, unlike many others, includes specific information about procedures used in treatment.

Literature from FOTO states that data compiled will be shared on a confidential basis with the American Physical Therapy Association and with researchers and educators (FOTO, 1996). The system is designed for use in organizations' program evaluation and quality improvement efforts. Graphic reports are made available at several levels of analysis, including individual, program or impairment groupings for an organization or practice, and companywide profiles. Comparative data are provided for subscribers, summarizing their own data compared with data aggregated for all users of the FOTO service.

Publicly Funded Databases

Spinal Cord Injury (SCI) and Traumatic Brain Injury (TBI) Model Systems The NIDRR has sponsored model systems in SCI (Stover, DeLisa, & Whiteneck, 1995) since the 1970s and for TBI since 1987 (Dahmer et al., 1993). These systems have contributed to an extensive database for the longitudinal study of SCI and TBI outcomes. These databases are much more detailed than most CPM databases. The SCI model systems database contains extensive data on numerous impairments and complications commonly seen after traumatic SCI. The TBI model systems database has data on numerous neuropsychologic tests. Both record data from annual follow-ups, and both are housed with a grantee university research group (Stover et al., 1995). Although the data are not available publicly, regular reports from the databases reach the public via the scientific literature.

Other Databases Other public databases contain valuable, if limited, data on rehabilitation. Medicare patient-level claims records are contained in MEDPAR, which is maintained by the Health Care Financing Administration. Although functional status and other health outcomes measures are not included, MEDPAR files can be studied for diagnosis, service delivery, resource utilization, and rehospitalization trends for patients served in rehabilitation facilities.

Clinical interest groups with a common diagnostic focus also have developed their own databases. An example is the Patient Data Management System (PDMS/fx) developed for the International Myelodysplasia Study Group (Shurtleff, 1991). It has been adapted for other patient groups (e.g., brain injury, myelomeningocele, spina bifida). These data systems contain a great deal of clinically relevant impairment data and are comparable in detail to model systems databases. Such databases have been the basis for many significant research publications and for program evaluation and quality improvement efforts (Shurtleff, 1991). Dozens of programs in the United States and around the world have collaborated in PDMS/fx data collection efforts. Such a collaborative approach, in which concerned clinicians collaborate to obtain insight into how to treat patients more effectively, is in many ways a model for improvement in the quality and effectiveness of rehabilitative interventions.

Past Research Contributions of CPM Systems in Rehabilitation

CPM data systems have been the source of a number of very important research findings in medical rehabilitation. Some illustrative highlights include the following:

- Groundbreaking work on outcomes norms and prognosis in rehabilitation was conducted by Carey, Posavac and Siebert using the LORS by Parkside Associates (Carey & Posavac, 1978, 1982; Carey, Siebert, & Posavac, 1988). Age, LOS, and admission function (disability) were found to predict rehabilitation outcomes, although curvilinear relationships were observed for some impairment groups.
- Using FIM/UDSMR data, Linacre, Heinemann, Wright, Granger, and Hamilton (1994) established that the FIM can be scaled to have equal-interval characteristics. The measure has at least two distinct dimensions: 1) a motor subscale measuring independence in adaptive activities and mobility and 2) a cognitive subscale measuring social interaction, cognition, and communication.
- Stineman and colleagues (Stineman, Escarce, et al., 1994) showed that rehabilitation costs are highly associated with severity of disability, not just with diagnosis. A classification model containing 53 function-related groups (FRGs) was found to explain 31% of the variance in LOS. Predictor variables are diagnosis, admission motor and cognitive function as measured by the FIM, and patient age. This research has also led to the development of a prototype classification system that could be used in prospective payment for medical rehabilitation (FIM-FRGs) (Stineman, Escarce, et al., 1994; Stineman, Hamilton, et al., 1994; Wilkerson, Batavia, & DeJong, 1992).
- Also using the UDSMR database, Heinemann and colleagues found that admission disability as measured by the FIM consistently predicted LOS and discharge function (Heinemann, Linacre, Wright, Hamilton, & Granger, 1994). Heinemann's work also established that subtle differences in these relationships exist depending on impairment group (Heinemann et al., 1993), making it essential to analyze rehabilitation outcomes within impairment group.

- Using program evaluation data, Johnston and Miller (1986) conducted work showing that imposition of the Medicare regulation requiring an increase in therapy to 3 hours per day had no detectable positive effect on patient functional gain in inpatient rehabilitation, although it did increase costs. Implications for rehabilitation service delivery include the need to scale the intensity of services to patient need rather than to an arbitrary minimum of therapy.
- Granger, Hamilton, and Fiedler (1992) examined outcomes for people with stroke using the UDSMR database. Independence at both admission to and discharge from rehabilitation and the likelihood of community discharge were negatively associated with age and bilateral paresis.
- In another study of stroke patients, Granger, Cotter, Hamilton, and Fiedler (1993) found that the FIM predicted minutes of help needed and, to a limited degree, life satisfaction. Depression was clearly linked with life satisfaction. The FIM, however, did not satisfactorily predict supervision needs (Disler, Roy, & Smith, 1993).
- Harvey et al. (1992) and Silverstein et al. (1991, 1992) reported on the psychometric criteria of functional status scales using the PECS. Fisher, Harvey, Taylor, Kilgore, and Kelly (1995) showed that the FIM and PECS motor ADL items measure the same dimension. It is technically possible to derive a measure of general physical independence in mobility and self-care that is independent of the particular rating scales used to measure it. Fisher et al. proposed calling units of this scale-free measure "Rehabits."
- Keith, Wilson, and Gutierrez (1995) compared stroke patients in a free-standing medical rehabilitation hospital with patients in a subacute unit. The study relied on ongoing program evaluation data and found that patients in acute medical rehabilitation experienced greater functional gains, but their costs also were higher.

Many studies have been based on ongoing clinical data systems supplemented by data collected specially for the research. For instance

- Computed tomography results were found to predict return to independent functioning for people with stroke and brain injury in studies using the PECS system (Chaudhuri, Harvey, Sulton, & Lambert, 1988; Rao, Jellinek, Harvey, & Flynn, 1984).
- Johnston's work (Johnston, 1991; Johnston & Lewis, 1991) demonstrated that patients with severe TBI improve substantially in function and independence in specialized postacute rehabilitation programs, especially in home productivity and instrumental ADL. Predictors of improvement were also identified.

Much of what we know of rehabilitation in practice is based on extensive data systems developed by programs for research purposes, usually funded by the federal government.

- The TBI model systems database has been the basis of substantial research on the outcomes in TBI. For example, an entire issue of the *Journal of Head Trauma Rehabilitation* was devoted to such studies (e.g., Dahmer et al., 1993).
- The SCI model systems database has contributed to understanding and treatment of SCI since the 1970s (Stover et al., 1995). Although the SCI model systems is primarily a longitudinal predictive database, it has provided data elements for numerous studies of clinical SCI interventions.

CPM databases have enabled rehabilitation to define basic outcomes. The field now has good data on average outcomes across broad patient groups (Fiedler, Granger, & Ottenbacher, 1996; Granger & Hamilton, 1992), and there has been learning about prognosis (Stover et al., 1995). However, only a little about effective treatment has been learned from these databases. The chief reasons for this lack of information about effective treatment can be discerned.

First, there is the too-common assumption that outcomes observed after rehabilitation are outcomes *due to* rehabilitation. Many factors impinge on an individual's use of skills learned in rehabilitation, such as social and physical environment and accessibility, individual motivations and values, finances, and resource availability, many of which are not in the control of the rehabilitation program and also are not assessed in typical databases. However, if these extra-rehabilitation variables are included, substantially better analyses can be conducted.

Second, many comparisons used in program outcomes management fail to control sufficiently for patient severity. Programs are often compared with averages from a group of programs without detailed control for case mix in terms of severity of disease, impairment, disability, chronicity (onset–admission interval), or comorbid conditions. Potentially important differences in treatment protocols and treatment objectives are typically not part of the database. More accurate methods of severity adjustment, communicated broadly to the field and operationalized in reporting systems, would help substantially. Development and standardization of data elements reflecting program content will also be an important step.

Third, access to private databases is difficult due to the competitive business environment of U.S. health care, even though many private databases ultimately, albeit indirectly, derive most of their funding from public sources. The issue of research uses of databases for the public good versus business uses for individual competitive facilities requires resolution if CPM databases are to be of maximal utility.

ESSENTIAL METHODS OF INFERENCE

Advocates of CPM systems sometimes speak as if knowledge will flow directly from description of outcomes per se, thereby resulting in many improvements to the service system. Although there is merit to these enthusiastic arguments, it is limited. Documentation of clinical program improvements attributable to many CPM systems, although not nonexistent (Forer & Everett, 1989), is scarce. CPM systems can be expensive and can yield disappointing results. However, CPM systems also can provide invaluable information, obtainable in essentially no other way. CPM systems are much more likely to be useful if attention is paid to principles of valid scientific inference. In designing a data CPM system, it should be understood the focused questions it may be able to answer, provided certain data patterns occur, and what questions cannot really be answered, unless large assumptions are made.

There is a continuum of scientific rigor, ranging from judgments, necessary in practice, of what is probably true to results of randomized clinical trials. If one insists on certitude, the embarrassment of a Type 1 error, the error of asserting as true something that is really false, is avoided, but numerous Type 2 errors, the error of identifying as false that which is really true, are committed. The rehabilitation literature may already be replete with Type 2 errors, given the low experimental power of most rehabilitation studies (Ottenbacher, 1995). Similarly, there is a trade-off between internal validity, or correctness of conclusions for the study sample itself, and external validity, or correctness of conclusions for the wider population that is being generalized.

Moreover, there is a valid distinction between uses of CPM for formative evaluation and summative evaluation (Posavac & Carey, 1989). Formative evaluation provides feedback on outcomes, number of clients served, and so forth to assist administrators and clinicians in developing and managing a program. Summative evaluation aims to make a more definitive judgment of whether the program is worthwhile. Existing CPM systems may have both formative and summative features. For instance, the main use of most existing program evaluation systems in rehabilitation is feedback to staff to improve services (CARF, 1995; Johnston et al., 1993; Wilkerson, 1991). At the same time, summative judgments of the program can be based on outcomes "expectancies" or on norms for functional gain supplied by a data service (Granger, Ottenbacher, & Fiedler, 1995). Keith and colleagues' comparison of acute versus subacute rehabilitation provides a potent example of a summative use of CPM data (Keith et al., 1995).

In the final analysis, both formative and summative uses of data need to be grounded in knowledge. Even granting that data systems have multiple uses and that some individuals seem to have a talent for interpreting and using CPM data, CPM systems need to be structured to enable some type of definite inferences. There are at least three essential methods of inference from CPM data systems: 1) inferences based on prior knowledge,

2) nonequivalent comparison groups and statistical control methods, and 3) time-series designs.

Inferences Based on Prior Knowledge

Without explicit control procedures, inferences from CPM data systems can be based only on existing knowledge or beliefs regarding causal processes. CPM systems gain a great deal of power when interpreted in the context of existing knowledge. Their main administrative use is to determine how known causal processes work in practice.

As an example of a well-grounded inference, a clinical data system may identify patients with symptomatic infections associated with a particular microorganism. This knowledge implies a particular course of antibiotic treatment and prophylaxis in the affected ward. As an example involving a reasonable but not completely tested assumption, Wennberg accumulated substantial data indicating that variations in treatment provided correlates with availability of treatment programs more than with indices of morbidity (Wennberg et al., 1987). The argument gains persuasiveness from the highly plausible assumption that financial incentives affect U.S. clinical practices.

In rehabilitation, however, a typical example would involve comparison of a program's average functional gain rates with norms provided by the UDS<small>MR</small> (Granger et al., 1995). If the program's functional gain rates are above average, is it justifiable to assume that the program is better than others? Or does the program merely admit patients with less severe impairment or fewer comorbidities? A number of factors, other than the program itself, affect functional gain rates; thus, the inference of superior (or inferior) treatment in the absence of other knowledge is quite suspect.

Formative evaluation can be expected to work only with the knowledge of causal relationships. When such relations are known, input-process-outcomes patterns may be judged on whether they reflect one known causal chain, as opposed to another. The effectiveness of treatment can in principle be inferred from deviations from outcomes known to be attainable in predicted circumstances. The problem is that prediction is rarely so accurate or independent of confounding factors as to permit such an inference. Many existing CPM data systems in rehabilitation involve observations (e.g., functional changes) whose causal basis is unclear, complex, or unknown. Existing CPM data systems commonly have input and outcomes data, but no control group. Such data systems can inform about prognosis but not reliably about treatment effectiveness without making grand assumptions. Can it really be assumed that improvement in rehabilitation is entirely or even mostly due to rehabilitative treatment? If not, what proportion of outcomes is due to treatment? Simple pre–post data systems, and even longitudinal data systems, cannot answer the crucial question of what aspects of outcomes are due to rehabilitation. CPM data systems need to incorporate a comparison group or stable baseline to obtain knowledge of effectiveness and relative cost–benefits (Johnston, 1987).

Nonequivalent Comparison Groups and Statistical Control Methods

Efforts to strengthen inference from CPM systems usually involve matching, analysis of covariance, path analysis, or variations of these (Cohen & Cohen, 1983; Reichardt, 1979). The essential logic is this: Effective treatment is inferred from large variations in outcomes that are highly associated with variations in treatment but not associated with variations in patient characteristics, despite excellent measurement of relevant case severity factors. These methods benefit greatly from knowledge of predictive factors, which enables the determination of whether groups being compared are really comparable. Alternatively, variations in outcomes need to 'be great to compensate for small differences between caseloads. Data systems therefore need to be structured to maximize chances for such patterns to be examined. Similar patients who receive different treatments must be found, and sophisticated analyses should be performed to determine whether the treatment variations made a difference.

Time-Series Designs

CPM data systems are not commonly based on time series, but there is no essential reason why they should not be. (An exception is claims data, which is structured as a time series but lacks a tie to clinical data.) Time-series designs, especially multiple time series with stable baseline and interventions whose effects are likely to be rapid or distinct, can be logically tight research designs (Johnston, Ottenbacher, & Reichardt, 1995). Data structures involving time series are very often applicable to the study of treatment of individuals or small numbers of individuals. Time-series logics are also applicable to larger databases. For instance, if a new rehabilitation method could be implemented in one region, and then another, and so on, a multiple time-series analysis could determine if the same change in average outcomes occurred repeatedly for similar patients despite local variations.

Valid inference of treatment effects requires a stable baseline, which requires multiple measures. This is often difficult in the clinical practice in independent rehabilitation settings. Large integrated health delivery corporations or multiprovider collaborations, however, could more easily establish systems that assess trends in patient function before referral to rehabilitation.

The Real-World Laboratory: What We Can Gain

Laboratory research and randomized clinical trials are essential to determine the efficacy or potential benefit of specific rehabilitation treatments and modalities and to develop new interventions, but the actual effects, and costs, of treatment in real-world practice must be verified. Clinical program monitoring systems reflect what happens in the real world under varied conditions, both those found in clinical trials and those that are not. Only operational real-world data systems can provide actual as opposed to theoretical outcomes and costs.

CPM databases should be able to detect a relationship between type and amount of treatment effort and outcome. CPM data can also provide information about access to services. When CPM data are combined with information on service setting and intensity, appropriateness and cost-effectiveness of different levels or categories of care can potentially be ascertained, as can clues as to what works best, and for whom, by studying how similar patients fare across settings.

CPM systems in rehabilitation have been used as the scaffolding for more detailed controlled research. At least a minimal CPM system is needed to know whether a site has patients with the diagnostic and functional characteristics necessary to support controlled research in rehabilitation. Program evaluation systems have provided the basis for more insightful research than can be cited in this chapter. Yet, to be worth the expense, CPM systems need to be based on a scientifically justifiable methodology for inference.

STRENGTHS AND LIMITATIONS OF CPM SYSTEMS

Strengths of CPM Databases

Chief among the assets of well-designed CPM databases is the routine use of a valid, reliable outcomes measure. Purely administrative charge databases (e.g., Medicare claims data) do not contain health status data and thus are very limited for outcomes research unless linked to outcomes databases. Common language, definitions, and coding schemes are often used in CPM databases to allow data to be pooled across programs. Such pooling of data yields large data samples (e.g., approaching 1 million cases in UDSmr, 50–60 or more facilities in the databases of large corporations) and data for comparisons across programs. Even though large data samples by themselves do not imply the presence of needed statistical control, they do increase the stability of statistical estimates.

Well-crafted CPM databases can and should be integrated into clinical processes. When clinical professionals believe in the utility of measures for their patients, they can become stalwart sources of accurate data for use in the aggregate.

Data collection cost is an increasingly important issue as health care providers cut costs. Even though good information systems have become more critical, administrators are loathe to spend money on non–revenue-generating activities. Economies of scale for CPM data systems range from substantial to enormous: It is only a little more work to analyze data on 100,000 patients than on 1,000 patients. Large samples and multifacility systems help to make CPM data systems more efficient.

With well-designed computer systems, outcomes data can be linked to already-collected financial and service intensity data from billing systems and consumer surveys to create a powerful database for analysis of program operations.

Limitations of CPM Databases

Limitations of CPM systems are always present and must be avoided by design and training, or at least considered in research and interpretation. Reliability of the data is usually a prime issue, especially when there are many individuals contributing data. Simplicity, clarity, training, and perhaps credentialing are needed even in the best of circumstances.

Completeness of data, a substantial issue even in controlled research, is a major issue in CPM data systems (see Donaldson & Lohr, 1994). Patients can easily be excluded from databases, even inadvertently (e.g., because of unexpected discharge or absence of usual staff). It is easy to design a CPM with functional status items that are difficult to test, or at least rather irrelevant, for some patients, leading busy clinicians to skip items. Medical instability, safety concerns, or time pressures can prevent completion of some items. Some standard items (e.g., stairs) may be too difficult for patients with severe disabilities or at any rate may not be clinical priorities. All these problems lead to missing data or missing cases.

It is often difficult to judge whether a database actually represents the population it claims to represent. CPM reports that do not specify percentage of missing data are prima facie suspect. A large data sample is in no way a cure for missing data, as the large sample may conceal severe sampling biases. A smaller sample, with fewer missing data and less sampling bias, will represent a population better than a large data sample per se.

Clinical data systems can also lack key variables needed for interpretation. For instance, severity of impairment and comorbidities may be poorly measured. Social and environmental factors are often neglected in operational data systems, largely because simple, valid measures have not been developed. Insufficient data on treatment processes and objectives will limit the studies of outcomes. Medical rehabilitation has not systematically included detailed process data in multi-institutional databases. Billing systems that contain therapy codes are a practical source of charge data but are usually not linked with functional status data. Systems that code the objective of therapeutic interventions, such as "PT for range of motion" or "transfer training," could be enormously more informative than systems that primarily code hours or units of therapy. Uniform process code schemes, defined in terms of their objective and/or nature, are needed.

RESEARCH USES OF CPM SYSTEMS IN REHABILITATION

Despite their limitations, clinical data systems can address many important research questions. Most of these are descriptive of the course of patient change, changes in the service delivery system, and prediction or prognosis. CPM databases can serve as a foundation for the following analyses:

- *Describe a historical baseline of patient groups served in various rehabilitation settings.* Such baselines are often the primary way of assessing the impact of major changes in the service delivery system.
- *Describe regional variation and trends over time in access, outcomes, and cost of care.* Access to and utilization of rehabilitation may vary geographically for patients with similar impairments (University of Minnesota, 1994). For those who do receive rehabilitation, level or setting of rehabilitation also varies (Keith et al., 1995; Kramer, Eilertsen, Hrincevich, & Schlenker, 1994; University of Minnesota, 1994). Rehabilitation CPM databases could be very instrumental in documenting changes in the rehabilitation service delivery system as the health care environment evolves, functioning as a ready-made data collection system for before-and-after analyses of health reform measures.
- *Describe relationships between rehabilitation processes and outcomes.* Such knowledge should assist with the efforts of rehabilitation providers to compare their performance to a benchmark themselves and to improve the quality and effectiveness of their care.
- *Predict outcomes in practice.* The prediction of outcomes is one of the key, valid products of CPM data systems. Prediction of costs and outcomes to the patient is becoming increasingly important in practice. Providers must predict outcome and cost to adjust to demands of the marketplace and may even find themselves reimbursed partly on the basis of outcomes. Rehabilitation teams must project attainable outcomes and costs to justify admission to some case managers and to prioritize their interventions. More accurate prediction also would enable more realistic consumer expectations and ensure the planning of safe, nonstressful discharge arrangements.
- *Describe the course of disabling conditions in practice.* CPM data systems can describe improvement curves, when repeated measures over time are available. Degree of retention of benefits after discharge can be analyzed using follow-up data already collected by rehabilitation program evaluation systems.
- *Help develop practice guidelines or treatment protocols for rehabilitation.* Practice parameters must work in practice, and CPM data sys-

tems are invaluable in testing their implementation and identifying ways in which they work or do not work. Determining geographic variations in outcomes while controlling for severity of impairment is an essential step in identifying the need for practice guidelines. Sensible practice guidelines involve assessment of patient function. Critical elements of CPM data systems can then be embedded in practice guidelines.

- *Extend assessment of rehabilitation outcomes toward independent living, community integration, and handicap reduction.* Rehabilitation outcomes goals should stretch beyond disability into reduction of handicap, independent living, and community integration, at the macro level of function (Johnston & Wilkerson, 1992; Whiteneck, 1988, 1992, 1994; Wilkerson, 1992; Willer, Ottenbacher, & Coad, 1994). The field could benefit from maturation of databases that contain measures of handicap, community integration, and independent living (Whiteneck, 1994). There is more to be learned about correlates of independent discharge disposition for various impairment groups, productivity at follow-up, and reduction of downstream medical costs after rehabilitation, all outcomes such as those described by DeJong (1979). Less likely to be available, but equally intriguing, are outcomes in self-direction and other elements of independent living philosophy such as the concept of personal independence described by Nosek, Fuhrer, and Howland (1992).

- *Determine characteristics of rehabilitation programming associated with better outcomes and with cost-effectiveness in practice.* In medical rehabilitation, many alternative treatments can *only* be tested using clinical databases because randomization is unethical or infeasible. Correlational methods can be used to distinguish rehabilitative treatments and strategies associated with better outcomes while controlling statistically for case severity. Again, the basic logic is the comparison of outcomes of very similar patient subgroups that receive very different treatments. Such studies would usually require collection of additional treatment processes not included in most CPM databases.

- *Detail the costs and outcomes of different service delivery settings or types of care.* The array of settings for provision of medical rehabilitation services has expanded rapidly. Several studies have explored outcomes and costs for alternative rehabilitation environments (Harvey et al., 1992; Keith et al., 1995; Kramer, Eilertson, Hrincevich, & Schlenker, 1994; University of Minnesota, 1994). Such studies involve, to a greater or lesser degree, access to existing documentation and data systems. A great deal more needs to be known about the retention of outcomes across different settings and what types of patients do best in what types of settings.

- *Provide a framework for more in-depth studies.* This is one of the main, valid uses of CPM data systems. Without a data system, the most appropriate site for a controlled study is not known. CPM systems can also provide essential parts of the data needed by controlled studies. To answer questions about the effectiveness or cost-effectiveness of interventions, however, CPM data systems usually must be augmented with additional data or explicitly designed to permit valid comparison of very similar patient groups that receive distinctly different interventions.

DATA SYSTEMS IN A HEALTH CARE BUSINESS ENVIRONMENT

Applications of CPM Systems to Clinical Management

The application of CPM data to practical clinical management is challenging, but essential. Unless clinicians contributing to CPM databases learn something relevant from them, such as information about their own performance, clues to improving clinical strategies, or relief from other documentation, data quality is likely to suffer. Although most rehabilitation programs have become accustomed to collection of data on outcomes at discharge, organizations find themselves collecting data without using it, sometimes because the system is too elaborate and attempts to address too many issues, or sometimes because it is too simplistic. In either case, such systems are likely to be underfunded, leading to poor data quality and even poorer utility.

This data-collection-without-application syndrome may derive from a fundamental ambivalence about evaluation itself. On the one hand, programs have a sincere desire to improve. They wish to be the best and to provide high-quality service, and they want data to demonstrate their superiority. On the other hand, programs may be threatened by the very evaluation findings they seek. They worry about comparing poorly with other programs and fear losing referrals or managed care contracts if performance is less than standard or even less than superior.

The Business versus Research Conundrum

Business and competition have become intertwined with outcomes research, putting pressures on CPM databases. Large corporations and provider networks are the primary entities able to afford the development of large databases. Although these databases present opportunities for outcomes research, they can also be problematic. Business motivations can put pressure on them to ensure positive findings. Data can be "gamed" in numerous ways, explicitly or by shrewd indirection, and perhaps even by hidden biases. Innocent logistical problems in data recording by busy clinicians can be as serious if the end point is a biased database.

Ownership of the data is not always clearly established, but for the most part CPM data belong to private organizations and are not in the public domain. This frequently prevents access to the data by independent researchers and slows progress. How can honest clinical data systems be developed in a business-oriented health care industry? Honesty and credibility are essential, for if data are not believed, the data system is of no use. Business executives will demand strict budget limits and clear payoffs and ask to use data for marketing. Such requests, however, lead to incentives for "gaming" of the data and put concerned clinicians and scientists in a conflict-of-interest position. The following are some partial solutions to the problem:

- *Ensure program confidentiality with strict standards and procedures, while allowing access to data by qualified independent investigators.* There are already strict standards to ensure patient confidentiality. The usual bottleneck in outcomes research is ensuring program confidentiality. Database holders would feel less constrained in sharing data if they could be assured of confidentiality.
- *Implement new accreditation requirements.* JCAHO (1995) requires that programs compare their outcomes and processes to objective standards. CARF (1995) accreditation standards give CARF the right to ask for outcomes and process data from accredited programs. CARF, because of its position in the rehabilitation field, could use this power to lead programs to actually compare their outcomes to those known to be attainable by similar patients.
- *Develop an institutional forum to promote study and publication of results from privately held databases.* Accrediting bodies, the National Center for Medical Rehabilitation Research, or respected private non-profit organizations could join together to create such an institution. Until then, database owners should be encouraged to allow their data to be used, with appropriate confidentiality protections, for research purposes.
- *Obtain agreement on methods of interpretation.* Programs have little to fear from research-level analyses and interpretations that take into account the full complexity of rehabilitation and the multitude of non-treatment factors that affect outcomes. Interpretation of outcomes needs to take case severity and exogenous factors, such as amount of funding available, family support, and preinjury history, into account in analysis and interpretation of outcomes.
- *Implement objective data-auditing procedures.* Ultimately, data on quality and outcomes need to be objective and trustworthy rather than subjective or totally controlled by the local program without effective oversight. If functional status were to become essential to a classification system for prospective payment in rehabilitation, pressures for data gaming would be multiplied, and audit procedures would be mandatory.

The problems of integrity and efficiency of access to CPM data systems can be solved, but only by the concerted actions of many.

FEASIBLE IMPROVEMENTS IN REHABILITATION CPM DATABASES

The following is a listing of a number of ways in which current CPM systems could be improved at little long-term cost:

- Adding information on processes of care (treatment type and quantity) is needed but would require uniform ways of coding treatment type. Embedding information about the treatment objective in the coding scheme could be extremely valuable.
- Obtaining accurate cost data at the patient level will be necessary if one is to truly understand the relationship between cost and outcomes and to maintain patient outcomes while controlling costs. Integrating outcomes data with billing systems would provide a powerful basis for cost-effectiveness analyses.
- Adding measures of handicap, community integration, life satisfaction, and consumer satisfaction would strengthen current rehabilitation CPM data systems. Consumer satisfaction data are already routinely collected by most rehabilitation providers, albeit in a nonstandardized and irregular way that is not linked to clinical data.
- Linking of databases can be expedited through coding schemes and identifiers. Important insights can be obtained by linking data in one segment of the treatment continuum (e.g., acute care) to data in another segment (e.g., inpatient and outpatient rehabilitation). Studies in a single setting can provide a very incomplete or biased picture of outcomes and cost-effectiveness.

    The need to protect confidentiality sometimes creates unnecessary insistence on absolute secrecy. Confidentiality issues can be dealt with reasonably so that patients are protected and data access is possible and reasonably efficient (Donaldson & Lohr, 1994). To accomplish efficient data linkages, common patient identifiers must be available across multiple settings and episodes of care. At a minimum, care organizations should use a common patient identifier throughout their organization. Rehabilitation databases should be modified to contain a unique patient identifier, so that readmissions of the same person can be distinguished from that of a new person.
- Precise severity adjustment is needed for scientifically valid inference of treatment effectiveness. Any meaningful distinction among outcomes for different groups should control for the risk of poor outcomes. Severity or risk adjustment is a way to remove or reduce the effects of confounding factors in studies where the cases are not randomly assigned to different treatments. The key confounding factors are those aspects of health status that are causally related to the outcome under study.

Risk is a multidimensional concept that may include genetic predisposition, comorbid conditions, lifestyle, family support, and many other variables unknown or unmeasurable (Iezzoni, 1994). Most CPM databases contain primary diagnosis, but severity or stage of disease or impairment may not be assessed. Fortunately, functional limitations or disability (e.g., FIM) at admission is commonly recorded. However, without description of disease stage or severity of impairments, severity or risk assessment for medical rehabilitation is limited.

Numerous severity adjusters for rehabilitation—factors causally related to rehabilitation outcomes—have been suggested in the literature. Analysts of the FIM (Granger, Hamilton, et al., 1993; Heinemann et al., 1993, 1994; Linacre et al., 1994; Stineman, Hamilton, et al., 1994), for instance, have found that admission functional status (disability level) is a strong predictor of discharge disability and may be curvilinearly related to gain in function. Level and completeness of spinal lesion is the central severity adjuster for study of physical disability outcomes in SCI (Stover et al., 1995). Severity of motor impairment—for example, as measured by the Fugl–Meyer (Duncan, Goldstein, Matchar, Divine, & Feussner, 1992)—and cognitive impairment—for example, as measured by the Neurobehavioral Cognitive States Exam (NCSE) (Galski, Bruno, Zorowitz, & Walker, 1993)—are outstanding severity adjusters in stroke. Risk- and severity-adjustment data systems have been developed by a number of vendors, providers, and agencies (Iezzoni, 1994). Most contain detailed clinical measures predictive of outcomes for disease. Medical rehabilitation is in the position of having functional status data, which are rarely available in other medical databases. Valid and reliable measures of environmental risk factors need to be further developed and would be a valuable addition to rehabilitation CPM databases.

• Data systems should be structured to enable comparison of outcomes across different programs that treat similar patients. This approach is the essence of ascertaining information on effectiveness and cost-effectiveness. Fear of misuse of data makes for a reluctance to allow comparative analyses, but without comparative analyses the question "What programs work?" cannot be answered. Agreements on proper interpretation of data and on protection of patient and program confidentiality can ameliorate the reluctance. Perhaps only accreditation requirements or laws requiring public disclosure can solve the problem.

• The CPM needs to be integrated with treatment guidelines or protocols. Rehabilitation facilities across the United States are developing clinical paths, and treatment guidelines have been developed for rehabilitation (e.g., for stroke rehabilitation, see Post-Stroke Rehabilitation Guideline Panel, 1995). Emerging rehabilitation clinical pathways entail measurement of function at key points. If key points of guidelines or clinical paths are documented, there will be valuable data on the methods by which superior outcomes are, or are not, attained.

- A great deal of progress can be made if clinical professionals will incorporate standardized assessment of impairments, disabilities, and objectives into their clinical documentation. Whether automated or not, clinical documentation provides a rich basis for research, if the system is systematically designed and implemented (Shields, Leo, Miller, Dostal, & Barr, 1994). Standardization of clinical assessment according to scientific measurement standards would be a step forward (Johnston et al., 1992).

- Methods of minimizing missing data elements can be further developed. Databases can be made simpler. Attention to details of administrative implementation results in better data, provided there is actual commitment to record the data. Items that are routinely collected for clinical purposes are more likely to be completed than items only for research or administrative purposes. Systems can be developed to require testing of some items only in highly clinically relevant conditions, rather than across all patients.

- As a corollary, methods of determining the representativeness of the sample can and should be implemented. As a first step, simple registries listing *all* admitted cases can be implemented, so that the percentage of lost cases will at least be known.

Although many improvements to CPM systems are needed, CPM systems also have great potential. The continuing automation of clinical and business records and pressures for standardization and for accountability to the consumers of rehabilitation services make CPM systems fertile grounds for research.

CONCLUSIONS

The new health care order in the United States during the 1990s has stimulated a dramatic rise in attention to cost-cutting strategies and realignments of provider arrangements, as well as to the use of information to manage and market programs. Although outcomes research continues to be important to establish the efficacy of rehabilitation interventions under controlled scientific circumstances, real-world effectiveness of rehabilitation programs must be established to respond to this new health care environment. The cost-reduction environment also begs for cost-effective information and research strategies.

Clinical program monitoring systems have been, and, it is argued here, will continue to be, an important basis for these investigations. The field of medical rehabilitation has a solid foundation of outcomes measurement and the building of pooled databases from which a number of research findings have been garnered. These findings are limited, however, by several problems with the use of CPM databases in outcomes research. Most of the systematic work pertains to traditional hospital-based inpatient medical rehabilitation; more work is needed in other venues of rehabilitation service provision such as subacute skilled nursing facilities, outpatient rehabilitation, and home-based settings.

CPM data systems can be improved to respond to these needs, and several ways of doing so are suggested in this chapter. Some improvements relate to technical matters of data element definitions, linking of records, and the use of uniform measures across settings. However, there are other, more global issues that must be addressed, including confidentiality and public disclosure of pooled data, access to privately held data for research purposes, and the confrontation between business competition and research or intellectual motivations for the use of CPM and outcomes databases. Again, several ways around these dilemmas are suggested. If these problems can be solved, there is much to be learned from using CPM databases in medical rehabilitation outcomes research.

REFERENCES

Batalden, P.B., Nelson, E.C., & Roberts, J.S. (1994). Linking outcomes measurement to continual improvement: The serial "V" way of thinking about improving clinical care. *Journal of Quality Improvement, 20*(4), 167–180.

Carey, R.G., & Posavac, E.J. (1978). Program evaluation of a physical medicine and rehabilitation unit: A new approach. *Archives of Physical Medicine and Rehabilitation, 59*(7), 330–337.

Carey, R.G., & Posavac, E.J. (1982). Rehabilitation program evaluation using a revised Level of Rehabilitation Scale (LORS-II). *Archives of Physical Medicine and Rehabilitation, 63*(8), 367–370.

Carey, R.G., Siebert, J.H., & Posavac, E.J. (1988). Who makes the most progress in inpatient rehabilitation? An analysis of functional gain. *Archives of Physical Medicine and Rehabilitation, 69*(5), 337–343.

CARF . . . The Rehabilitation Accreditation Commission (CARF). (1995). *1995 standards manual and interpretive guidelines for medical rehabilitation.* Tucson, AZ: Author.

Chaudhuri, B., Harvey, R.F., Sulton, L.D., & Lambert, R.W. (1988). Computerized tomography head scans as predictors of functional outcome of stroke patients. *Archives of Physical Medicine and Rehabilitation, 69*(7), 496–498.

Cohen, J., & Cohen, P. (1983). *Applied multiple regression/correlation analysis for the behavioral sciences* (2nd ed.). Hillsdale, NJ: Lawrence Erlbaum Associates.

Dahmer, E.R., Shilling, M.A., Hamilton, B.B., Bontke, C.F., Englander, J., Kreutzer, J.S., Ragnarsson, K.T., & Rosenthal, M. (1993). A model systems database for traumatic brain injury. *Journal of Head Trauma Rehabilitation, 8*(2), 12–22.

DeJong, G. (1979). *The movement for independent living: Origins, ideology, and implications for disability research.* East Lansing MI: University Centers for International Rehabilitation.

DesHarnais, S., Marshall, B., & Dulski, J. (1994). Information management in the age of managed competition. *Journal of Quality Improvement, 20*(11), 631–638.

Disler, P.B., Roy, C.W., & Smith, B.P. (1993). Predicting hours of care needed. *Archives of Physical Medicine and Rehabilitation, 74*(2), 139–143.

Donaldson, M.S., & Lohr, K.N. (Eds.). (1994). *Health data in the information age: Use, disclosure, and privacy.* Washington, DC: National Academy Press.

Duncan, P.W., Goldstein, L.B., Matchar, D., Divine, G.W., & Feussner, J. (1992). Measurement of motor recovery after stroke. Outcome assessment and sample size requirements. *Stroke, 23*(8), 1084–1089.

Ellwood, P. (1988). Outcomes management: A technology of patient experience. (Shattuck Lecture). *New England Journal of Medicine, 31*(23), 1549–1556.

Fiedler, R.C., Granger, C.V., & Ottenbacher, K.J. (1996). The Uniform Data System for Medical Rehabilitation: Report of first admissions for 1994. *American Journal of Physical Medicine and Rehabilitation, 75*(2), 125–129.

Fisher, W.P., Jr., Harvey, R.F., Taylor, P., Kilgore, K.M., & Kelly, C.K. (1995). Rehabits: A common language of functional assessment. *Archives of Physical Medicine and Rehabilitation, 76,* 113–122.

Focus on Therapeutic Outcomes, Inc. (FOTO). (1996). *Data report services, version 3.1.* Knoxville, TN: Author.

Forer, S.K. (1987). Outcome analysis for program service management. In M.J. Fuhrer (Ed.), *Rehabilitation outcomes: Analysis and measurement* (pp. 115–136). Baltimore: Paul H. Brookes Publishing Co.

Forer, S.K., & Everett, J. (1989). Marketing program quality: The California Association of Rehabilitation Facilities. In B. England, R.M. Glass, & C.H. Patterson (Eds.), *Quality rehabilitation: Results-oriented patient care* (pp. 95–101). Chicago: American Hospital Publishing, Inc.

Formations in Healthcare, Inc. (1993). *Rehabilitation outcomes reports.* Chicago: Author.

Fuhrer, M.J. (Ed.). (1987). *Rehabilitation outcomes: Analysis and measurement.* Baltimore: Paul H. Brookes Publishing Co.

Galski, T., Bruno, R.L., Zorowitz, R., & Walker, J. (1993). Predicting length of stay, functional outcome, and aftercare in the rehabilitation of stroke patients: The dominant role of higher-order cognition. *Stroke, 24*(12), 1794–1800.

Gennarelli, T.A., Champion, H.R., Copes, W.S., & Sacco, W.J. (1994). Comparison of mortality, morbidity, and severity of 59,713 head injured patients with 114,447 patients with extracranial injuries. *The Journal of Trauma, 37*(6), 962–968.

Glaser, J. (1994). Developing a clinical information system: The role of the chief information officer. *Journal of Quality Improvement, 20*(11), 614–621.

Glueckauf, R.L. (1990). Program evaluation guidelines for the rehabilitation professional. In M.G. Eisenberg & R.C. Grzesiak (Eds.), *Advances in clinical rehabilitation* (Vol. 3, pp. 250–264). New York: Springer-Verlag.

Granger, C.V., Cotter, A.C., Hamilton, B.B., & Fiedler, R.C. (1993). Functional assessment scales: A study of persons after stroke. *Archives of Physical Medicine and Rehabilitation, 74*(2), 133–138.

Granger, C.V., & Gresham G. (Eds.). (1984). *Functional assessment in rehabilitation medicine.* Baltimore: Williams & Wilkins.

Granger, C.V., & Hamilton, B.B. (1992). UDS Report: The Uniform Data System for Medical Rehabilitation report of first admissions for 1990. *American Journal of Physical Medicine and Rehabilitation, 71*(2), 108–113.

Granger, C.V., Hamilton, B.B., & Fiedler, R.C. (1992). Discharge outcome after stroke rehabilitation. *Stroke, 23*(7), 978–982.

Granger, C.V., Hamilton, B.B., Linacre, J.M., Heinemann, A.W., & Wright, B.D. (1993). Performance profiles of the Functional Independence Measure. *American Journal of Physical Medicine and Rehabilitation, 72*(2), 84–89.

Granger, C.V., Ottenbacher, K.J., & Fiedler, R.C. (1995). The Uniform Data System for Medical Rehabilitation: Report of first admissions for 1993. *American Journal of Physical Medicine and Rehabilitation, 74*(1), 62–66.

Hamilton, B.B., Granger, C.V., Sherwin, F.S., Zielzny, M., & Tashman, J.S. (1987). A uniform national data system for medical rehabilitation. In M.J. Fuhrer (Ed.), *Rehabilitation outcomes: Analysis and measurement* (pp. 137–150). Baltimore: Paul H. Brookes Publishing Co.

Harvey, R.F., & Jellinek, H.M. (1981). Functional performance assessment: A program approach. *Archives of Physical Medicine and Rehabilitation, 62*(9), 456–460.

Harvey, R.F., & Jellinek, H.M. (1983). Patient profiles: Utilization in functional performance assessment. *Archives of Physical Medicine and Rehabilitation, 64*(6), 268–271.

Harvey, R.F., Silverstein, B., Venzon, M.A., Kilgore, K.M., Fisher, W.P., Steiner, M., & Harley, J.P. (1992). Applying psychometric criteria to functional assessment in medical rehabilitation: III. Construct validity and predicting level of care. *Archives of Physical Medicine and Rehabilitation, 73*(10), 887–892.

Heinemann, A.W., Linacre, J.M., Wright, B.D., Hamilton, B.B., & Granger, C.V. (1993). Relationships between impairment and physical disability as measured by the Functional Independence Measure. *Archives of Physical Medicine and Rehabilitation, 74*(6), 566–573.

Heinemann, A.W., Linacre, J.M., Wright, B.D., Hamilton, B.B., & Granger, C.V. (1994). Prediction of rehabilitation outcomes with disbability measures. *Archives of Physical Medicine and Rehabilitation, 75*(2), 133–143.

Horn, S. (1993, December). *Great expectations: Fulfilling the potential of outcomes findings and practice guidelines.* Presented at the Medical Outcomes Research Conference III: The Remaking of a Revolution, Arlington, VA.

Horn, S.D., & Horn, R.A. (1986). The Computerized Severity Index: A new tool for case-mix management. *Journal of Medical Systems, 10*(1), 73–78.

Iezzoni, L. (Ed). (1994). *Risk adjustment for measuring health care outcomes.* Ann Arbor, MI: Health Administration Press.

Johnston, M.V. (1987). Cost–benefit methodologies in rehabilitation. In M.J. Fuhrer (Ed.), *Rehabilitation outcomes: Analysis and measurement* (pp. 99–113). Baltimore: Paul H. Brookes Publishing Co.

Johnston, M.V. (1991). Outcomes of community re-entry programmes for brain injury survivors. Part 2: Further investigations. *Brain Injury, 5*(2), 155–168.

Johnston, M.V., & Granger, C. V. (1994). Outcomes research in medical rehabilitation: A primer and introduction to a series. *American Journal of Physical Medcine and Rehabilitation, 73*(4), 296–303.

Johnston, M.V., Keith, R. A., & Hinderer, S. (1992). Measurement standards for interdisciplinary medical rehabilitation. *Archives of Physical Medicine and Rehabilitation, 73*(Suppl 12-S), S6–S23.

Johnston, M.V., & Lewis, F.D. (1991). Outcomes of community re-entry programmes for brain injury survirors. Part 1: Independent living and productive activities. *Brain Injury, 5*(2), 141–154.

Johnston, M.V., & Miller, L.S. (1986). Cost-effectiveness of the Medicare three-hour regulation. *Archives of Physical Medicine and Rehabilitation, 67*(9), 581–585.

Johnston, M.V., Ottenbacher, K., & Reichardt, K. (1995). Strong quasi-experimental designs for research on the effectiveness of rehabilitation. *American Journal of Physical Medicine and Rehabilitation, 74*(5), 383–392.

Johnston, M.V., & Wilkerson, D.L. (1992). Program evaluation and quality improvement systems in brain injury rehabilitation. *Journal of Head Trauma Rehabilitation, 7,* 68–82.

Johnston, M.V., Wilkerson, D.L., & Maney, M. (1993). Evaluation of the quality and outcomes of medical rehabilitation programs. In J.A. DeLisa & B. Gans (Eds.), *Rehabilitation medicine: Principles and practice* (2nd ed., pp. 240–268). Philadelphia: J.B. Lippincott.

Joint Commission on Accreditation of Healthcare Organizations (JCAHO). (1995). *Accreditation manual for hospitals: Vol. I. Standards.* Oakbrook Terrace, IL: Author.

Keith, R.A., Wilson, D.B., & Gutierrez, P. (1995). Acute and subacute rehabilitation for stroke: A comparison. *Archives of Physical Medicine and Rehabilitation, 76*(6), 495–500.

Kilgore, K.M., Fisher, W.P., Silverstein, B., Harley, J.P., & Harvey, R.F. (1993). Application of Rasch analysis to the Patient Evaluation and Conference System. *Physical Medicine and Rehabilitation Clinics of North America, 4*(3), 493–515.

Kramer, A.M., Eilertsen, T.B., Hrincevich, C.A., & Schlenker, R.E. (1994). Rehabilitation of Medicare patients in rehabilitation hospitals and skilled nursing facilities. Study Paper 5 of *Study of the cost-effectiveness of subacute care alternatives and services.* Denver: Center for Health Services Research, University of Colorado Health Sciences Center.

Krousel-Wood, M.A., McCune, T.W., Abdoh, A., & Re, R.N. (1994). Predicting work status for patients in an occupational medicine setting who report back pain. *Archives of Family Medicine, 3*(4), 349–355.

Linacre, J.M., Heinemann, A.W., Wright, B.D., Granger, C.V., & Hamilton, B.B. (1994). The structure and stability of the Functional Independence Measure. *Archives of Physical Medicine and Rehabilitation, 75*(2), 127–132.

Marianjoy Rehabilitation Hospital & Clinics (Marianjoy). (1992). *The rehabilitation outcome reporting system with PECS©: Manual for managers.* Wheaton, IL: Author.

Nosek, M.A., Fuhrer, M.J., & Howland, C.A. (1992). Independence among people with disabilities. II: Personal Independence Profile. *Rehab Counseling Bulletin, 36*(1), 21–36.

Ottenbacher, K.J. (1995). Why rehabilitation research does not work (as well as we think it should). *Archives of Physical Medicine and Rehabilitation, 76,* 123–129.

Phelps, C.E. (1993). The methodologic foundations of studies of the appropriateness of medical care. *New England Journal of Medicine, 329,* 1241–1245.

Pope, A.M., & Tarlov, A.R. (Eds.). (1991). *Disability in America: Toward a national agenda for prevention.* Washington, DC: National Academy Press.

Posavac, E.J., & Carey, P.G. (1989). *Program evaluation: Methods and case studies* (3rd ed.). Englewood Cliffs, NJ: Prentice Hall.

Post-Stroke Rehabilitation Guideline Panel. (1995). *Clinical practice guideline number 16: Post-stroke rehabilitation.* Rockville, MD: U.S. Department of Health and Human Services, Public Health Service, Agency for Health Care Policy and Research. (AHCPR Publication No. 95-0662)

Rao, N., Jellinek, H.M., Harvey, R.F., & Flynn, M.M. (1984). Computerized tomography head scans as predictors of rehabilitation outcome. *Archives of Physical Medicine and Rehabilitation, 65*(1), 18–20.

Rehabilitation Institute of Chicago (RIC). (1989). *RIC-FAS II: Rehabilitation Institute of Chicago Functional Assessment Scale.* Chicago: Author.

Rehabilitation Institute of Chicago (RIC). (1996). *Rehabilitation Institute of Chicago Functional Assessment Scale manual, version IV.* Chicago: Author.

Reichardt, C.S. (1979). The statistical analysis of data from non-equivalent group designs. In T.D. Cook & D.T. Campbell (Eds.), *Quasi-experimentation: Design and analysis issues for field settings* (pp. 147–206). Boston: Houghton Mifflin.

Shields, R.K., Leo, K.C., Miller, B., Dostal, W.F., & Barr, R. (1994). An acute care physical therapy clinic practice database for outcomes research. *Physical Therapy, 75*(5), 463–470.

Shurtleff, D.B. (1991). Computer data bases for pediatric disability: Clinical and research applications. *Pediatric Rehabilitation: Physical Medicine and Rehabilitation Clinics of North America, 2*(4), 665–687.

Silverstein, B., Fisher, W.P., Kilgore, K.M., Harley, J.P., & Harvey, R.F. (1992). Applying psychometric criteria to functional assessment in medical rehabilitation: II. Defining interval measures. *Archives of Physical Medicine and Rehabilitation, 73*(6), 507–518.

Silverstein, B., Kilgore, K.M., Fisher, W.P., Harley, J.P., & Harvey, R.F. (1991). Applying psychometric criteria to functional assessment in medical rehabilitation: I. Exploring unidimensionality. *Archives of Physical Medicine and Rehabilitation, 72*(9), 631–637.

State University of New York at Buffalo. (1993). *Guide for the Uniform Data Set for Medical Rehabilitation (Adult FIM), version 4.0.* Buffalo, NY: Author.

Stewart, A.L., & Ware, J.E., Jr. (Eds.). (1992). *Measuring functioning and well-being.* Durham, NC: Duke University Press.

Stineman, M.G., Escarce, J.J., Goin, J.E., Hamilton, B.B., Granger, C.V., & Williams, S.V. (1994). A case-mix classification system for medical rehabilitation. *Medical Care, 32*(4), 366–379.

Stineman, M.G., Hamilton, B.B., Granger, C.V., Goin, J.E., Escarce, J.J., & Williams, S.V. (1994). Four methods for characterizing disablty in the formation of function related groups. *Archives of Physical Medicine and Rehabilitation, 75*(12), 1277–1283.

Stover, S.L., DeLisa, J.A., & Whiteneck, G.G. (1995). *Spinal cord injury: Clinical outcomes from the model systems.* Rockville, MD: Aspen Publishers.

University of Minnesota. (1994). *Final report, executive summary, Post-Acute Care Project.* HCFA #17-C98891. Minneapolis: Author.

Wade, D.T. (1992). *Measurement in neurological rehabilitation.* New York: Oxford University Press.

Wagner, K.A. (1987). Outcome analysis in comprehensive medical rehabilitation. In M.J. Fuhrer (Ed.), *Rehabilitation outcomes: Analysis and measurement* (pp. 19–28). Baltimore: Paul H. Brookes Publishing Co.

Ware, J.E., & Sherbourne, C.D. (1992). The MOS 36-item short-form health survey (SF-36). *Medical Care, 30*(6), 473–483.

Wennberg, J.E. (1987). Population illness rates do not explain population hospitalization rates. *Medical Care, 25*(4), 354–359.

Wennberg, J.E. (1990a). Outcomes research, cost containment, and the fear of health care rationing. *New England Journal of Medicine, 323*(17), 1202–1204.

Wennberg, J.E. (1990b). Small area analysis and the medical care outcome problem. In L. Sechrest, E. Perrin, & J. Bunker (Eds.), *AHCPR conference proceedings: Research methodology: Strengthening causal interpretations of nonexperimental data* (pp. 177–206). Rockville, MD: U.S. Department of Health and Human Services, Agency for Health Care Policy and Research.

Wennberg, J.E., Freeman, J.L., & Culp, W.J. (1987). Are hospital services rationed in New Haven or over-utilized in Boston? *Lancet, 1,* 1185–1189.

Wennberg, J.E., Freeman, J.L., Shelton, R.M., & Bubolz, T.A. (1989). Hospital use and mortality among Medicare beneficiaries in Boston and New Haven. *New England Journal of Medicine, 321,* 1168–1173.

Wennberg, J.E., & Gittelsohn, A. (1982). Variations in medical care among small areas. *Scientific American, 246,* 120–134.

Whiteneck, G.G. (1994). Measuring what matters: Key rehabilitation outcomes. *Archives of Physical Medicine and Rehabilitation, 75*(10), 1073–1076.

Whiteneck, G.G., Charlifue, S.W., Gerhart, K.A., Overholser, J.D., & Richardson, G.N. (1988). *Guide for use of the CHART: Craig Handicap Assessment and Reporting Technique.* Englewood, CO: Craig Hospital.

Whiteneck, G.G., Charlifue, S.W., Gerhart, K.A., Overholser, J.D., & Richardson, G.N. (1992). Quantifying handicap: A new measure of long-term rehabilitation outcomes. *Archives of Physical Medicine and Rehabilitation, 73*(6), 519–526.

Whyte, J. (1994). Toward a methodology for rehabilitation research. *American Journal of Phyiscal Medicine and Rehabilitation, 73*(6), 428–435.

Wilkerson, D. (1991). Program and outcome evaluation: Opportunity for the 1990's. *Occupational Therapy Practice, 2*(2), 1–15.

Wilkerson, D. (1992). *Level-of-function as an organizing framework for functional assessment applications.* Paper presented at annual meeting of the American Congress of Rehabilitation Medicine, San Francisco, CA, November 1992 [Abstract]. *Archives of Physical Medicine and Rehabilitation, 73,* 977.

Wilkerson, D. (1996). *Level of function as an organizing framework for functional assessment applications.* Manuscript submitted for publication.

Wilkerson, D.L., Batavia, A.I., & DeJong, G. (1992). Use of functional status measures for payment of medical rehabilitation services. *Archives of Physical Medicine and Rehabilitation, 73*(2), 111–120.

Willer, B., Ottenbacher, K.J., & Coad, M.L. (1994). The Community Integration Questionnaire: A comparative examination. *American Journal of Physical Medicine and Rehabilitation, 73,* 103–111.

World Health Organization (WHO). (1980). *International classification of impairments, disabilities, and handicaps.* Geneva, Switzerland: Author.

CHAPTER 13

Characterizing Rehabilitation Interventions

Pamela W. Duncan, Helen Hoenig,
Gregory Samsa, and Byron Hamilton

The increasing focus on the cost and effectiveness of medical care places additional emphasis on outcomes. More and more frequently, answers are required for questions such as the following:

1. Which treatments work?
2. Which providers offer the most clinically effective and cost-effective care?
3. Which settings are most efficacious?

Rehabilitation shares with other aspects of medical care the challenge of establishing the success of its outcomes. Rehabilitation practitioners must be prepared to define interventions and demonstrate where, when, and how they work. This chapter presents models for defining the "black box" of rehabilitation practices. Evaluation of stroke rehabilitation outcomes is used as an example to demonstrate the usefulness of the models.

DEFINING REHABILITATION INTERVENTIONS

Even experienced researchers may sometimes address their subjects in terms that are too general. They may begin with a broad question, such as, "Does rehabilitation make a difference in minimizing disability?" Posing this question is similar to asking, "Does carotid endarterectomy prevent

This chapter was supported by the Center for Medical Effectiveness Research, Agency for Health Care Policy Research, Contract No. 282-91-0028. This chapter also was supported in part by the National Institutes of Health, National Institute on Aging, Geriatric Research and Training Centers, National Grant 1 P30 AG09463, and the Claude D. Pepper Older Americans Independence Center, Grant 5 P60 AG11268.

stroke?" Research questions need to be targeted to a specific type of patient for whom a certain intervention is used with the purpose of producing predefined outcomes. Using this approach, stroke researchers very effectively demonstrated that although carotid endarterectomy was not a cost-effective way to prevent all strokes, it was highly effective in preventing strokes in patients who have carotid distribution transient ischemic attacks and carotid stenosis greater than 70% (Matchar, Pauk, & Lipscomb, 1996). Similarly, in rehabilitation research, interventions must be targeted to certain patient types. Researchers must ask, "For a given patient type with specific causes for existing impairments, functional limitation, or disability, what specific interventions are effective?"

One approach to defining rehabilitation interventions is to meticulously characterize rehabilitation services by considering collectively and individually all of the components involved. For this approach, a micro level and a macro level of characterization are recommended. The micro level concerns the patient and the immediate factors related to the patient and his or her care (Figure 1). The macro level deals with group-level effects and addresses the process of structuring care and providing services (Figure 2).

The components of the micro level may be identified by asking three questions:

1. Why is the intervention being selected?
2. What is the structure of the intervention?
3. How is the intervention being done?

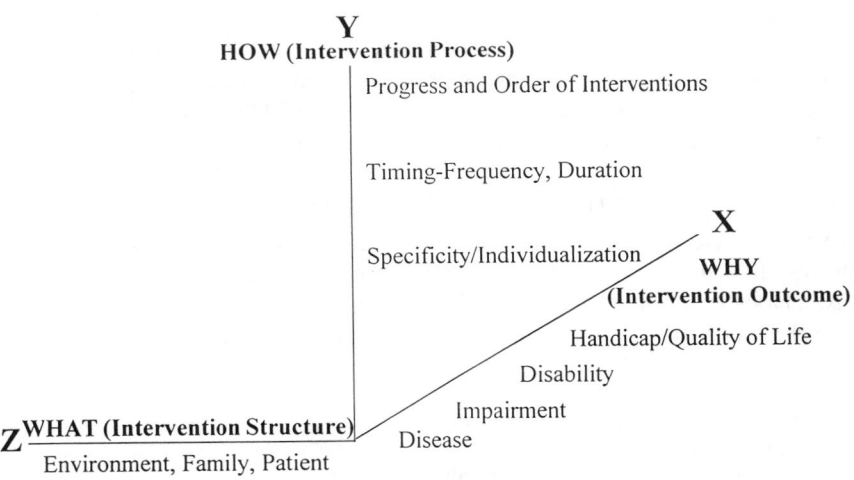

Figure 1. Micro (individual) level.

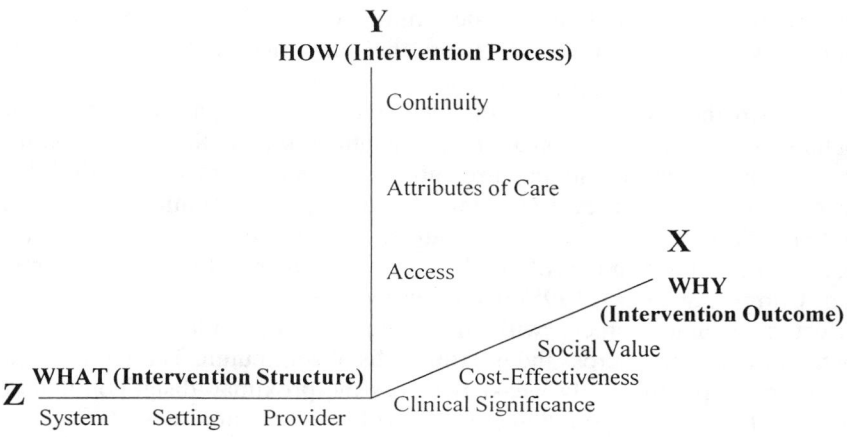

Figure 2. Macro (group) level.

In Figure 1, the why is represented on the *x* axis, the what on the *z* axis, and the how on the *y* axis.

The why question addresses the outcomes that interventions are expected to produce. These outcomes may be classified by using a conceptual framework, the *International Classification of Impairments, Disabilities, and Handicaps* (ICIDH) model of the disabling process (see Figure 3) (World Health Organization, 1980). This model categorizes a proximal–distal continuum of outcomes. The most proximal outcomes are the impairments, the physiologic or psychologic consequences, and the signs and symptoms of the disease at the organ level. The more intermediate outcomes involve the disability (functional limitations in areas of performance, such as mobility, activities of daily living). The most distal outcomes refer to handicaps (limitations in role function and health-related quality of life). The expected outcome of the rehabilitation program has major implications for selecting and defining the interventions. For example, if the expected outcome is to increase strength, the intervention may be rather straightforward, such as a progressive resistance exercise program. However, if the expected outcome is to decrease falls, the intervention may need to include programs of strengthening exercises, modification of the environment, modification of the patient's risk-taking behavior, and development of social support. Specifically, determining the point in the continuum of the disablement model where the effects of the

Disease ⟶ Impairment ⟶ Disability ⟶ Handicap

Figure 3. ICIDH model.

intervention are desired helps to determine the complexity of the intervention as well as the number of factors that may modify the effects of the intervention.

When the intervention is directed only at the impairment level, the outcomes of the intervention are mostly captured only at the more proximal levels. The effects of an impairment-level intervention on the disability level or the handicap level are more than likely to be minimal, unless the initial illness is severe and the treatment is very curative or unless the pretreatment function is profoundly altered. Brenner and colleagues (Brenner, Curbow, & Legro, 1995) demonstrated this principle in a study of the effect of cataract surgery with intraocular lens implantations on patient outcomes variables across the proximal–distal continuum. The effect of the intervention progressively weakens across the proximal–distal continuum, but it is larger at all points in patients with greater initial deficits.

When the outcomes are more distal (instrumental activities of daily living or quality of life), myriad factors (e.g., depression, social support, environment) may modify the effects of the interventions or may become part of the interventions themselves (Figure 4). As the interventions are selected, these factors must be considered as part of the intervention or as important modifiers of the intervention. For example, if the goal of the intervention is to improve instrumental activities of daily living (IADL) (disability level), the intervention may need to include both 1) interventions targeted at specific impairments and modifications of the environment to improve accessibility and 2) family counseling to ensure that the family encourages the patient's independence.

Thus, defining the nature of the treatment requires a proximal–distal continuum of specification. For example, the therapist must consider

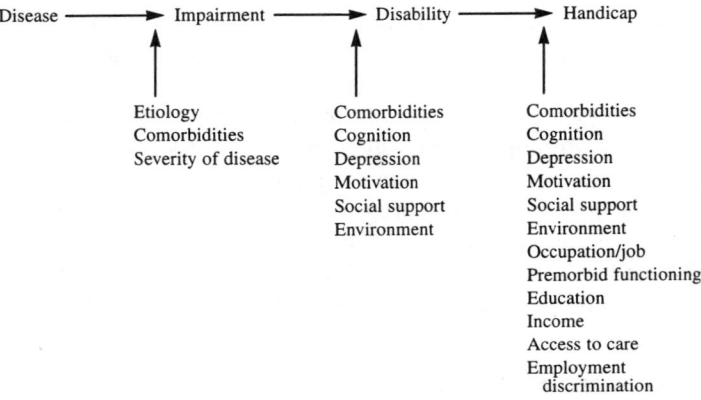

Figure 4. Factors that affect the disablement process.

whether the treatment is rendered to the patient only or whether it includes family and environmental interventions. As we move along the proximal–distal continuum of the nature of the intervention (the z axis in Figure 1), the number of variables becomes greater and the characterization of the interventions also becomes more complex.

As Figure 1 illustrates, the nature of the rehabilitation intervention may be characterized at multiple levels: the patient, the family, and the environment. At the patient level, interventions can be defined by types of exercises, modalities, activities, education programs, or equipment selected to address specific problems. At the family level, interventions selected must be appropriate for those providing informal care and must include family education and caregiver support groups. At the environmental level, the patient's physical surroundings can be modified to remove dangers or to increase access. The social and psychological environment also can be changed to provide additional patient support and to minimize caregiver burden.

IMPLEMENTING REHABILITATION INTERVENTIONS

How the intervention is implemented (the y axis in Figure 1) is another major characterization of the intervention. This category defines the duration, frequency, and intensity of treatments; their progression; and their specificity. For example, if the patient exercises or practices skills only during supervised therapy sessions, the benefits obtained may be substantially less than the benefits accrued by the patient who also practices at home in his or her usual environment. The patient whose regimen is progressive (i.e., requires increasingly more difficult exercises and activities) may benefit more than the patient whose regimen remains static.

The more proximal the variables of interest for characterizing the why, the what, and the how of the intervention, the more easily the intervention can be defined (see Figure 1). Moving distally on each axis of the intervention profiles, the characterization of the interventions becomes increasingly more complex. The complexity is a challenge but should not be a deterrent to evaluating the success of rehabilitation interventions.

As interventions are developed and characterized at the micro level, flexibility is an essential part of the profiles of the interventions. As in all good medicine, the treatment should be appropriate for the illness. There are multiple causes of seemingly similar problems, and it is likely that interventions will be most effective if they target the underlying factors contributing to the problem; that is, rehabilitation programs should be individualized for each patient. This individualization needs to be accounted for in rehabilitation research.

For example, in a randomized trial comparing therapy in stroke patients managed in stroke rehabilitation units with those managed in general medical wards, the percentage of patients who received individualized programs was significantly greater in the rehabilitation unit compared with the general medical ward (Kalra, Dale, & Crome, 1993). Although the general medical ward patients received more therapy, the rehabilitation patients demonstrated better outcomes and reduced hospital stay. The individualized rehabilitation program was the only variable that significantly differentiated the therapeutic interventions for the two groups.

Another study demonstrated that development of individualized intervention programs has good interclinician reliability (Koch, Gottschalk, Baker, Palumbo, & Tinetti, 1994). The effectiveness of these individualized intervention programs in reducing falls and improving mobility in community-living older adults was also evaluated in a randomized trial (Tinetti et al., 1994).

At the macro level (Figure 2), the provision of rehabilitation services may be characterized by asking the following questions:

1.   What are the expected outcomes (x axis)?
2.   What are the characteristics of the provider, setting, and system of care (z axis)?
3.   How are the rehabilitation services provided (y axis)?

The outcomes of rehabilitation services are judged by three criteria: clinical significance, cost-effectiveness, and social value. An intervention that improves a person's health is considered clinically significant. However, it is considered cost-effective only if it demonstrates economic value. An intervention may be very effective clinically, but the cost of the services may be so large that the economic costs outweigh the clinical benefits. Finally, an intervention may have little potential for restoring function but retain a high social value. For example, patients with severe cognitive impairment may not function independently, but exercises may be offered to the particular groups to maintain mobility and minimize complications of immobility. These types of services are provided because society has decided that they are needed to ease transition, to support the groups, and to demonstrate social caring.

Numerous other factors in the provision of rehabilitation services may influence the outcomes of care. Provider qualifications and skills are factors that should be considered in the effectiveness of rehabilitation interventions. Is the intervention more effective when performed by a professional than when performed by a less trained individual or a family member? Is any increase in effectiveness sufficient to justify the additional cost of the professional's services?

The organization of providers and their relationships have been demonstrated to be predictors of outcomes and utilization of services in geriatrics (Applegate et al., 1990; Rubenstein et al., 1984). Yet there are few data on the value of interdisciplinary providers in rehabilitation. It must be ascertained not only what provider characteristics are associated with positive outcomes but also the best way to organize providers.

Characterizing the intervention is especially complicated because of the many different types of settings (e.g., home, nursing facility, inpatient rehabilitation hospital, outpatient setting) in which rehabilitation services may be provided. The organization of services across these varied settings is very different. For example, in a nursing facility, the interventions may be rendered by independent contractors who have little knowledge of what other team members are doing. In rehabilitation facilities, therapy is coordinated by a multidisciplinary team, and the patient is required to receive at least 3 hours of therapy per day. It is very likely that the organization of services in these various settings may modify the effects of the intervention.

Provision of rehabilitation in the home is expanding. It has been suggested that, in select patients, home health care may be more clinically effective and cost-effective than care provided in other settings (Pryor & Williams, 1989; Young & Forster, 1992). The site of care must be a component of characterization of rehabilitation interventions, and it should not be assumed that demonstrated benefit in one setting is generalizable to another.

An important factor in structuring care is the system of health care delivery, which may have profound effects on the nature of the intervention. Access to care and availability of resources vary among systems. For example, the intervention effects may be modified if the intervention is rendered in a managed health care environment in which access to and frequency of care are controlled, as opposed to a fee-for-service environment, where there is less regulation of the providers and the types and frequency of treatments.

Regulation by prospective payment systems has defined rehabilitation services in some settings, such as inpatient rehabilitation units. For example, the Medicare prospective payment system mandates at least 3 hours of therapy each day for each client. The Tax Equity and Fiscal Responsibility Act of 1982 (PL 97-248), which reimburses exempt diagnosis-related group units at a single rate per patient discharged, creates incentives to admit patients with less severe impairments and encourages shorter lengths of stay.

Finally, there is tremendous variability in use and availability of rehabilitation settings across the United States. For example, the percentage of stroke survivors admitted to skilled nursing facilities varies from 17% in the southern states to 32% in the Pacific states. The utilization of home health services for stroke survivors varies from 25% in the northern midwest states to 42% in both the New England and central southeastern states

(Gresham et al., 1995). The accessibility of rehabilitation services, the co-ordination of these services, and the continuity with which they are rendered across settings and over time are all important characteristics that will affect outcomes.

CONCLUSIONS

The conceptual models presented in this chapter provide a framework for defining the "black box" of rehabilitation practices. The structure and process of rehabilitation practices can be defined at the micro and macro levels. Evaluation of stroke rehabilitation outcomes serves as an example to demonstrate the utility of the models.

At the micro level (i.e., individual), an important question in stroke rehabilitation is, "Does therapeutic exercise improve motor recovery and subsequently functional independence?" Figure 5 represents the variables that must be defined in a randomized clinical trial to determine the efficacy of therapeutic exercise. The therapeutic intervention is at the patient level and is expected to improve motor control, balance, and endurance. The benefits of the program may be modified by engaging the family in the

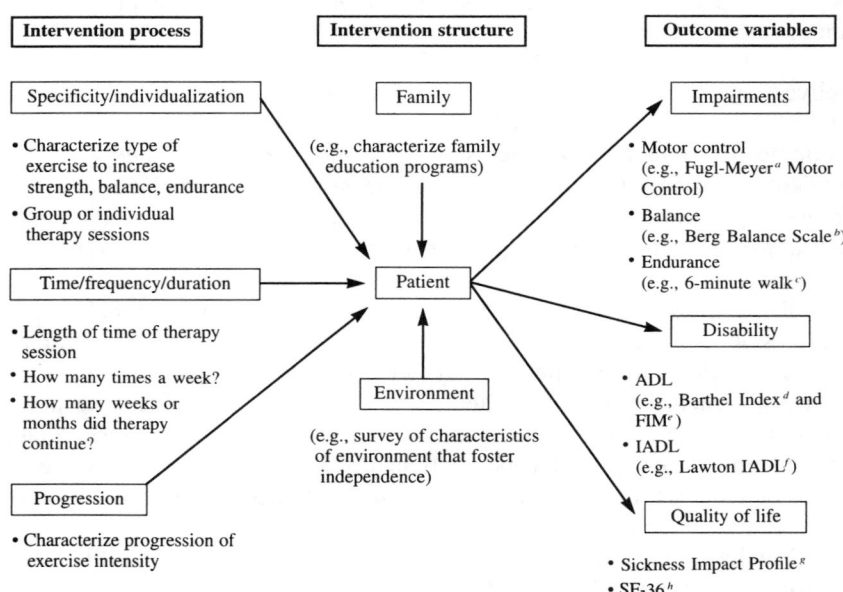

Figure 5. Evaluating the efficacy of therapeutic exercise for stroke patients at the micro level. (ADL = activities of daily living, FIM = Functional Independence Measure, IADL = instrumental activities of daily living.) ([a]Fugl-Meyer et al., 1975; [b]Berg, 1988; [c]Guyatt & Thompson, 1985; [d]Mahoney & Barthel, 1965; [e]State University of New York at Buffalo, 1993; [f]Lawton, 1988; [g]Bergner, Bobbitt, Carter, & Gilson, 1981; [h]Ware & Sherbourne, 1992.)

exercise program and educating them to promote patient exercise compliance. The ability of the patient to translate improved motor control, balance, and endurance into improved activities of daily living and improved quality of life will be modified by the ability of the environment to foster independence.

Evaluation of stroke rehabilitation services at the macro (i.e., group) level may be exemplified by comparison of outcomes across various rehabilitation settings (e.g., inpatient rehabilitation units, nursing facilities, home health care), different providers, or different financial systems. Figure 6 represents examples of variables necessary to characterize process and measure outcomes. Evaluation of the effectiveness of stroke rehabilitation services at the macro level should be done with prospective data collection. In the absence of randomized trials, comparisons of services will always be subject to selection bias. Yet a prospective study will offer many advantages over a retrospective study. In the prospective study the variables can be well defined and measured, making covariance adjustment much easier.

Intervention structure	Intervention process	Outcome variables
Settings	**Access**	**Clinical significance**
• Inpatient rehabilitation units or hospitals	• Characterized patient mix across settings	• Activities of daily living (e.g., Barthel[c] or FIM[d])
• Nursing facilities		• Instrumental activities of
• Home health care	**Attributes of care**	daily living
• Outpatient services		(e.g., Lawton IADL[e])
	• Team care (e.g., Baggs[a] measure of team coordination)	• Quality of life (e.g., SF-36[f])
Provider		• Days living in the community
	• Intensity of services (e.g., direct patient care time, frequency and duration of services, wage rate for different caregivers, group vs. individualized)	• Mortality
• Education		
• Specialty		**Cost-effectiveness**
• Contract vs. noncontract		
• Professional/paraprofessional		• Direct/indirect costs
	• Compliance with Clinical Practice Guidelines[b] for post-stroke rehabilitation	• Estimating marginal costs and outcome functions
System		• Cost-effectiveness ratios
		• Cost–utility analyses
• Fee for service	**Continuity**	
• Managed health care		**Social Value**
• Private insured	• Utilization of health care services after discharge	
• Medicaid	• Referral for community services	• Survey of public's willingness to pay for stroke rehabilitation services

Figure 6. Evaluating stroke rehabilitation services at the macro level. (FIM = Functional Independence Measure, IADL = instrumental activities of daily living.) ([a]Baggs, 1994; [b]Gresham, Duncan, & Stason, 1995; [c]Mahoney & Barthel, 1965; [d]State University of New York at Buffalo, 1993; [e]Lawton, 1988; [f]Ware & Sherbourne, 1992.)

The emphasis on establishing the effectiveness of rehabilitation care foreshadows increasing numbers of randomized trials and epidemiologic analyses. The micro model of the why, what, and how of rehabilitation interventions, combined with the macro model for characterizing rehabilitation services, will provide some basis for framing research questions and defining the structures and process of care that are sufficiently specific and targeted to find the answers that consumers and payers will demand.

REFERENCES

Applegate, W.B., Miller, S.T., Graney, M.J., Elam, J.T., Burns, R., & Akins, D.E. (1990). A randomized, controlled trial of a geriatric assessment unit in a community rehabilitation hospital. *New England Journal of Medicine, 71,* 1572–1578.

Baggs, J.G. (1994). Development of an instrument to measure collaboration and satisfaction about care decisions. *Journal of Advanced Nursing, 20,* 176–182.

Berg, K. (1988). *Measuring balance in the elderly: Validation of an instrument.* Unpublished doctoral dissertation, McGill University, Montréal, PQ, Canada.

Bergner, M., Bobbitt, R.A., Carter, W.B., & Gilson, B.S. (1981). The Sickness Impact Profile: Development and final revision of a health status measure. *Medical Care, 19,* 787–805.

Brenner, M.H., Curbow, B., & Legro, M.W. (1995). The proximal–distal continuum of multiple health outcomes measures: The case of the cataract surgery. *Medical Care, 4*(Suppl.), AS236–AS244.

Fugl-Meyer, A.R., Jaasko, I., Leyman, I., Olsson, S., & Steglind, S. (1975). The post-stroke hemiplegic patient: A method for evaluation of physical performance. *Scandinavian Journal of Rehabilitation Medicine, 7*(1), 13–31.

Guyatt, G., & Thompson, P.J. (1985). How should we measure function in patients with chronic heart and lung diseases. *Journal of Chronic Disease, 38,* 517–524.

Gresham, G., Duncan, P.W., Stason, W.B., et al. (1995). *Post-stroke rehabilitation guideline technical support.* Rockville, MD: U.S. Department of Health and Human Services, Public Health Service, Agency for Health Care Policy and Research.

Kalra, L., Dale, P., & Crome, P. (1993). Improving stroke rehabilitation: A controlled study. *Stroke, 24*(10), 1462–1467.

Koch, M., Gottschalk, M., Baker, D.I., Palumbo, S., & Tinetti, M.E. (1994). An impairment and disability assessment and treatment protocol for community-living elderly persons. *Physical Therapy, 74*(4), 286–294.

Lawton, M.P. (1988). Instrumental Activities of Daily Living. *Psychopharmacology Bulletin, 24*(4), 785–787.

Mahoney, F.I., & Barthel, D.W. (1965). Functional evaluation: The Barthel Index. *Maryland State Medical Journal, 14,* 61–65.

Matchar, D.B., Pauk, J.S., & Lipscomb, J. (1996). A health policy perspective on carotid endarectomy: Cost, effectiveness, and cost-effectiveness. In W. Moore (Ed.), *Surgery for cerebrovascular disease* (pp. 680–689). Philadelphia: W.B. Saunders.

Pryor, G.A., & Williams, D.R.R. (1989). Rehabilitation after hip fractures: Home and hospital management compared. *Journal of Bone and Joint Surgery, 71,* 471–474.

Rubenstein, L.Z., Josephson, K.R., Wieland, D., English, P.A., Sayre, J.A., & Kane, R.L. (1984). Effectiveness of a geriatric evaluation unit. *New England Journal of Medicine, 311*, 1664–1670.

State University of New York at Buffalo. (1993). *Guide for the Uniform Data Set for Medical Rehabilitation (Adult FIM), version 4.0.* Buffalo, NY: Author.

Tax Equity and Fiscal Responsibility Act of 1982, PL 97-248. *Statutes at Large, 96*, 324 *et seq.*

Tinetti, M.E., Baker, D.I., McAvay, G., Claus, E.B., Garrett, P., Gottschalk, M., Koch, M.L., Trainor, K., & Horwitz, R.I. (1994). A multifactoidal intervention to reduce the risk of falling among elderly people living in the community. *New England Journal of Medicine, 331*(13), 821–827.

Ware, J.E., & Sherbourne, C.D. (1992). The MOS 36-Item Short-Form Health Survey (SF-36): I. Conceptual framework and item selection. *Medical Care, 30*(6), 473–483.

World Health Organization (WHO). (1980). *International classification of impairments, disabilities, and handicaps.* Geneva, Switzerland: Author.

Young, J.B., & Forster, A. (1992). The Bradford community stroke trial: Results at six months. *British Medical Journal, 304*, 1085–1089.

CHAPTER 14

Central Nervous System Conditions

J. Scott Richards, W.T. Jackson, and T.N. Novack

Delimiting the status of central nervous system (CNS) conditions outcomes research is a daunting task. CNS dysfunction can result from trauma, disease, or congenital developmental causes and affects every age and segment of society. Although physical limitation is the most common defining characteristic of disability in general and CNS disorders specifically, it is not always present or the major source of limitation (e.g., acquired brain injury [ABI], certain psychiatric diseases, mental retardation). Onset can be gradual or sudden and recovery can be complete or near-complete to minimal, and, when recovery does occur, it can take place rapidly or over many years. In some cases, a fluctuating course of disability and recovery can occur (e.g., multiple sclerosis). In others, improvements in recovery are compromised by concomitant losses due to aging and unknown environmental factors. Risk factors run the gamut from genetic to environmental and behavioral. What this means is that outlining the necessary and sufficient boundaries of outcomes research in CNS disorders is not likely to result in a uniform set of measures or domains that apply to all conditions. Specificity is likely to be more productive in defining the outcomes domains of greatest importance to each CNS condition, with further delineation based on the demographics of the sample under consideration (e.g., vocational outcomes are irrelevant to retired people who sustain a stroke, but not to those of working age). Defining the state of outcomes research for all CNS conditions in such a way, however, is beyond the scope of this chapter. With this caveat in mind, this chapter utilizes representative CNS disorders to describe the problems and limitations of rehabilitation outcomes research as of 1995 and delineate needs for future research.

TYPES OF CENTRAL NERVOUS SYSTEM DISORDERS

The following schema is adapted from deGrott and Chusid (1988, p. 383) and is illustrative of the broad range of disorders and etiologies of the central nervous system.

1. *Vascular disorders*: These typically involve occlusion or rupture of blood vessels that supply the central nervous system. The most prominent example is stroke involving cortical or subcortical structures. Less common are vascular disruptions to the spinal cord.

2. *Trauma*: Injuries to the skull and meninges or to the spine may destroy neural tissue or cause vascular lesions. Spinal cord injury and acquired brain injury are the most prominent examples.

3. *Infections and inflammations*: These may be accompanied by fever, especially in acute onset. Examples are meningitis, abscess formation, and encephalitis.

4. *Toxic, deficiency, and metabolic disorders*: Examples include poisoning, vitamin deficiency, and enzyme defects leading to disruption of neural cell function.

5. *Demyelinating diseases*: Multiple sclerosis is a prominent example.

6. *Degenerative diseases*: These include spinal, cerebellar, subcortical, and cortical degenerative disorders.

7. *Congenital malformations and perinatal disorders*: Exogenous factors (e.g., infection, radiation) or genetic and chromosomal factors may result in abnormalities of the brain or spinal cord in newborn infants. Hydrocephalus, Chiari malformation, and cerebral palsy are examples.

8. *Neuromuscular disorders*: Includes muscular dystrophies, congenital myopathies, neuromuscular junction disorders, transmitter deficiencies, and neuropathies.

With this diversity of etiologies, CNS disorders can be tremendously diverse in how they manifest themselves regarding levels of injury or disease, impairment, disability, and handicap. Table 1 presents three representative CNS examples and ways in which they vary across those different levels. These three CNS disorders—spinal cord injury, ABI, and cerebrovascular accident (CVA)—were chosen to provide a representative cross-section of etiologies (traumatic and nontraumatic), sequelae (primarily cognitive versus primarily physical), and age ranges. Although neuronal cell injury or death may be the common starting point, the ultimate end points—disability and handicap—can be quite different, depending on whether those cells were cortical, subcortical, or spinal and at what age and to what extent they were injured. Outcomes research in CNS disorders, therefore, is also not likely to follow a single common pathway, but needs to be defined by the specific, unique characteristics of the disorder being

Table 1. Levels of disease, impairment, disability, and handicap for three representative CNS conditions

Injury/Disease	Impairment	Disability	Handicap
Interruption or interference of normal physiologic and developmental processes or structures	Loss and/or abnormality of cognitive, emotional, physiologic, or anatomic structure or function	Restriction or lack of ability (from an impairment) to perform an activity in the manner or within the range considered normal for a human	Disadvantage resulting from an impairment or disability that limits or prevents the fulfillment of a role that is normal for that person
		Levels of Reference	
CNS neuronal cell dysfunction or death	Brain or spinal cord dysfunction	Individual: task performance within the social and cultural context	Society
1. *Spinal cord injury*: Trauma producing incomplete or complete lesions	Muscle atrophy; loss of voluntary control of movement; bowel, bladder, sexual dysfunction	Physical interference with activities of daily living	Unlikely to be able to perform prior job and participate in society fully because of attitudinal and physical barriers
2. *Acquired brain injury*: Trauma producing focal or diffuse cortical and/or subcortical damage	Information processing deficits; lack of insight, awareness, self-control; paresis, spasticity, seizure	Cognitive (and/or physical) interference with activities of daily living	May be unable to perform prior job; difficulty in interpersonal relations, generally; educational/vocational barriers
3. *Cerebrovascular accident*: Bleeding, thrombosis, or embolus causing localized or diffuse CNS cell death	Information-processing deficits; lack of awareness, visuospatial neglect; speech disturbance, hemiplegia	Cognitive (and/or physical) interference with activities of daily living; communication problems	Unlikely to be able to perform prior job; difficulty in interpersonal relations; communication/social integration problems

Adapted from World Health Organization (1980).

studied. The rest of this chapter is devoted to a description of spinal cord injury, ABI, and CVA; their epidemiology, functional consequences, and behavioral sequelae; typical rehabilitation management; and the status of outcomes research.

SPINAL CORD INJURY

Spinal cord injury (SCI) typically affects young males four times more often than females (Stover & Fine, 1986) and is becoming a disproportionately prevalent problem for African Americans (DeVivo, Rutt, Black, Go, & Stover, 1992). Leading causes of SCI are motor vehicle crashes, falls (more frequent in older individuals), sporting injuries, and acts of violence (Stover & Fine, 1986). However, in some spinal cord injury centers in the United States, acts of violence have become the leading cause (Go, DeVivo, & Richards, 1995). Spinal cord injury is at this point considered a permanent source of paralysis, the extent of which depends on the level and extent of destruction of the spinal cord. A number of basic and applied investigations are ongoing that attempt to minimize the cascade of physiologic events causing cell death immediately postinjury. Other attempts are ongoing to repair or bridge the damaged spinal cord in acute and chronic injuries. However, SCI is still considered a permanent source of paralysis. With tetraplegia, all four limbs are involved; with paraplegia, there is sparing of upper-extremity function. Bowel, bladder, and sexual function are often profoundly disrupted; ability to return to the former type of employment is also often limited. Pain and a number of other debilitating secondary complications can occur both in the acute and chronic phases with negative consequences for quality of life.

Initial rehabilitation efforts are most often interdisciplinary and typically include occupational therapy, physical therapy, recreational therapy, psychology, social work, nursing, and vocational counseling, as well as obvious input and direction from a variety of medical specialties, including physiatry. The goal is maximization of physical independence through strengthening of remaining functional muscle groups and the use of adaptive equipment. When the patient cannot be made completely independent, family members or other help surrogates are trained to provide the additional assistance needed for discharge to home. In the SCI model system of care, 92.3% of people with SCI are ultimately discharged to home (Dijkers, Abela, Gans, & Gordon, 1995). Outpatient rehabilitation services, if available, are provided either in the home or in an institutional setting postdischarge but are typically limited to physical therapy and sometimes occupational therapy. If the person with SCI is receptive and deemed appropriate, he or she may be referred to state vocational rehabilitation personnel for evaluation and potential retraining for work. However, the ultimate return-to-work rate for many of these individuals is still quite low. People with SCI require lifelong follow-up because of the high prevalence of secondary complications including those involving the urinary tract and skin, as well as behavioral and environmental problems such as substance abuse, marital discord, and poor coping and adjustment. Some of these individuals experience severe pain. In addition, the aging process has an impact on people with SCI. The length of stay for rehabilitation of people with SCI has been dramatically shortened, with an increasing emphasis on outpatient services. The impact of that trend is not yet well documented.

SCI Rehabilitation Outcomes

The most productive source of rehabilitation outcome information for people with SCI has come from Spinal Cord Injury Model Systems of Care, funded by the National Institute on Disability and Rehabilitation Research (NIDRR). This effort began in 1970, when the southwestern regional system for the treatment of SCI was established at the Good Samaritan Hospital in Phoenix, Arizona. One of the initial objectives of that project was to develop a database to document the results of a system of care, including rehabilitation outcomes and cost-effectiveness. As the model systems program has grown, the collaborative database has evolved with it and remained a viable NIDRR-funded activity in 1995. The number of model systems that were funded at any one time has varied since 1970, but, in 1995, 18 such systems were funded. One of their mandates is to continue contributing data to the national data set, now maintained and managed at the University of Alabama at Birmingham National Spinal Cord Injury Statistical Center (NSCISC). Of the current variables, 72% have been part of the database since 1975. A smaller percentage has been a part of the database since its inception. This continuity has allowed for exploration of longitudinal outcomes for particular patient cohorts and for a variety of investigations examining trends in rehabilitation practices and outcomes. What follows are outcomes results derived from this extensive longitudinal database and information gleaned from other outcomes studies that shed light on the effectiveness of SCI rehabilitation.

A review of the SCI rehabilitation outcomes literature not surprisingly reveals a lack of studies conducted using what amounts to a "gold standard" for experimental design: randomized controlled trials. Ethical considerations have precluded, and will continue to effectively preclude, such a pure experimental approach. If the question, for example, is simply whether SCI rehabilitation works, this would necessitate a randomized assignment of newly injured persons with SCI, some to rehabilitation treatment centers and some to no treatment or some form of waiting-list control. No institutional review board (IRB) would allow such an experiment to be carried out. Even if such a design passed an IRB review, it would be difficult to conceive of any patient agreeing to potentially be randomized to a no-treatment condition.

Information from the NSCISC database represents a convenience sample; therefore, it is not likely to be representative of all people with SCI in the United States. In fact, there is evidence that the model systems, through their particular referral and practice patterns, treat people with neurologically complete injuries, particularly high-level complete injuries, non-Caucasians, males, and people injured by violence more frequently than non–model systems treatment centers (Go et al., 1995). Given those limitations in generalizability of the NSCISC sample, the next sections of this chapter divide the existing outcomes studies in the literature into three categories and characterize results in each: 1) descriptive, 2) quasi-experimental, and 3) additive designs.

Descriptive Studies

Although descriptive studies may bear the stigma of being primitive forms of research, in fields such as SCI care even descriptive studies may be difficult to carry out in many settings because of the extremely low incidence rate of SCI, making sufficient sample sizes for any kind of investigation, descriptive or otherwise, difficult to obtain (Go et al., 1995). Accordingly, the NSCISC database, with its very large sample of individuals with SCI treated across a variety of centers over many years, provides the richest resource available in terms of describing who receives this type of injury, what kinds of complications occur, and the nature of immediate and remote outcomes. A book published in 1995 by Stover, DeLisa, and Whiteneck (1995) is essentially a compilation of descriptive analyses of the entire database through 1992 and builds on earlier descriptive works using that same database (Stover & Fine, 1986; Young, Burns, Bowen, & McCutchen, 1982). This chapter does not summarize the results of the Stover et al. (1995) book; however, several trends are discussed.

A primary emphasis of this book is the epidemiology of SCI, early medical management and complications, functional outcomes, psychosocial outcomes, the economic impact of SCI, the impact of aging, and long-term survival and causes of death. As improvements in acute medical management have led to increased survival, there has been increasing emphasis on long-term care rather than acute care and initial rehabilitation outcomes and also an increased awareness of the impact of aging on people with SCI. Increased consumer involvement in research is also driving outcomes research in terms of requirements for increased accountability and relevance to consumers, as well as an increased focus on improving quality of life through whatever intervention is possible: legislation, personal and group empowerment, public policy activism, and so forth. Descriptive studies are a necessary first step in the development of a new field; however, outcomes research designs, which are more theoretically driven and designed to yield insight into causation and possible interventions, are necessary to advance any field. In the absence of the ability to perform most pure types of randomized controlled studies, quasi-experimental designs have provided a reasonable alternative for rehabilitation researchers.

Quasi-Experimental Studies

A longitudinal database such as that provided by the NSCISC allows for examination of improvement in outcomes over time as a function of changes in rehabilitation service delivery. For example, it has been determined that there has been a gradual increase over time in the percentage of incomplete injuries from 44.3% in 1973–1977 to as high as 56.7% in 1987–1989 (Go et al., 1995). This increase probably resulted from better accident site and acute care management. Preserved neurologic function likely translates to improved functional outcomes, although this relation is not definitively proved. Mean lengths of stay for both acute care and rehabilitation have decreased over time in the model systems, despite the increase in the percentage of people with quadriplegia and those requiring ventilator assistance (Waters, Apple, Meyer, Cotler, & Adkins, 1995). The percentage of people rehospitalized during the second postinjury year has decreased substantially, and there has been a 66% decrease in the risk of dying within the first 2 years of injury over those same time periods (DeVivo et al., 1992). Renal failure and urinary tract complications were reported to be the leading causes of death among people with SCI. However, with improved attention and care for urinary tract complications, the morbidity and mortality associated with those complications have been reduced to the point that respiratory complications, primarily pneumonia, are now the leading cause of death in people with tetraplegia (DeVivo & Stover, 1995). Time from injury to admission to a model system of care also appears to have an important impact on ultimate rehabilitation outcomes. Heinemann et al. (1989) compared rehabilitation outcomes among patients initially admitted to a specialized short-term care unit versus those initially treated at general hospitals. All patients were eventually transferred to the Rehabilitation Institute of Chicago and received the same rehabilitation program. Demographic and entry characteristics between the two groups were similar. However, the duration from injury to rehabilitation was more than twice as long for noncenter patients. Although both groups made equivalent gains across rehabilitation, the rate of gain for patients admitted to the specialized acute care units was greater than that for patients initially admitted to a general hospital. In a similar study, Yarkony and Heinemann (1995) demonstrated that patients admitted to a model system of care within 24 hours, as opposed to those with delayed admissions, were less likely to have costly, debilitating, and rehabilitation-impeding complications, such as pressure ulcers.

Some rudimentary comparisons between model systems and other SCI systems of care are possible with the existence of the Uniform Data System, which gathers general outcomes data, including functional outcomes, for many rehabilitation hospitals in the United States. Local, regional, and national comparisons can be made. During the period from 1973 to 1992, more than 92% of people with SCI treated in the model systems program were discharged to private residences in the community, which represents a substantial gain over discharges of 82% reported from non–system hospitals (Stover, Hall, DeLisa, & Donovan, 1995). Analysis of functional outcomes data also suggests a greater efficiency in the model systems compared with nonmodel systems, meaning greater functional gains per day of rehabilitation stay. These are obviously not perfectly controlled studies, because not all of the characteristics of nonsystem patients as compared with system patients are known; these might have an impact on outcome, as could other factors such as type of sponsorship, availability of equipment resources, postdischarge community support services, and so forth. Thus, all such comparisons, even those that might favor a model systems approach, must be evaluated with some caution.

In the absence of the availability of true control populations, other quasi-experimental design approaches have used age- and sex-matched able-bodied norms to examine rehabilitation outcomes. For example, using this approach, it is apparent that marriage and divorce rates, both pre-injury and postinjury, are higher in the model systems population than in the general population (Dijkers et al., 1995). The percentage of people with SCI working 1–7 years postinjury is also lower compared with norms for age-matched peers (Dijkers et al., 1995). Considerably more effort is needed from funding agencies to acquire longitudinal rather than cross-sectional designs, focusing on long-term coping and adjustment in the population with SCI. There is appropriate concern being expressed for the need to measure the elusive concept of quality of life (Dijkers et al., 1995), coupled with the realization that the best medical care may be inconsequential if access to full participation in society is not granted or available.

Additive Designs

Additive designs, used by some to establish rehabilitation effectiveness, are much less frequently evident in the literature than the descriptive and quasi-experimental designs previously described. With this approach, attempts are made to hold rehabilitation constant or assume that it is constant across two comparison groups and that the only difference between the groups is the independent variable being manipulated. The attempt, therefore, is to assess the impact of the addition of a particular rehabilitation service or therapy to the existing panoply of services provided. A good example of this approach is by Klose and colleagues (Klose, Needham, Schmidt, Broton, & Green, 1993), in which one group of people with tetraplegia was provided upper-extremity biofeedback and their functional outcomes were compared with those who received standard physical and occupational therapy. No differences were found in this case, but it is an excellent demonstration of the additive design approach to research. Unfortunately, there are very few studies of this sort in the SCI literature. Effect size with such approaches is likely to be small, but this represents one method for attempting to determine the relative benefits of the individual components of the rehabilitation process.

ACQUIRED BRAIN INJURY

Like spinal cord injury, ABI is typically a young male phenomenon, although obviously not exclusively so, and one that is often associated with motor vehicle crashes, risk-taking behavior, or substance abuse (Callon & Jackson, 1995). Although there may be profound physical dysfunction following ABI, often the most problematic and persistent difficulties are in the realms of cognition and behavior. Recovery can be minimal and people can be left essentially in a vegetative state after many years, despite rehabilitation efforts. In contrast, recovery can also be dramatic and rapid, with minimal problematic residual deficits after a period of months or years. Rehabilitation efforts for people with ABI, in contrast to the physically oriented modalities useful in SCI rehabilitation such as physical therapy, may be more focused on cognitive and behavioral dysfunction. Cognitive remediation, behavior modification, and individual and family education and counseling are the primary methods of treatment in a rehabilitation setting. These are most often provided by a speech pathologist, occupational therapist, and psychologist. Psychopharmacologic management of behavioral difficulties is often needed, but, in many facilities, the philosophy is to minimize the use of pharmacologic methods for managing agitation or behavioral acting out because such chemical interventions often further compromise an already impaired sensorium. Serial assessment of readiness to return to school, work, or vocational training is a necessity. Rehabilitation efforts are also directed toward the well-being of caregivers (typically family members), who bear the brunt of managing these individuals after they are discharged to home. Care requirements are likely to be more behavioral and emotional than physical, but the burden of what often amounts to 24-hour supervision during some stages of recovery can be tremendous.

ABI Rehabilitation Outcomes

Individuals with ABI represent a unique rehabilitation population. With severe ABI, there are often significant physical deficits; but, unlike SCI, there are also cognitive difficulties. The cognitive difficulties are persistent in many cases and represent the greatest barrier, along with behavioral problems, to full resumption of daily activities. The combination of physical and cognitive problems is similar to that seen in stroke; but, in the case of ABI it is in a much younger population. Among the population with ABI, issues such as return to employment and independent living must be addressed more often than with the stroke population. The peak incidence of ABI is during the 20s, and rehabilitation services must take into account the longevity of such individuals. Of the many studies examining outcome following ABI, few have provided a comparison or control group to judge the effectiveness of rehabilitation efforts. In general, it has been difficult to establish control groups in rehabilitation studies. Those who do not receive rehabilitation differ from those receiving such treatment in ways that might influence recovery and thus confound results (Wrigley, Yoels, Webb, & Fine, 1994). The breadth of services provided to individuals with ABI also complicates the issue. Rehabilitation in the broad sense is no longer meaningful, and researchers must address specific interventions, from coma stimulation to community and vocational reentry.

There have been two excellent reviews published on ABI rehabilitation, particularly focusing on effectiveness (Cope, 1995; High, Boake, & Lehmkuhl, 1995), which also highlight many of the pitfalls of rehabilitation effectiveness research. For instance, there is disagreement between studies with regard to how severity of injury is measured, the duration of rehabilitation efforts, and when rehabilitation is initiated. Each of these factors can have a significant impact on outcome, and together they make comparison of studies extremely difficult. In addition, there is limited consistency in how outcome is defined and measured. In many studies, the focus is on measurement of deficit or disability and not on the ultimate handicap associated with ABI. As noted by Cope (1995), this leaves open to question whether rehabilitation services are worthwhile from a financial perspective, which in the 1990s is carrying increasing weight in determining whether particular interventions will be provided.

Acute Rehabilitation

For the purposes of this chapter, acute rehabilitation is defined as treatment from the time of injury to discharge from an inpatient rehabilitation program with a focus on physical recovery and performance of daily functions. Cope and Hall (1982) examined the effectiveness of acute rehabilitation for those receiving early versus late intervention. In separating patients into those who received acute rehabilitation before or after 35 days from onset of injury, a significant time effect was detected with late admissions re-quiring longer acute rehabilitation stays (89 days versus 44 days). The subjects were matched on the basis of severity and demographic variables. It is interesting to note that 2–3 years postinjury, the Disability Rating Scale (DRS) (Hall, Cope, & Rappaport, 1985) scores were comparable for the two groups, thus indicating that delayed onset of rehabilitation did not have a long-term impact, at least in terms of DRS scores.

In a widely cited study, Aronow (1987) compared 61 individuals with ABI receiving acute rehabilitation to 68 people who received appropriate neurologic care but no rehabilitation. The participants were matched for age, gender, race, posttraumatic amnesia (PTA) duration, and time post-onset. The follow-up interval was not directly specified but apparently was several years after injury. Outcome was measured in terms of living ar-rangements, functional status, amount of care required, and vocational status. The treatment group was found to be more severely injured but exhibited equivalent outcome. Aronow concluded that this supported the impact of rehabilitation because the more severely injured individuals would not be expected to do as well. Aronow also examined the savings associated with rehabilitation, noting that individuals experiencing up to 1 month of PTA who received rehabilitation exhibited a projected savings of more than $11,000 per year. Those with 2–3 months of PTA who under-went rehabilitation exhibited savings of more than $3,000 per month. Total savings attributed to rehabilitation for the 61 treatment cases was $335,000 annually.

Heinemann et al. (1990) followed 66 individuals with ABI for 3 months after discharge from acute rehabilitation. There was a significant improvement in activities of daily living (ADL) during acute rehabilitation, which was maintained at follow-up. Individuals were admitted 47 days after injury on average, but recovery was unrelated to the delay between injury and admission, implying that spontaneous recovery was not the pri-mary factor in the progress noted. Blackerby (1990) examined the results of 149 individuals in two treatment centers providing acute rehabilitation. The study compared individuals receiving 5 hours of therapy a day with those receiving 8 hours. The subjects were matched based on time postin-jury as well as level of functioning on admission. Blackerby reported a 31% decrease in length of stay for those receiving 8 hours of rehabilitation per day. There was no follow-up after discharge. It is not clear if the discharge was based on progress exhibited or on payer characteristics, which may have necessitated the increase in the number of hours of therapy per day.

In a clever use of naturally occurring populations, Mackay, Bernstein, Chapman, Morgan, and Milazzo (1992) compared 38 individuals with se-vere ABI who received rehabilitation services during acute medical care before admission to a rehabilitation hospital with 21 individuals who did not receive such rehabilitation care until arriving at a rehabilitation hospital. Those receiving early rehabilitation care had hospital stays half as long as those with later onset of rehabilitation care. The overall range of outcomes scores and the percentage of patients discharged to home also were better for the early rehabilitation group. The authors regarded coma length as an outcomes variable and noted that, for the early intervention group, length of coma was one third of that noted for the late intervention group. However, this raises the possibility that the early intervention group was less severely injured, and, for that reason alone, a better outcome and shorter length of stay might be anticipated. The authors did not follow subjects after discharge from acute rehabilitation.

Spivack, Spettell, Ellis, and Ross (1992) followed 95 individuals with severe ABI receiving acute rehabilitation and reported improvements in functional behavior and performance on physical and cognitive tasks. For those with more severe deficits on admission, lengths of stay were increased but outcomes were comparable, suggesting that rehabilitation had an impact on that particular group. There was no extended follow-up of individuals. Spivack et al. (1992) also found that, in contrast to several other studies, the longer the length of stay, the better the outcome. A report by McLaughlin and Peters (1993) represents the only attempt to examine subcomponents of the entire acute rehabilitation process. Thirty-one severely injured people were followed for 6–18 months postinjury. A comparison was made between individuals who had participated in the standard acute rehabilitation program and those who had received the same care and in the last week of their hospital stay were placed in a transitional living situation. The authors noted more independence in terms of ADLs in the latter group. There was also a significant cost savings due to the lessened supervision and care required by the transitional living group after discharge.

In contrast to the results already reviewed, Putnam and Adams (1992) found that rehabilitation services did not affect outcome among individuals with severe ABI. The study was a retrospective examination of 100 randomly selected files from a statewide listing of individuals with ABI. The severity of injury ranged from very mild to extremely severe based on duration of coma, which was the only measure of severity available. Records indicated the duration of involvement in activities such as physical therapy, occupational therapy, speech therapy, neurologic care, and psychological services. There was no indication whether subjects actually participated in comprehensive programs; only an indication whether they received these specific services. Outcome was based on independent living status, degree of improvement since injury, general neuropsychologic functioning, prognosis, and psychological outcome. The authors found no relationship between therapy services and outcome, and there was an inverse relationship between years since injury and ultimate outcome. The best predictors of outcome were injury severity and age at the time of injury. However, generalizability of the study results to the effectiveness of comprehensive acute rehabilitation programs appears to be very limited. The breadth of injury severity among the population studied also clouds the results.

Despite the results of Putnam and Adams (1992), the studies reviewed suggest that acute rehabilitation is associated with improvement in functioning overall, which is maintained several months or even years after completion of treatment. However, the potential confounding factor of spontaneous recovery cannot be dismissed. There are aspects of several studies suggesting that rehabilitation offers improvement beyond that anticipated with spontaneous recovery, but the test has not been definitive. There has been no determination of which components in an acute rehabilitation program may be most important in determining outcome. Clinicians should be aware of innovative approaches that might improve overall outcome, such as those described by McLaughlin and Peters (1993).

Postacute Rehabilitation

Postacute rehabilitation in this chapter refers to treatment received beyond acute rehabilitation, in either day treatment or residential postacute programs. Postacute rehabilitation has been studied more extensively than any other component of rehabilitation following ABI, perhaps due to the need to justify the expense involved. Postacute rehabilitation also represents a nonstandard rehabilitation approach in that the focus is not on medical recovery, but on improvement in community functioning.

In a widely cited article, Prigatano et al. (1984) compared 18 individuals in a day treatment program with 17 controls, who averaged 22 months since injury. Outcome was judged at discharge from the program and 1 year later. Treatment resulted in increased productivity, including return to work (50% versus 36% in the control group). Decreased emotional distress was also noted among the treatment group. Scherzer (1986) focused on improvement in cognitive abilities in postacute day treatment for 32 individuals. At the time of the program, the mean length of time since onset of the participants' injuries was 5 years. Outcome was measured 3–12 months after treatment. Improvement was noted in attention, memory, complex reasoning, and visual information processing. Ninety-four cases of ABI were followed by Ben-Yishay, Silver, Piasetsky, and Rattok (1987) an average of 3 years after trauma. Following a day treatment program, the authors noted a significant increase in employment (0% to 63%) that was maintained in a subsample 3 years later. Mills, Nesbeda, Katz, and Alexander (1992) and Malec, Schafer, and Jacket (1992) obtained similarly

positive results in day treatment programs. Both studies followed participants for 1 year or more after discharge and found that improvements in
functional status and employment were maintained.

Several studies have shown that residential postacute rehabilitation is
associated with improvement in functioning as measured by several parameters and that progress is maintained in the year following treatment. For
instance, Eames and Wood (1985) reported on 24 severely injured individuals who entered treatment a minimum of 12 months postonset of trauma
and exhibited significant improvement in their living situation (e.g., living
alone) and independence in ADLs. These individuals spent an average of
15 months in treatment. Evans and Ruff (1992) examined a larger sample
($N = 248$) and obtained similarly positive results for a group under treatment an average of 1.5 years postonset of trauma. At 1 year follow-up,
38% of the individuals were employed, whereas before treatment 6% had
been employed. It should be noted that 13% of this sample was mildly
injured.

Using another large sample ($N = 433$), Jones and Evans (1992) found
place of residence, productivity, and amount of supervision required to be
improved following participation in a postacute residential program.
Follow-up was conducted an average of 12 months after treatment. Involvement in productive activities (referring to competitive employment, volunteer work, or school activities) improved from 6% to 51% of the sample,
whereas those living independently increased from 33% to 84%. Johnston
(1991) and Johnston and Lewis (1991), examining the results from 9
postacute residential programs, detected significant gains in independent
living and productivity among participants that were maintained 1 year
after discharge. The average length of stay for this population was just
under 9 months. The authors noted that progress was equally likely among
those admitted later than 1 year postonset of injury compared with those
admitted earlier, suggesting that spontaneous recovery was not the determining factor. Cope, Cole, Hall, and Barkan (1991a, 1991b) also emphasized that significant gains were noted in productivity and diminished need
for attendant care among individuals admitted to a postacute program
within 1 year after injury. Improvement was evident in all severity groups
and was maintained for up to 2 years postonset of injury. However, it
should be noted that the population followed appeared to diminish precipitously as the time since injury increased. Twenty-seven percent of the
population was also mildly injured and 30% had been admitted within 3
months of injury.

In addition to addressing significant gains in functional status as a
result of postacute treatment, Ashley, Persel, and Krych (1993) and Cope
et al. (1991b) addressed the costs involved in such treatment relative to
the gains obtained. Cope et al. (1991b), focusing on the decreased need

for supervision among program participants, noted a savings of $2,600–$41,000 when examining mild to severe trauma. Judging from diminished supervision as well as a lesser need for public assistance, Ashley et al. (1993) estimated an annual savings of $180,000 per patient in the postacute program.

As noted with acute rehabilitation, there are numerous studies indicating that improvement in functional status, as measured by employment, independent living, and general productivity, is associated with participation in postacute rehabilitation. It has not been proved, however, that the improvement can be directly attributed to the treatment received. The studies reviewed are encouraging, but their characteristics raise questions about the generalizability of the results, particularly to individuals who are severely traumatized. For instance, in several of the studies reviewed, a significant proportion of people in postacute rehabilitation were mildly injured or admitted within a few months of injury. It should also be noted that enrollment in a postacute program can be selective. For instance, in the Cope et al. (1991a, 1991b) studies, participants exhibited higher levels of employment before injury (more than 90%) and education than are found in the typical ABI population. Thus, although the results with regard to postacute rehabilitation are encouraging, close examination of the studies confirms the need for ongoing research.

Cognitive Remediation

A discussion of rehabilitation activities would not be complete without mention of cognitive remediation. On the one hand, cognitive remediation is very specific in that it focuses on thinking skills and not on physical recovery; on the other hand, it is extremely broad in that it can be addressed in numerous settings, such as occupational therapy, a psychology clinic, or speech therapy. The studies examining recovery in response to treatment following the onset of deficits in areas such as language functioning, memory abilities, spatial and constructional skills, and problem-solving skills, to name a few, are too numerous to review in this chapter. There have been excellent reviews published, such as Ben-Yishay and Diller (1993); Gordon, Hibbard, and Kreutzer (1989); Rimmele and Hester (1987); and Wilson (1991).

In addition to providing coverage of existing literature in specific areas, these reviews also focus on the rationale of cognitive remediation. There is no question that neural plasticity plays a role in recovery from ABI, but it is not clear if cognitive remediation influences neuroplasticity to a greater extent than everyday living. It is possible that the effect of cognitive remediation is less on the neural substrate and the cognitive abilities than on the level of confidence exhibited by the person. Rimmele and Hester (1987), for instance, noted that, in general, cognitive remediation appears to improve academic skills and diminishes helplessness, even though the actual changes in cognitive abilities are often rather modest. The issue of generalizability of treatment effects to everyday living skills is only beginning to be addressed. Evidence that early treatment gains in cognitive remediation are matched by control subjects at a later time suggests that cognitive remediation expedites, but does not extend, recovery.

Some areas of cognition, such as perceptual skills, seem to be more responsive to intervention than others, such as memory functioning. In some instances, the effort required for training and the limited changes that result (particularly when viewed in terms of return to productivity) draw into question the overall effectiveness of the treatment. A rapid and clear resolution of issues related to cognitive remediation should not be anticipated. In many respects, cognitive functioning is more complex than physical functioning in that it is more varied and difficult to measure. However, the absence of a smoking gun with respect to the effectiveness of cognitive remediation should not be construed as a condemnation of cognitive remediation and an allowance to discontinue the treatment. It should not be overlooked that deficits in cognition and behavior cause greater handicap than physical problems for survivors of ABI. Therefore, it would be unconscionable to ignore cognitive difficulties and minimize treatment to address such deficits.

Vocational Rehabilitation

Return to employment is one of the most important measures of rehabilitation outcomes. However, return to employment, particularly a previous job, is not a common occurrence following severe ABI. In a sample of 366 individuals, Dikmen et al. (1994) found that only 8% of those unable to follow commands within 29 days were able to return to employment following ABI. The authors noted that those who were unable to return to employment were more likely to be over age 50, to have less than a high school education, and to exhibit poor stability in their employment before injury. The results reported by Wehman et al. (1993) were slightly more positive and also included individuals with moderate ABI. The authors reported that, of the population studied, 10% were able to return to previous jobs and 30% to less demanding jobs.

Several postacute rehabilitation programs address return to work and report positive findings. There appear to be two general models of vocational rehabilitation following ABI. Wehman et al. (1990) emphasized the supported employment approach, in which individuals are placed in competitive jobs with a support person in place to help train the injured person on-site. Twenty weeks of staff involvement is common for such an approach, beginning with full-time supervision of the client. Specifically, 291 hours of staff time were required on average, at a total cost of $8,700 per placement. Wehman et al. (1990) noted that 36% of the individuals in their sample had returned to work following ABI without the supported employment program. Seventy percent were able to return to some kind of employment following participation in this program, and 71% reported continuing employment at follow-up. One of the most impressive figures is that, for the entire duration of time since program completion, subjects were able to maintain employment for 75% of the total months compared with 15% of months before treatment. This result was obtained with a sample of individuals with severe ABI (Glasgow Coma Score less than 9; Teasdale & Jennett, 1974) an average of 7 years postonset of injury. With this degree of success, the cost of the program does not appear exorbitant.

Haffey and Abrams (1991) argued that such extensive staff involvement is not necessary. Their approach is to carefully develop jobs, place individuals in jobs in the hospital setting under supervision, and then place those individuals in the community. In a controlled study comparing those who received this treatment to individuals who received acute rehabilitation or day treatment only, 68% of the vocational training clients were placed in competitive employment compared with 34% and 39% for the acute rehabilitation and day treatment programs, respectively. They also reported 71% job retention for the vocational rehabilitation individuals, although the specific follow-up interval was not indicated. It should also be noted that, of the individuals who achieved competitive employment after the vocational program, 67% were working at less than full time. Haffey and Abrams (1991) emphasized that this program involved approximately 60 hours of staff time on average compared with the 291 hours in the Wehman et al. (1990) program.

The results with regard to vocational rehabilitation following ABI, whether using supported employment or in-hospital placement approaches, are very encouraging. In this particular situation, the status of individuals without intervention has been clearly established, meaning that a direct comparison of treatment effects is possible. Not only is there initial success as a result of the treatment, but there is also indication that the impact is durable. The initial expense involved in providing such rehabilitation may seem prohibitive until the dividends of that investment (both economically and in terms of lifestyle) are considered (Abrams, Barker, Haffey, & Nelson, 1993).

CEREBROVASCULAR ACCIDENT

In contrast to SCI and ABI, CVA more typically occurs in older adults who may well have a substantial history of cardiovascular and other ongoing medical complications. The site and extent of damage are associated with the particular constellation of physical, cognitive, and behavioral difficulties that follow, and these deficits in turn dictate the kinds of rehabilitation services provided. For example, left-hemisphere lesions are more typically associated with expressive and receptive language difficulties than are right-hemisphere lesions; therefore, in the former case, speech therapists are an integral part of rehabilitation care. Cognitive remediation activities are increasingly provided to people following CVA, and these may be provided by speech pathologists, occupational therapists, or psychologists, depending on the setting. The emphasis is on improving cognitive abilities such as attention and concentration, memory, and reasoning, either through direct practice or through adaptive techniques that bypass the deficit (e.g., learning to use memory aids). Physical therapists and occupational therapists provide services to address the functional deficits following CVA. Education of family caregivers is a task for all. There is evidence of spontaneous recovery following CVA, with differing opinions and bodies of evidence regarding the length of time over which that recovery occurs (Nakayama, Jorgensen, Reaschou, & Olsen, 1994; Taub et al., 1993). But for a large number of these individuals, the process of recovery may be compromised by the process of aging and its increasing constellation of medical complications. Length of rehabilitation for people with CVA has also been dramatically reduced since the 1970s, and availability of follow-up services can often be quite limited due to transportation, insurance coverage, physical accessibility, and other factors.

Stroke Outcomes Research
The epidemiologic characteristics of stroke may explain the substantial attention this condition has received from outcomes researchers. Terent (1993) reported the average age-adjusted incidence rate of stroke to be 114 per 100,000, with reports ranging from 81 to 150 per 100,000, depending on study characteristics. Not only does stroke have a uniquely high incidence rate, but there is also a high rate of survival among stroke patients left with substantial residual disability (Gresham, 1990). It was estimated that more than 1.5 million Americans are disabled because of stroke (Ottenbacher & Jannell, 1993). These individuals compose one of the largest rehabilitation patient groups in the United States. Rusin (1990) noted that stroke primarily affects geriatric patients, with 43% of new strokes occurring after age of 74 (Hartunian, Smart, & Thompson, 1980).

The field of stroke rehabilitation has evolved to the point that clinical practice guidelines have been developed based on systematic evaluation and synthesis of the treatment outcomes research. A panel of nationally recognized experts in each of the allied disciplines that provide stroke rehabilitation services was assembled by the Agency for Health Care Policy and Research (AHCPR) of the Public Health Service under the auspices of the U.S. Department of Health and Human Services. The task of the panel was to review existing research and current standards of clinical practice, with the goal of developing a set of recommended guidelines for stroke rehabilitation. The results of the panel's work were published in May 1995 (Gresham et al., 1995). Copies of these guidelines are now available to rehabilitation professionals. (To order single copies of guideline products or to obtain further information on their availability, call the AHCPR Publications Clearinghouse toll-free at 1-800-358-9295, or write to AHCPR Publications Clearinghouse, P.O. Box 8547, Silver Spring, MD 20907.)

Support for each recommendation of the Post-Stroke Rehabilitation Guideline Panel is characterized by both research evidence and expert opinion. Research evidence was divided into three tiers: 1) "A," evidence supported by the results of two or more randomized controlled trials (RCTs) with good internal and external validity; 2) "B," evidence supported by a single A-level RCT, by two or more less-rigorous RCTs, or by two or more case control or cohort studies; and 3) "C," evidence supported by a single B-level study, by studies using historical controls, or by studies using quasi-experimental design (e.g., pre- to posttreatment comparison). Expert opinion was operationalized into two categories: 1) *strong consensus,* defined as agreement among 90% or more of panel members and expert reviewers; and 2) *consensus,* defined as agreement among 75%–89% of panel members and expert reviewers. In addition to summarizing reviews of the literature and providing interpretive conclusions, the *Clinical Practice Guideline* reports new results of meta-analyses of the benefits of stroke units, biofeedback, and functional electrical stimulation. The remainder of this section surveys some of the major conclusions based on meta-analyses of the stroke treatment literature, updated where necessary with new findings.

The foremost question that investigators endeavor to answer about stroke rehabilitation concerns the nature of the interaction between the treatments provided and the natural spontaneous recovery of neurologic functioning. Does rehabilitation contribute to patients' gains in functional ability? As of 1995, the results suggested a resounding "probably so." The utility of coordinated management and rehabilitation of acute strokes on stroke units by stroke teams is supported by A-level research and consensus of expert opinion, as defined by the Post-Stroke Rehabilitation Guideline Panel. Four RCTs with reasonably rigorous methods and fairly large sample sizes (mean $N = 228$) support the benefits of treatment of acute deficits on stroke units that are staffed with specifically trained physicians, nurses, and rehabilitation therapists (Gresham et al., 1995). However, one RCT conducted in Canada that compared stroke team care with traditional care at a medical unit showed no significant differences in mortality, motor functioning, or ADL functioning in a sample of 126 acute stroke patients (Wood-Dauphinee et al., 1984).

Such equivocal results are also found among meta-analyses that attempt to evaluate the overall effectiveness of stroke rehabilitation programs. One meta-analysis of 20 RCTs reported mixed results on the effectiveness of stroke unit rehabilitation versus medical ward rehabilitation or no rehabilitation, as measured by ADL level and motor functioning on follow-up (De Pedro-Cuesta, Widen-Holmqvist, & Bach-y-Rita, 1992). These authors noted that the results were particularly inconclusive regarding life in the home environment postdischarge. Ottenbacher and Jannell (1993) conducted a meta-analysis on 36 clinical trials that pooled data on more than 3,700 stroke patients. Based on the resulting effect size index, they reported that the average stroke patient receiving a program of focused rehabilitation performed better on follow-up than approximately 65% of those patients in comparison groups. The strongest findings, however, relate to decreased mortality rather than appreciable functional differences. Langhorne and colleagues (Langhorne, Williams, Gilchrist, & Howie, 1993) showed in their meta-analysis of controlled trials that stroke patients who were treated with comprehensive, coordinated rehabilitation services had reduced mortality for up to 1 year poststroke.

Studies have begun to compare the treatment outcomes and relative costs of subacute rehabilitation in skilled nursing facilities with that of more traditional, acute, hospital-based inpatient rehabilitation programs. The subacute care model involves the same rehabilitation treatment team found in acute rehabilitation, but it is less aggressive in the amount of therapy provided (Keith, Wilson, & Gutierrez, 1995). This form of treatment may better meet the needs of deconditioned patients who cannot initially meet the standard Medicare rehabilitation admission requirements of undergoing at least 3 hours of therapy each day. Keith and colleagues found that subacute rehabilitation was more cost-effective than acute rehabilitation in their retrospective analysis of the billing records of 428 stroke patients; 331 patients received acute rehabilitation and 97 patients received subacute rehabilitation. Further research is needed in this important area.

A majority of outcomes studies have not attempted to evaluate the overall effectiveness of stroke rehabilitation but rather have focused on component parts of the treatment package. Such unbundling methods have been used to evaluate specific treatment techniques for most of the major deficit areas, such as sensorimotor deficits (e.g., hemiplegia), cognitive and perceptual deficits (e.g., spatial neglect), and speech and language disorders (e.g., aphasia). The evidence supporting treatment of sensorimotor deficits are considered first here.

According to the Post-Stroke Rehabilitation Guideline Panel, rehabilitation of sensorimotor deficits is supported by C-level research and strong consensus of expert opinion (Gresham et al., 1995). Five RCTs with sample sizes ranging from 42 to 432 reported no differences in functional outcomes on follow-up when different types of physical therapy (PT) were compared. In the most ambitious RCT ($N = 432$) of these five studies, an enhanced PT program was compared with an orthodox PT program. At 6-month follow-up, the stroke patients who received the enhanced PT demonstrated more improvement in upper-extremity function; however, the treatment effect was no longer present at the 1-year follow-up interval (Sunderland et al., 1994).

A number of studies have unbundled PT interventions even further. Neither research evidence nor expert opinion have differentially supported the use of biofeedback, functional electrical stimulation, balance training, sensory retraining, or different types of exercise (e.g., isokinetic versus resisted versus active). Biofeedback technology has been by far the most heavily studied. Despite the amount of research attention it has received, the results of biofeedback studies are inconclusive (Gresham et al., 1995). In addition, a 1995 meta-analysis of RCTs does not support the efficacy of biofeedback therapy in restoring the range of motion in hemiparetic joints during poststroke rehabilitation (Glanz et al., 1995). One unconventional approach to improving use of hemiparetic limbs among stroke patients has demonstrated very good maintenance of treatment effects at 2-year follow-up. Taub and colleagues (1993) used restraint of the unimpaired upper extremity to increase use of the hemiparetic limb in a very small sample of patients ($N = 9$). Their results are interesting, but they require replication.

Of the various cognitive and perceptual deficits that may result from stroke, spatial neglect has received the most research attention (for reviews, see Chatterjee & Mennemeier, in press; Gouvier, Webster, & Warner, 1986). The effectiveness of treatments for spatial neglect are supported only by the strong consensus of experts on the Post-Stroke Rehabilitation Guideline Panel. Early RCTs with modest sample sizes (mean $N = 55$) conducted by Weinberg et al. (1977, 1979) showed significant treatment effects on multiple tests of perceptual ability at 4-week follow-up; however, no study has demonstrated that these improvements on clinical tests are maintained or that they generalize to functional activities (Gresham et al., 1995).

A sizable amount of investigation also has been conducted in the area of treating speech and language disorders after stroke. The Post-Stroke Rehabilitation Guideline Panel recommends that patients with aphasia should be offered treatment to improve their level of functional communication. This recommendation is supported by C-level research and consensus of expert opinion. Overall, the evidence from RCTs on the effectiveness of speech therapy is inconclusive (Gresham et al., 1995). Some studies fail to document sustained improvements on follow-up, but a meta-analysis conducted by De Pedro-Cuesta and colleagues (1992) concluded that treatment for aphasia is effective for several months after acute stroke. These conclusions must be tempered because there are no studies that have systematically examined the relation between patient characteristics and treatment effectiveness. In addition, there are no good studies that pinpoint the interaction between the natural course of recovery of language functioning and the provision of treatment.

These findings represent the most credible scientific evidence for the effectiveness of stroke rehabilitation. The following additional areas need substantial research attention: 1) emotional and behavioral sequelae of stroke, such as depression, anxiety, agitation, and sleep disturbances; 2) psychosocial factors, such as patient–family education, caregiver stress, and sexuality; and 3) functional issues, such as competence to live independently and driving. In addition, rapid advances in the acute medical management of stroke are taking place alongside developments in basic neuroscience. Numerous neurochemical interventions to lessen the brain damage associated with stroke (e.g., calcium channel blockers, excitatory amino acid antagonists) are being tested in clinical trials. The latter developments have much promise in affecting the severity of stroke symptoms that ultimately require rehabilitative treatment. The complexion of stroke unit patient populations may change considerably from the mid-1990s to the 21st century, necessitating adaptation of current models of stroke rehabilitation to the changing needs of patients and the developments in managed health care.

CONCLUSIONS

Development of rehabilitation as a field is beyond asking and answering in a scientifically rigorous way, Does rehabilitation work? It is unlikely that a true experimental design with random assignment of newly injured or impaired individuals to no treatment or even delayed treatment is possible. Patients, families, and IRBs obviously would not allow such a design to exist. In the absence of that possibility, there are a number of outcomes research designs that have been pursued and continue to need to be pursued to ascertain the relatively effective and ineffective components of rehabilitation. If individuals and organizations could be required or encouraged to participate in evaluative studies, outcomes from different systems of care could be compared. For example, inpatient program outcomes could be compared with those of a subacute unit, or those from specialized rehabilitation hospitals versus those from smaller units in general medical hospitals. In theory, it appears possible to randomize patient distribution to participating systems in such a study, but this would require true randomization at the point of emergency medicine or referral for rehabilitation. Although such an approach is theoretically feasible, political and economic forces are likely to prevent it from being worked out. More feasible are studies that attempt to unbundle various aspects of the rehabilitation process. Small effect sizes should be expected with this approach, given that the question being asked is what the impact is of the addition of one service to standard rehabilitation approaches. Where techniques being evaluated are relatively new or nonstandard aspects of the rehabilitation process, true randomized designs are ethically feasible. Such techniques should be scrutinized via randomized controlled designs before they become accepted practice and ethically beyond reach for experimental designs. In some cases, delayed rehabilitation to evaluate specific techniques by ruling out spontaneous recovery also appears feasible (Taub et al., 1993). Once stability of function is achieved, the impact of an additional technique can be evaluated. In this way, spontaneous recovery, initial rehabilitation, and other factors are controlled by allowing the patient to reach maximal gains with standard rehabilitation practices before a new technique is added. Within-system designs are also useful and continue to be possible. More effort needs to be placed on longitudinal designs with outcomes reflecting not just medical status but quality-of-life issues for people with disability. Single-subject multiple-baseline designs are also a reasonable approach to be used in assessing rehabilitation outcomes.

Advances in statistical analysis may help to establish the efficacy of rehabilitation techniques where strict experimental techniques are not feasible. A number of investigators have begun to apply hierarchical linear models to measure change and study the correlates of change (Bryk & Raudenbush, 1987) using a two-stage conceptualization. In the within-subject stage, a patient's status on some variable is modeled as a function of an individual growth curve plus random error. In the between-subject stage, the parameters of the individual growth curves vary as a function of between-subject differences in background characteristics and treatment experiences. By using such an approach, investigators can model individual change, predict future change, evaluate measures for distinguishing between growth curves, and study trends in growth curves as a function of background and treatment variables. Individual growth curve analysis lends itself to the study of rehabilitation outcomes. Several investigators have begun to apply this statistical technology in clinical neuropsychology research to the study of developmental trends among children with learning disabilities and recovery of cognitive function following pediatric head injury (Francis, Fletcher, Stuebing, Davidson, & Thompson, 1991; Francis, Shaywitz, Stuebing, Shaywitz, & Fletcher, 1993).

No discussion of methodologic considerations in outcomes research would be complete without a brief mention of measurement issues. The state of the art of outcomes measurement is quite unsophisticated. "First generation" functional measures are quite coarse and they are limited by commonly occurring floor and ceiling effects. Often they include poorly operationalized cognitive and psychosocial indices. Qualitative aspects of outcome, such as quality of life, are frequently neglected. In addition, the functional validity of many widely used neuropsychologic tests is unknown. The argument can be made that rehabilitation has much better treatment efficacy than clinicians and researchers in the field have been able to measure using first generation assessment techniques (for a review, see Wade, 1992). In sum, treatment outcome is only as good as the instruments used to measure it. The ability of rehabilitation team members to adequately document their treatment effectiveness has strong implications for the future of rehabilitation in the burgeoning world of managed care. Furthermore, the elusive construct of quality of life is fundamental to health care outcomes across medical and applied disciplines.

Finally, there is at least one major policy implication. Funding agencies need to require the most scientifically valid methods of investigating the efficacy of rehabilitation in terms of requests for proposals they publish. In a meta-analysis of the impact of psychosocial interventions on SCI outcomes, it was noted that of the very few true experimental designs discovered, virtually all were dissertations and not studies completed postdoctorate (M.A. McAweeney, personal communication, 1995). What this suggests is that with sufficient external force, scientifically valid experimental designs can be developed and executed, but in the absence of such contingencies, many investigators of rehabilitation outcomes succumb to more expedient approaches. If federal grant funds are made available only for scientifically rigorous investigations of rehabilitation outcomes and not expeditious ones, the relatively effective and ineffective components of the rehabilitation process will more rapidly become apparent.

REFERENCES

Abrams, D., Barker, L.T., Haffey, W., & Nelson, H. (1993). The economics of return to work for survivors of traumatic brain injury: Vocational services are worth the investment. *Journal of Head Trauma Rehabilitation, 8*(4), 59–76.

Aronow, H.U. (1987). Rehabilitation effectiveness with severe brain injury: Translating research into policy. *Journal of Head Trauma Rehabilitation, 2*(3), 24–36.

Ashley, M.J., Persel, C.S., & Krych, D.K. (1993). Changes in reimbursement climate: Relationship among outcome, cost, and payor type in the postacute rehabilitation environment. *Journal of Head Trauma and Rehabilitation, 8*(4), 30–47.

Ben-Yishay, Y., & Diller, L. (1993). Cognitive remediation in traumatic brain injury: Update and issues. *Archives of Physical Medicine and Rehabilitation, 74*, 204–213.

Ben-Yishay, Y., Silver, S.M., Piasetsky, E., & Rattok, J. (1987). Relationship between employability and vocational outcome after intensive holistic cognitive rehabilitation. *Journal of Head Trauma Rehabilitation, 2*(1), 35–48.

Blackerby, W.F. (1990). Intensity of rehabilitation and length of stay. *Brain Injury, 4,* 167–173.

Bryk, A.S., & Raudenbush, S.W. (1987). Application of hierarchical linear models to assessing change. *Psychological Bulletin, 101*(1), 147–158.

Callon, E.B., & Jackson, W.T. (1995). Traumatic brain injury. In A.J. Goreczny (Ed.), *Handbook of health and rehabilitation psychology* (pp. 431–456). New York: Plenum.

Chatterjee, A., & Mennemeier, M. (in press). Diagnosis and treatment of spatial neglect. In R. Lazar (Ed.), *Principles of neurorehabilitation.* New York: McGraw-Hill.

Cope, D.N. (1995). The effectiveness of traumatic brain injury rehabilitation: A review. *Brain Injury, 9*(7), 649–670.

Cope, D.N., Cole, J.R., Hall, K.M., & Barkan, H. (1991a). Brain injury: Analysis of outcome in a post-acute rehabilitation system. Part 1: General analysis. *Brain Injury, 5*(2), 111–125.

Cope, D.N., Cole, J.R., Hall, K.M., & Barkan, H. (1991b). Brain injury: Analysis of outcome in a post-acute rehabilitation system. Part 2: Subanalyses. *Brain Injury, 5*(2), 127–139.

Cope, D.N., & Hall, K. (1982). Head injury rehabilitation: Benefit of early intervention. *Archives of Physical Medicine and Rehabilitation, 63,* 433–437.

deGrott, J., & Chusid, J.G. (1988). *Correlative neuroanatomy* (20th ed.). Englewood Cliffs, NJ: Prentice Hall.

De Pedro-Cuesta, J., Widen-Holmqvist, L., & Bach-y-Rita, P. (1992). Evaluation of stroke rehabilitation by randomized controlled studies: A review. *Acta Neurologica Scandinavia, 86,* 433–439.

DeVivo, M.J., Rutt, R.D., Black, K.J., Go, B.K., & Stover, S.L. (1992). Trends in spinal cord injury demographics and treatment outcomes between 1973 and 1986. *Archives of Physical Medicine and Rehabilitation, 73,* 424–429.

DeVivo, M.J., & Stover, S.L. (1995). Long-term survival and causes of death. In S.L. Stover, G.G. Whiteneck, & J.A. DeLisa (Eds.), *Spinal cord injury: Clinical outcomes from the model systems* (pp. 289–316). Rockville, MD: Aspen Publishers, Inc.

Dijkers, M.P., Abela, M.B., Gans, B.M., & Gordon, W.A. (1995). The aftermath of spinal cord injury. In S.L. Stover, G.G. Whiteneck, & J.A. DeLisa (Eds.), *Spinal cord injury: Clinical outcomes from the model systems* (pp. 185-209). Rockville, MD: Aspen Publishers, Inc.

Dikmen, S.S., Temkin, N.R., Machamer, J.E., Holubkov, A.L., Fraser, R.T., & Winn, H.R. (1994). Employment following traumatic head injuries. *Archives of Neurology, 51,* 177–186.

Eames, P., & Wood, R. (1985). Rehabilitation after severe brain injury: A follow-up study of behavior modification approach. *Journal of Neurology, Neurosurgery, and Psychiatry, 48,* 613–619.

Evans, R., & Ruff, R. M. (1992). Outcome and value: A perspective on rehabilitation outcomes achieved in acquired brain injury. *Journal of Head Trauma Rehabilitation, 7,* 24–36.

Francis, D. J., Fletcher, J. M., Stuebing, K. K., Davidson, K. C., & Thompson, N. M. (1991). Analysis of change: Modeling individual growth. *Journal of Consulting and Clinical Psychology, 59*(1), 27–37.

Francis, D.J., Shaywitz, S.E., Stuebing, K.K., Shaywitz, B.A., & Fletcher, J.M. (1993). The measurement of change: Assessing behavior over time and within a developmental context. In G.R. Lyon (Ed.), *Frames of reference for the assessment of learning disabilities: New views on measurement issues* (pp. 29–58). Baltimore: Paul H. Brookes Publishing Co.

Glanz, M., Klawansky, S., Stason, W., Berkey, C., Shah, N., Phan, H., & Chalmers, T.C. (1995). Biofeedback therapy in poststroke rehabilitation: A meta-analysis of the randomized controlled trials. *Archives of Physical Medicine and Rehabilitation, 76,* 508–515.

Go, B.K., DeVivo, M.J., & Richards, J.S. (1995). The epidemiology of spinal cord injury. In S.L. Stover, G.G. Whiteneck, & J.A. DeLisa (Eds.), *Spinal cord injury: Clinical outcomes from the model systems* (pp. 21–51). Gaithersburg, MD: Aspen Publishers, Inc.

Gordon, W.A., Hibbard, M.R., & Kreutzer, J.S. (1989). Cognitive remediation: Issues in research and practice. *Journal of Head Trauma Rehabilitation, 4*(3), 76–84.

Gouvier, W.D., Webster, J.S., & Warner, M.S. (1986). Treatment of acquired visuoperceptual and hemiattentional disorders. *Annals of Behavioral Medicine, 8*(1), 15–20.

Gresham, G.E. (1990). Past achievement and new directions in stroke outcome research. *Stroke, 21*(Suppl. II), II1–II2.

Gresham, G.E., et al. (1995). *Post-stroke rehabilitation: Clinical practice guideline no. 16.* Rockville, MD: U.S. Department of Health and Human Services, Public Health Service, Agency for Health Care Policy and Research. (AHCPR Publication No. 95-0662)

Haffey, W.J., & Abrams, D.L. (1991). Employment outcomes for participants in a brain injury work reentry program: Preliminary findings. *Journal of Head Trauma Rehabilitation, 6*(3), 24–34.

Hall, K., Cope, D.N., & Rappaport, M.R. (1985). Glasgow Outcome Scale and Disability Rating Scale: Comparative usefulness in following recovery in traumatic brain injury. *Archives of Physical Medicine and Rehabilitation, 66,* 35–37.

Hartunian, N.S., Smart, C.N., & Thompson, M.S. (1980). The incidence and economic costs of cancer, motor vehicle injuries, coronary heart disease, and stroke: A comparative analysis. *American Journal of Public Health, 70,* 1249–1260.

Heinemann, A.W., Saghal, V., Cichowski, K., Ginsburg, K., Tuel, S.M., & Betts, H.B. (1990). Functional outcome following traumatic brain injury rehabilitation. *Journal of Neurorehabilitation, 4,* 27–37.

Heinemann, A.W., Yarkony, G.M., Roth, E.J., Lovell, L., Hamilton, B., Ginsburg, K., Brown, J.T., & Meyer, P.R. (1989). Functional outcome following spinal cord injury. *Archives of Neurology, 46,* 1098–1102.

High, W.M., Boake, C., & Lehmkuhl, L.D. (1995). Critical analysis of studies evaluating the effectiveness of rehabilitation after traumatic brain injury. *Journal of Head Trauma Rehabilitation, 10,* 14–26.

Johnston, M.V. (1991). Outcomes of community re-entry programmes for brain injury survivors. Part 2: Further investigations. *Brain Injury, 5*(2), 155–168.

Johnston, M.V., & Lewis, F.D. (1991). Outcomes of community re-entry programmes for brain injury survivors. Part 1: Independent living and productive activities. *Brain Injury, 5*(2), 141–154.

Jones, M.L., & Evans, R.W. (1992). Outcome validation in post-acute rehabilitation: Trends and correlates in treatment and outcome. *Journal of Insurance Medicine, 24,* 186–192.

Keith, R.A., Wilson, D.B., & Gutierrez, P. (1995). Acute and subacute rehabilitation for stroke: A comparison. *Archives of Physical Medicine and Rehabilitation, 76,* 495–500.

Klose, K.J., Needham, B.M., Schmidt, D., Broton, J.G., & Green, B.A. (1993). An assessment of the contribution of electromyographic biofeedback as an adjunct therapy in the physical training of spinal cord injured persons. *Archives of Physical Medicine and Rehabilitation, 74,* 453–456.

Langhorne, P., Williams, B.O., Gilchrist, W., & Howie, K. (1993). Do stroke units save lives? *Lancet, 342,* 395–398.

Mackay, L.E., Bernstein, B.A., Chapman, P.E., Morgan, A.S., & Milazzo, L.S. (1992). Early intervention in severe head injury: Long-term benefits of a formalized program. *Archives of Physical Medicine and Rehabilitation, 73,* 635–641.

Malec, J., Schafer, D., & Jacket, M. (1992). Comprehensive-integrated postacute outpatient brain injury rehabilitation. *Neurorehabilitation, 2*(3), 1–11.

McLaughlin, A.M., & Peters, S. (1993). Evaluation of an innovative cost-effective programme for brain injury patients: Response to a need for flexible treatment planning. *Brain Injury, 7*(1), 71–75.

Mills, V.M., Nesbeda, T., Katz, D.I., & Alexander, M.P. (1992). Outcomes for traumatically brain injured patients following post-acute rehabilitation programmes. *Brain Injury, 6,* 219–228.

Nakayama, H., Jorgensen, H.S., Reaschou, H.O., & Olsen, T.S. (1994). Recovery of upper extremity function in stroke patients: The Copenhagen stroke study. *Archives of Physical Medicine and Rehabilitation, 75,* 394–398.

Ottenbacher, K.J., & Jannell, S. (1993). The results of clinical trials in stroke rehabilitation research. *Archives of Neurology, 50,* 37–44.

Prigatano, G.P., Fordyce, D.J., Zeiner, H.K., Roueche, J.R., Pepping, M., & Wood, B.C. (1984). Neuropsychological rehabilitation after closed head injury in young adults. *Journal of Neurology, Neurosurgery, and Psychiatry, 47,* 505–513.

Putnam, S.H., & Adams, K.M. (1992). Regression-based prediction of long-term outcome following multidisciplinary rehabilitation for traumatic brain injury. *The Clinical Neuropsychologist, 6*(4), 383–405.

Rimmele, C.T., & Hester, R.K. (1987). Cognitive rehabilitation after traumatic head injury. *Archives of Clinical Neuropsychology, 2,* 353–384.

Rusin, M.J. (1990). Stroke rehabilitation: A geropsychological perspective. *Archives of Physical Medicine and Rehabilitation, 71,* 914–922.

Scherzer, B.P. (1986). Rehabilitation following severe head trauma: Results of a three-year program. *Archives of Physical Medicine and Rehabilitation, 67,* 366–374.

Spivack, G., Spettell, C.M., Ellis, E.W., & Ross, S.E. (1992). Effects of intensity of treatment and length of stay on rehabilitation outcomes. *Brain Injury, 6*(5), 419–434.

Stover, S.L., DeLisa, J.A., & Whiteneck, G.G. (Eds.). (1995). *Spinal cord injury: Clinical outcomes from the model systems.* Rockville, MD: Aspen, Publishers, Inc.

Stover, S.L., & Fine, P.R. (Eds.). (1986). *Spinal cord injury: The facts & figures.* Birmingham: University of Alabama at Birmingham.

Stover, S.L., Hall, K.M., DeLisa, J.A., & Donovan, W.H. (1995). System benefits. In S.L. Stover, J.A. DeLisa, & G.G. Whiteneck (Eds.), *Spinal cord injury: Clinical outcomes from the model systems* (pp. 317–326). Rockville, MD: Aspen Publishers, Inc.

Sunderland, A., Tinson, D.J., Bradley, E.L., Fletcher, D., Langton-Hewer, R., & Wade, D.T. (1994). Enhanced physical therapy for arm function after stroke: A one year follow-up. *Journal of Neurology, Neurosurgery, and Psychiatry, 57,* 856–858.

Taub, E., Miller, N.E., Novack, T.A., Cook, E.W., Fleming, W.C., Nepomuceno, C.S., Connell, J.S., & Crago, J.E. (1993). Technique to improve chronic motor deficit after stroke. *Archives of Physical Medicine and Rehabilitation, 74,* 347–354.

Teasdale, G., & Jennett, B. (1974). Assessment of coma and impaired consciousness: A practical scale. *Lancet, 2,* 81–84.

Terent, A. (1993). Stroke morbidity. In J. Whisnant (Ed.), *Stroke: Populations, cohorts, and clinical trials* (pp. 37–58). Boston: Butterworth-Heinemann.

Wade, D.T. (1992). *Measurement in neurological rehabilitation.* New York: Oxford University Press.

Waters, R.L., Apple, D.F., Meyer, P.R., Cotler, J.M., & Adkins, R.H. (1995). Emergency and acute management of spine trauma. In S.L. Stover, J.A. DeLisa, & G.G. Whiteneck (Eds.), *Spinal cord injury: Clinical outcomes from the model systems* (pp. 56–78). Rockville, MD: Aspen Publishers, Inc.

Wehman, P.H., Kreutzer, J.S., West, M.D., Sherron, P.D., Zasler, N.D., Groach, C.H., Stonnington, H.H., Burns, C.T., & Sale, P.R. (1990). Return to work for persons with traumatic brain injury: A supported employment approach. *Archives of Physical Medicine and Rehabilitation, 71,* 1047–1052.

Wehman, P., Sherron, P., Kregel, J., Kreutzer, J., Tran, S., & Cifu, D. (1993). Return to work for persons following severe traumatic brain injury. *American Journal of Physical Medicine and Rehabilitation, 72*(6), 355–363.

Weinberg, J., Diller, L., Gordon, W. A., Gerstman, L. J., Lieberman, A., Lakin, P., Hodges, G., & Ezrachi, O. (1977). Visual scanning training effect on reading-related tasks in acquired right brain damage. *Archives of Physical Medicine and Rehabilitation, 58,* 479–486.

Weinberg, J., Diller, L., Gordon, W. A., Gerstman, L. J., Lieberman, A., Lakin, P., Hodges, G., & Ezrachi, O. (1979). Training sensory awareness and spatial organization in people with right brain damage. *Archives of Physical Medicine and Rehabilitation, 60,* 491–496.

Wilson, B. (1991) Theory, assessment, and treatment in neuropsychological rehabilitation. *Neuropsychology, 5*(4), 281–291.

Wood-Dauphinee, S., Shapiro, S., Bass, E., Fletcher, C., Georges, P., Hensby, V., & Mendelsohn, B. (1984). A randomized trial of team care following stroke. *Stroke, 15*(5), 864–872.

World Health Organization. (1980). *International classification of impairments, disabilities, and handicaps.* Geneva, Switzerland: Author.

Wrigley, J.M., Yoels, W.C., Webb, C.R., & Fine, P.R. (1994). Social and physical factors in the referral of people with traumatic brain injuries to rehabilitation. *Archives of Physical Medicine and Rehabilitation, 75,* 149–155.

Yarkony, G.M., & Heinemann, A.W. (1995). Pressure ulcers. In S.L. Stover, J.A. Delisa, & G.G. Whiteneck (Eds.), *Spinal cord injury: Clinical outcomes from the model systems* (pp. 100–119). Rockville, MD: Aspen Publishers, Inc.

Young, J.S., Burns, P.E., Bowen, A.M., & McCutchen, R. (1982). *Spinal cord injury statistics: Experience of the regional model spinal cord injury systems.* Phoenix, AZ: Good Samaritan Medical Center.

CHAPTER 15

Cardiovascular Conditions

Nanette K. Wenger

The U.S. Public Health Service assessment defined cardiac rehabilitation as follows:

> Cardiac rehabilitation services are comprehensive, long-term programs involving medical evaluation, prescribed exercise, cardiac risk factor modification, education, and counseling. These programs are designed to limit the physiologic and psychological effects of cardiac illness, reduce the risk for sudden death or reinfarction, control cardiac symptoms, stabilize or reverse the atherosclerotic process, and enhance the psychosocial and vocational status of selected patients. (Feigenbaum & Carter, 1988)

A 1964 World Health Organization (WHO) report defined cardiac rehabilitation as "the sum of activities required to ensure patients the best possible physical, mental and social conditions so that they resume and maintain as normal a place as possible in the community" (WHO Expert Committee, 1964). In the WHO Expert Committee 1993 report, the goals of cardiac rehabilitation are to "improve functional capacity, alleviate or lessen activity-related symptoms, reduce untoward invalidism, and enable the cardiac patients to return to a useful and personally satisfying role in society" (p. 1).

The American College of Cardiology position report characterized cardiac rehabilitation as "those exercise and counseling services which will reduce symptoms or improve cardiac function in many patients with cardiovascular disorders" (Parmley, 1986, p. 451). Comparable definitions offered by the American College of Physicians (1988), and the American College of Sports Medicine (1991), emphasize the pivotal components of cardiac rehabilitation as exercise training and education, counseling, and behavioral interventions.

The author expresses appreciation to Julia C. Wright for expert assistance in the preparation of this chapter.

A 1995 Clinical Practice Guideline of the Agency for Health Care Policy and Research (AHCPR) and the National Heart, Lung, and Blood Institute, U.S. Department of Health and Human Services, entitled *Cardiac Rehabilitation*, provides broad recommendations for the application of cardiac rehabilitation services based on evaluation of the scientific evidence pertaining to various components of cardiac rehabilitation for patients with coronary heart disease, heart failure, and cardiac transplantation (Wenger et al., 1995).

OVERVIEW OF CARDIAC REHABILITATION

Enlarging the Scope of Eligible Patients

The pattern of delivery of cardiac rehabilitative care and the scope of patients considered eligible for cardiac rehabilitation services have changed substantially since the 1960s, reflecting changes in the demography and characteristics of the cardiac population, as well as in treatment strategies for these patients. These changes buttress the recommendations for medical outcomes research needed to ascertain the benefits of contemporary cardiac rehabilitation. In the early years, most patients enrolled in rehabilitative exercise training and in research studies of such training were middle-age men recovered from uncomplicated myocardial infarction. In recent years, many patients with serious complications of myocardial infarction, including angina pectoris, ventricular dysfunction, and cardiac arrhythmias, have been considered eligible for exercise training. Also new to cardiac rehabilitative care are patients who have had percutaneous transluminal coronary angioplasty (PTCA) and coronary artery bypass graft (CABG) surgery, as well as patients following valvular heart surgery and those with implanted cardiac pacemakers and defibrillators (AHCPR, 1991).

In the initial years of exercise rehabilitation, age 65 years was arbitrarily defined as the upper limit of eligibility for exercise training. In the 1990s, with the aging of the U.S. population, rehabilitative care, including exercise training, is provided to a sizable number of older adult patients, many of whom have severe and complicated coronary illness characterized by angina pectoris, myocardial ischemia, cardiac arrhythmias, compensated heart failure, implanted cardiac pacemakers, and so forth. Furthermore, in recent years, patients with compensated ventricular dysfunction and heart failure have been demonstrated to benefit from exercise training, which improves their functional capacity and symptomatic status. There has been convincing demonstration that ventricular ejection fraction correlates poorly with functional capacity; comparably, improvements in functional capacity with exercise training appear independently of baseline ventricular ejection fraction. As benefits and safety are increasingly documented, cardiac rehabilitation services for patients with heart failure and after cardiac transplantation are gaining increasing acceptance (AHCPR, 1991; Stevenson et al., 1995).

Changes in Exercise Training

A further advance has been the documentation that low- to moderate-intensity exercise training of longer duration can produce a comparable improvement in exercise tolerance as higher-intensity exercise training (Blumenthal et al., 1988; Goble et al., 1991; Rechnitzer et al., 1983). This approach, which results in similar enhancement of functional capacity and endurance, may translate into particular benefit when less supervised or unsupervised exercise training is undertaken and may promote long-term adherence to exercise training because of less discomfort during exercise. Finally, mild to moderate strength or resistive exercise training has been shown to safely and effectively improve both muscle strength and cardiovascular endurance, albeit predominantly in middle-age men who had already undergone aerobic exercise training after a coronary event (Kelemen, 1989; Sparling, Cantwell, Dolan, & Niederman, 1990; Stewart, Mason, & Kelemen, 1988; Wilke et al., 1991). Thus, there has been substantial change in not only the scope but also the pattern of exercise training.

Limitations of Outcomes Data

In a number of large studies of coronary patients, exercise rehabilitation has not been shown to lessen reinfarction, but meta-analyses suggest that mortality is favorably altered (O'Connor et al., 1989; Oldridge, Guyatt, Fischer, & Rimm, 1988). These data, however, were derived predominantly from middle-age men following relatively uncomplicated myocardial infarction before the advent of contemporary medical and surgical therapies. Further data are needed to examine current polar populations of coronary patients, that is, the large number of essentially asymptomatic patients at low risk and the increasing number of highly symptomatic, often elderly and impaired, individuals at high risk. In these populations, the morbidity and mortality associated with exercise training must be examined, as well as the potential beneficial effects of exercise training on long-term morbidity and mortality. An unmet need is the assessment of cardiac rehabilitation outcomes in women, because fewer women than men participate in cardiac rehabilitation, fewer are referred by their physicians, and even fewer have been enrolled in research studies (Ades, Waldmann, Polk, & Coflesky, 1992; Cannistra, Balady, O'Malley, Weiner, & Ryan, 1992).

Coronary Risk Reduction

In recent years, emphasis has been placed on coronary risk reduction as a component of cardiac rehabilitative care, with major attention to the control of elevated blood pressure, lipid disorders, cigarette smoking, overweight, and so forth. Innovative changes have occurred in the approaches to education and counseling. The changes were designed to enable the patient's acquisition of knowledge, skills, and behaviors that optimize adherence, with emphasis being placed on the behavioral approach. Furthermore, home-based rehabilitation, guided by nurse managers, has proved effective and may provide an alternate approach to the traditional, highly structured rehabilitation setting (DeBusk et al., 1994; Haskell et al., 1994).

Alternate Delivery Approaches

Alternate approaches to the delivery of cardiac rehabilitation services, other than the traditional supervised group and individual programs, have been examined in recent years in carefully selected clinically stable coronary patients. Data from randomized controlled trials suggest that these alternate approaches, often home-based, can be effectively and safely implemented for such patients (DeBusk et al., 1994; Haskell et al., 1994). Transtelephonic and other means of monitoring and surveillance of low- and moderate-risk coronary patients have the potential to extend cardiac rehabilitation services beyond the traditional supervised setting and to broaden the availability of such services.

Despite these advances, little comparative evaluation has been done of approaches to the delivery of rehabilitative care, its relationship to the return to work, and its effects on quality of life, an outcome variable particularly valued by cardiac patients who are sicker or older. Quality-of-life dimensions have received only limited assessment in studies of cardiac rehabilitation (Oldridge et al., 1991). Furthermore, instruments to measure this component must address the polar populations—those at low risk and with minimal symptoms compared with those at high risk and with substantial activity-limiting symptoms, such as patients with heart failure and those awaiting cardiac transplantation.

Return to Work, Disability, and Cardiac Rehabilitation

During the past decade, almost one fourth of the men and women receiving Social Security disability allowances were considered permanently disabled by coronary disease (Wenger, 1987). The indirect health care costs of disability, including lessened productivity, loss of income, welfare payments, and unemployment costs, must be considered when the cost-effectiveness of rehabilitative interventions is ascertained. However, return to work is not considered by many to be an acceptable outcomes variable to measure the efficacy of cardiac rehabilitation services in that it is not the rehabilitation services, but rather the employer, that often is the determinant of return to work. Additionally, economic incentives or disincentives for return to work and preillness employment status, among others, may profoundly influence the return to work (Walter, 1985).

Multidisciplinary Cardiac Rehabilitation

Finally, contemporary cardiac rehabilitation is multidisciplinary, whereas many of the prior studies addressed either exercise training as a sole intervention or exercise training with limited application of coronary risk reduction or other aspects of education and counseling. The outcomes variables that should be assessed are those that relate to multidisciplinary cardiac rehabilitation because many interventions are likely to be interactive. It appears more important to ascertain the benefit of a multidisciplinary approach, rather than to attempt to dissect the benefits related to each of the components. Additionally, contemporary cardiac rehabilitative care involves the tailoring of services to individual patient needs and preferences; it is this individualized approach that requires outcomes assessment.

Diagnostic Entities that Comprise Cardiovascular Disabling Conditions

In the early years of cardiac rehabilitation, this approach was applied predominantly to patients recovering from uncomplicated myocardial infarction. The predominant application in the 1990s is to patients with a variety of manifestations of coronary heart disease, ranging from angina pectoris, to silent ischemia, to myocardial infarction, and to patients recovering from CABG surgery and PTCA and other transcatheter interventions (AHCPR, 1991; Parmley, 1986; Wenger et al., 1990; Wenger & Hellerstein, 1992).

Although fewer data are available on specific outcomes (AHCPR, 1991), cardiac rehabilitation services have been applied to patients recovering from surgery for valvular heart disease (Wenger et al., 1990) and to patients with heart failure and after cardiac transplantation (Wenger, Haskell, Kanter, Squires, & Yusef, 1991). Although rehabilitative interventions have been applied to patients with implanted cardiac pacemakers and defibrillators, with surgical correction of congenital heart disease, and others, only limited descriptive outcomes are available (Superko, 1983).

A combination of the frequency of occurrence of the cardiovascular disorders and the data available regarding outcomes of cardiac rehabilitative care has contributed to the selection of diagnostic entities highlighted in this chapter (Wenger et al., 1995).

CORONARY HEART DISEASE

Cardiovascular disease is the leading cause of morbidity and mortality in the United States, with coronary heart disease being the major category of cardiovascular illness. Coronary heart disease is manifest as angina pectoris, myocardial infarction, silent myocardial ischemia, and sudden death and also may be categorized by the invasive therapeutic interventions PTCA and other transcatheter procedures and CABG. More than 6 million adults in the United States have a history of myocardial infarction or have stable angina pectoris. About 1½ million episodes of myocardial infarction occur each year, of which almost 500,000 are fatal. More than half of all acute myocardial infarctions occur in those ages 65 and older. It is estimated that the almost 1 million survivors of myocardial infarction each year are candidates for cardiac rehabilitation services, as are the more than 3 million patients with stable angina pectoris, the more than 300,000 patients who annually undergo CABG, and the approximately 360,000 patients following PTCA and other transcatheter interventional procedures (Wenger et al., 1995). Although beneficial outcomes from cardiac rehabilitation can be expected for most of these patients, only 11%–38% (Leon et al., 1990; Mark et al., 1994) participate in cardiac rehabilitation programs, with no major recent increase in this trend (Harlan, Sandler, Lee, Lam, & Mark, 1995).

Pathophysiology, Overall Health Status, Impairment, and Disability

Patients with coronary heart disease are often encountered for rehabilitative care in the early weeks after an episode of myocardial infarction. For many patients who have an uncomplicated myocardial infarction and a short hospital stay, their physical limitations are modest, their risk for proximate coronary events is low, and the major rehabilitative interventions are designed to stabilize or reverse the atherosclerotic process and limit the psychologic effects of cardiac illness. Patients with complications of myocardial infarction, many of whom are older adults, may have recurrent symptomatic myocardial ischemia, ventricular dysfunction, or serious cardiac arrhythmias. They often have a more prolonged hospital stay and have more severe symptomatic limitations relating either to the ischemia, the ventricular dysfunction, or the cardiac arrhythmias. The initial approach of risk stratification is designed to identify those individuals at high risk of a proximate coronary event for whom myocardial revascularization procedures may be appropriate. Among patients for whom myocardial revascularization is not indicated or not feasible, their functional status and symptoms may be improved by exercise training, and intensive education, counseling, and behavioral interventions are indicated for coronary risk reduction.

Patients who undergo elective myocardial revascularization with CABG or PTCA are often at low to moderate risk of subsequent coronary events because of the limitation of myocardial ischemia and ventricular dysfunction; however, patients who have residual myocardial ischemia and ventricular dysfunction, as well as many older adult patients, may continue to be limited following myocardial revascularization, although to a lesser degree, by symptoms of their illness. Of concern is the potential for restenosis in patients following successful PTCA—up to 50% during the initial 6 months—and their requirement for subsequent procedures. Although there is no evidence that exercise training alters the risk of restenosis, the supervision of exercise rehabilitation may provide added surveillance to that given by the patient's treating physician; earlier detection of restenosis during periods of physical activity may increase the likelihood of successful repeat PTCA. Patients with stable angina pectoris without recent myocardial infarction, who make up almost one fourth of the total coronary population, often have substantial symptomatic manifestations of myocardial ischemia and are at risk for progression of the underlying coronary disease, including the development of unstable angina, myocardial infarction, heart failure, and cardiac arrhythmias (Fuster, Badimon, Badimon, & Chesebro, 1992).

Objectives and Desired Outcomes of Cardiac Rehabilitation

Exercise rehabilitation of coronary patients is designed to increase the physical work capacity that can be undertaken before the onset of symptoms, to lessen the physical activity barriers to the performance of activities of daily living and to employment, and to enhance the cardiac safety and effectiveness of exercise training by allowing patients to learn the exercise skills needed to perform physical activities of sufficient intensity to achieve benefit but below the level to engender risk. Education, counseling, and behavioral interventions aim to achieve the modification of coronary risk factors and are designed to prevent progression or induce regression of the underlying atherosclerotic process. They address the learning, practice, and reinforcement of personal skills for risk reduction to lower cholesterol levels, effect smoking cessation, control elevated blood pressure, and control or reduce weight; and they emphasize adherence to other aspects of the medical care plan. Additionally, emphasis is placed on improving psychosocial status and optimization of return to work (Walter, 1985).

The Ad Hoc Task Force of the American College of Cardiology (Wenger et al., 1990) recommended that rehabilitation services standards define the total number of rehabilitation sessions, rather than specify the number of weeks of program length. The emphasis was that greater benefit can often be derived from supervised exercise sessions at progressively longer intervals, particularly for patients who are more impaired or at higher risk and who require more gradual progression of their exercise intensity, as well as for implementation of coronary risk reduction and of other education and behavioral strategies. The type, intensity, and duration of cardiac rehabilitation services vary, depending on an individual patient's risk status (as determined by risk stratification procedures); the baseline level of function before the coronary event; and individual patient needs and goals such as return to work, maintenance of independent living, and so forth.

Outcomes of Cardiac Rehabilitation

Based on reports in the scientific literature, the most substantial benefits of cardiac rehabilitation services (Wenger et al., 1995) include improvement in exercise tolerance, improvement in symptoms, improvement in blood lipid levels, reduction in cigarette smoking, improvement in psychosocial well-being, reduction of stress, and reduction in mortality.

Cardiac rehabilitation exercise training improves exercise tolerance in patients with coronary heart disease, including older adult patients (Ades, Waldmann, & Gillespie, 1995; Lavie, Milani, & Littman, 1993). This functional improvement occurs without significant cardiovascular complications or other adverse outcomes, such that appropriately prescribed and conducted exercise training should be an integral component of cardiac rehabilitation services. Patients with decreased exercise tolerance derive particular benefit, but maintenance of exercise training is required to sustain the improvement in exercise tolerance. Cardiac rehabilitation exercise training also decreases symptoms of angina pectoris; the improvement in clinical measures of myocardial ischemia provides objective support for the reported symptomatic improvement. Multidisciplinary cardiac rehabilitation results in improved lipid and lipoprotein levels, with pharmacologic management often being required as well. Of those patients receiving multidisciplinary cardiac rehabilitation services, 16%–26% can be expected to stop smoking. Cardiac rehabilitation is also associated with improvement in psychologic status and functioning, including measures of emotional stress and reduction of the Type A behavior pattern.

Meta-analyses (O'Connor et al., 1989; Oldridge et al., 1988) of the randomized control trials of exercise rehabilitation in patients following myocardial infarction defined a reduction in mortality approximating 25% at 3-year follow-up, but these data antedate contemporary therapies for coronary heart disease. The safety of cardiac rehabilitation exercise training is established by the very low rates of occurrence of myocardial infarction and of cardiovascular complications during supervised exercise training (Haskell, 1978; Van Camp & Peterson, 1986).

Patients undergoing initial PTCA (Wenger et al., 1990) without prior myocardial infarction are less impaired than most patients following myocardial infarction or CABG (Raft, McKee, Popio, & Haggerty, 1985). Therefore, patients' exercise training can be initiated at a higher intensity and can progress rapidly after a few exercise orientation sessions if they have not previously exercised; most of these low-risk coronary patients can exercise independently, and their degree of improvement in functional capacity is related predominantly to their fitness level before PTCA. However, the brief illness of these patients often engenders denial of the potential seriousness of the underlying coronary atherosclerosis and may hamper efforts at coronary risk reduction (Ben-Ari et al., 1989). Although patients following PTCA may require more medication to attempt to avert restenosis than do patients following CABG, their return to work is usually more prompt than that of patients following myocardial infarction or

CABG. Patients with varying residual coronary obstruction and myocardial ischemia following PTCA and patients with prior or recent myocardial infarction and ventricular dysfunction, often including those who have had prior or multivessel PTCA, have an intermediate risk status; their training recommendations are comparable to those for patients following myocardial infarction. A small subset of patients following PTCA are older adults, often those considered too ill for CABG, and constitute the group of medically complex patients with frequent residual myocardial ischemia and severe ventricular dysfunction. This group includes some patients with failed PTCA. The recommendations for their exercise training are comparable to those for high-risk patients following myocardial infarction.

HEART FAILURE

Heart failure is the most common discharge diagnosis for hospitalized patients in those ages 65 and older and the fourth most common hospital discharge diagnosis for all U.S. patients. An estimated 2 million patients with heart failure in the United States may be eligible for cardiac rehabilitation services.

Pathophysiology, Overall Health Status, Impairment, and Disability

The prevalence of heart failure increases incrementally with age and, with the aging of the U.S. population, has become an escalating clinical problem. In the early years of exercise rehabilitation, cardiac enlargement and a decreased left ventricular ejection fraction, as well as overt heart failure, were considered relative or absolute contraindications to exercise training. Only in recent years has exercise training been undertaken in these patients, with the goal of improving their functional and symptomatic status. As previously noted, exercise capacity correlates poorly with ventricular ejection fraction and with the improvement that occurs in functional capacity with exercise training. Patients with heart failure are potentially at increased risk of arrhythmic complications (Konstam et al., 1994; Wenger et al., 1995).

Objectives and Desired Outcomes of Cardiac Rehabilitation

The prevalence of heart failure has increased, a fact related both to the aging of the U.S. population and to the improved survival of patients with a variety of cardiovascular illnesses due to the use of newer therapies (Konstam et al., 1994). Exercise training is designed to improve their exercise tolerance and to decrease symptoms; recent data suggest that skeletal muscle and peripheral circulatory adaptations mediate the improvement in exercise tolerance and that this improvement can be accomplished without further deterioration of ventricular function (Giannuzzi et al., 1993). Education, counseling, and behavioral interventions are designed to emphasize appropriate medication taking and care of the underlying cardio-vascular illness.

Outcomes of Cardiac Rehabilitation

Cardiac rehabilitation exercise training improves exercise tolerance in patients with heart failure (Wenger et al., 1995). The exercise training of patients with left ventricular systolic dysfunction provides added symptomatic improvement to that achieved by appropriate medication management, including use of angiotensin-converting enzyme inhibitors (Meyer et al., 1991).

CARDIAC TRANSPLANTATION

The approximately 2,000 patients who undergo cardiac transplantation in the United States each year may also benefit from cardiac rehabilitation services (Wenger et al., 1991, 1995).

Pathophysiology, Overall Health Status, Impairment, and Disability

Candidates for cardiac transplantation have end-stage heart failure of multiple etiologies. They typically have decreased ventricular ejection fractions of less than 25%, as well as signs and symptoms of heart failure compatible with New York Heart Association functional Class III–IV. These patients have very limited functional capacities; are often deconditioned, owing to their severe cardiac impairment; and have increased perception of breathlessness on exertion, increased pulmonary vascular pressures, and, at times, cardiac cachexia before cardiac transplantation (Wenger et al., 1991). Pre-transplantation patients are at increased risk of sudden death. A 1995 study of nonsupervised prescribed walking in clinically stable patients with heart failure listed for cardiac transplantation showed sufficient clinical improvement in a subset of these patients to enable removal from the transplant list (Stevenson et al., 1995). The mean patient age at transplantation in the United States approximates 45 years, and current data indicate a median patient survival of more than 5 years following cardiac transplantation.

Following cardiac transplantation, patients exhibit predisposition to the development of coronary atherosclerosis, susceptibility to transplant rejection, diastolic dysfunction of the transplanted heart, long-term effects of medication-related hypertension on cardiac function and exercise capacity, skeletal muscle wasting and weakness as a result of corticosteroid hormone therapy, a high risk for infection due to a variety of immunosuppressive medications, and a blunted heart rate response and lower cardiac output with exercise due to cardiac denervation. A number of psychosocial problems also complicate their functional status.

Objectives and Desired Outcomes of Cardiac Rehabilitation

Many patients with end-stage heart failure are candidates for cardiac transplantation surgery. Cardiac rehabilitation for cardiac transplantation candidates and for posttransplantation patients is designed to improve their clinical and functional status, enhance their quality of life, and potentially decrease their long-term need for medical services. These interventions can help to optimize the substantial effectiveness of cardiac transplantation surgery (Wenger et al., 1991).

The goal of exercise rehabilitation for pretransplantation patients is to prevent further systemic deconditioning and, in some patients, to improve skeletal muscle status. Standard exercise testing can aid in the formulation of physical activity recommendations; pretransplantation patients must be considered at high to intermediate risk for exercise rehabilitation. For patients who can exercise to a 3–4 metabolic equivalent units (MET) level without serious ischemia, high-grade ventricular arrhythmias, or hypotension—generally patients who do not require hospitalization—routine activities of daily living are appropriate to minimize the deconditioning effects of bed rest. Such patients also may undertake slow walking or stationary bicycle exercise. Most Class IV nonambulatory severely symptomatic pretransplantation patients require hospitalization; these are the patients at high risk. Physical activity should include in-hospital personal care, sitting and standing with assistance, and in-bed passive exercises. For patients with an exercise capacity of 1–2 METs, only routine daily living activities are appropriate between hospitalizations; if heart failure status improves to Class III, these patients can be considered at intermediate risk and can undertake more intensive exercise. Education, counseling, and behavioral interventions can introduce the concept of reducing coronary risk factors, improve motivation and psychologic status, encourage family support, and foster preparation for the future. Reducing the fear of physical activity is likely to improve the patient's compliance with exercise recommendations; it is recognized that pretransplantation patients often exhibit decreased libido, changes in body image, fear of death, and mood swings, and are at high risk of death.

Once the posttransplantation patient has stabilized following surgery, exercise rehabilitation is undertaken as a component of the intensive early postoperative treatment. Exercise training is designed to reverse or limit the effects of preoperative and perioperative deconditioning. Muscle strengthening exercises can help counteract the muscle wasting effects of corticosteroid hormones. Posttransplantation patients are at intermediate or low risk for exercise training and generally remain in a supervised formal rehabilitation program at the tertiary care center for the initial few weeks as a component of their intensive early postoperative treatment and rehabilitation. Because of the potential for transplant rejection and for infection, the low exercise capacity, the exercise limitations of the transplanted heart, and the complications of surgery, posttransplantation patients—even when free of major medical complications—are considered at intermediate risk for 2–3 months after the operation. Exercise training should follow the model for patients following CABG surgery who are free of major medical complications. Professional supervision can help guide the type, intensity, and duration of exercise, although continuous ECG monitoring may not be necessary for posttransplantation patients, owing to their low risk of serious arrhythmias. The usual increase in heart rate is delayed at the onset of exercise because the transplanted heart is denervated; thus, the heart rate response may not serve as a guide to the intensity of exercise. Use of the rating of perceived exertion (Borg Scale) is better to control exercise intensity. Warmup activities are important to gradually stimulate an increase in heart rate.

After 2–3 months following cardiac transplant surgery, patients are considered at low risk and can exercise without supervision; however, initial supervision facilitates a proper sequence of gradually increasing physical activity and fosters improvement in the confidence of the patient, spouse, and family. During periods of acute rejection or infection, physical activity must be curtailed or reduced. Continued improvement in physical work capacity and endurance can be anticipated for up to 1 year, subsequent to which a maintenance exercise regimen is recommended. The components of exercise training should be designed to increase muscle strength and mass, in addition to increasing endurance. During the initial months of exercise training, monitoring of blood pressure is of utmost importance because immunosuppressant medications are likely to increase blood pressure such that the patient requires antihypertensive therapy. Long-term maintenance exercise regimens must consider that the development of myocardial ischemia may not result in angina pectoris in the denervated heart; thus, annual exercise testing is recommended.

Although the initial rehabilitative services take place in the tertiary care center where cardiac transplantation is performed, subsequent rehabilitative care typically occurs where the patient receives primary long-term care. Thus, rehabilitative exercise training may be in a community-based facility or may be undertaken without supervision at home. In this setting, there is variable local access to transplant-specific counseling, but patients are generally followed by their referring community physician for risk factor modification and most other routine treatments, based on recommendations from the tertiary care transplantation center, where periodic visits are also scheduled.

Education, counseling, and behavioral interventions are designed to teach patients the importance of control of exercise intensity to optimize the safety of exercise training. Because patients feel better following surgery, supervision and counseling are important to prevent overexertion and to teach the patient use of the perception of exertion to guide exercise intensity and thereby increase exercise safety. Education and counseling are also needed for the long-term management of transplant rejection and prevention of transplant coronary atherosclerosis, as well as to help manage the hypertension and hyperlipidemia that often occur several months after surgery. An education and counseling format that involves other cardiac transplantation patients may help psychological well-being and limit the later onset of psychomorbidity. Educational and vocational counseling continue to be important in preparation for return to school or reemployment.

In summary, cardiac transplantation candidates and patients can benefit from multidisciplinary cardiac rehabilitation services, including individually prescribed physical activity, coronary risk modification, and psychosocial counseling. An effective program can improve clinical and functional status.

Outcomes of Cardiac Rehabilitation

A highly organized follow-up structure of frequent, formal medical evaluations is operative at most tertiary care centers that perform cardiac transplantation. Although this structure provides an optimal opportunity for the initiation and maintenance of all aspects of cardiac rehabilitation, most of the relevant data are based on clinical observations or small series of experimental studies, with none being derived from formal randomized controlled clinical trials (Wenger et al., 1991, 1995).

Many candidates for cardiac transplantation do not survive to receive such therapy; however, optimal medical management that includes cardiac rehabilitation services may improve the functional status of pretransplantation patients and the quality of their lives. Because of the stringent eligibility requirements and screening evaluations for cardiac transplantation, the candidates selected are a very compliant population, well motivated, with an excellent family support system, limited comorbidity, and a better chance of reemployment than other patients with heart failure.

VALVULAR HEART DISEASE

An estimated 58,000 patients (based on 1993 data) who have cardiac valvular surgery or transcatheter balloon valvuloplasty each year may benefit from cardiac rehabilitation services.

Pathophysiology, Overall Health Status, Impairment, and Disability

Wenger and colleagues (1990) discovered that patients who undergo cardiac valvular surgery often have had a prolonged, ongoing illness and varying severities of disability; valvular surgery is deferred for as long as possible because of the imperfect character and limited duration of function of prosthetic heart valves. With the current application of transcatheter balloon valvuloplasty or valvular repair technology, patients may be considered candidates for these valvular procedures earlier in their clinical course. Functional capabilities of patients with valvular heart disease are altered by pulmonary, musculoskeletal, and cardiovascular limitations related both to the underlying disease and to the surgical procedure. Their exercise capacity correlates poorly with either objectively determined ventricular ejection fraction or the presence of serious cardiac arrhythmias. Major postoperative concerns are the residual ventricular dysfunction and the risk for arrhythmias and sudden death. Additionally, a significant subset of these patients, particularly those undergoing valvular replacement for aortic stenosis, are older adults.

Patients following valvular surgery are often in greater need of exercise rehabilitation than are other patient groups, and exercise supervision may be more important for these patients because of their generally higher risk status, including the risk of arrhythmia and sudden death. In addition, the rate of return to work of patients following valvular surgery is substantially less than that for patients following CABG.

Objectives and Desired Outcomes of Cardiac Rehabilitation

Exercise rehabilitation is designed to improve functional status and enable return to reasonable activities of daily living and to remunerative employment when appropriate. The goals of exercise training include the achievement and maintenance of an independent lifestyle by a moderate percentage of older adult patients, an increased physical working capacity in a moderate percentage of all patients, and reversal of the deconditioning that often characterizes the presurgical status. The safety and effectiveness of exercise training involve a number of variables; for example, low-impact exercise may limit hemarthroses in anticoagulated patients. Additionally, longer-term exercise regimens, beginning at initially lower exercise intensities, are particularly appropriate for patients with limited functional capacity. ECG monitoring may be required for patients with serious arrhythmias (Wenger et al., 1990).

The risk stratification of patients following valvular surgery is more subjective than that of coronary patients. Patients with pulmonary hypertension, moderate to severe ventricular dysfunction, high-grade arrhythmias, renal or hepatic dysfunction, low-level exercise test abnormalities, and multiple concomitant medical problems are considered at high risk. These individuals require more gradual exercise rehabilitation, as does the frequently very aged population following aortic valve surgery. If exercise work capacity does not improve after 3 months of gradually progressive exercise training, the patient should be reassessed to ascertain if additional problems have developed that limit work capacity. Improvement in exercise capacity should be anticipated to be slow compared with that for coronary patients because of the frequent long-term presurgical disability and multiple medical problems related to valvular heart disease. The maintenance of functional capacity in older adult patients that permits them to continue independent living should prove cost-effective. By contrast, patients following valvular surgery with reasonable ventricular function and without arrhythmias are considered at low risk and may require only a few exercise sessions to learn exercise skills, subsequent to which independent exercise is often appropriate.

Education, counseling, and behavioral interventions are designed to decrease medication and procedure-related complications by teaching about anticoagulant therapy (when appropriate) and endocarditis prophylaxis. Weight and blood pressure control may help lessen myocardial work in patients with residual ventricular dysfunction. Vocational counseling may enable earlier and more appropriate return to work.

Outcomes of Cardiac Rehabilitation

In contrast to data available for the rehabilitation of patients with coronary heart disease, few or no randomized studies are available to document the results of cardiac rehabilitation interventions for patients after valvular surgery. The variation in disease severity renders it unwise to use the reports of small series to document, rather than to suggest, the efficacy of cardiac rehabilitation services (Wenger et al., 1990).

As more patients undergo balloon valvuloplasty or valvular repair, rather than valvular replacement at an earlier stage than is usual for prosthetic heart valve implantation, their substantially more optimal preoperative functional status is likely to enable faster exercise rehabilitation, more rapid return to normal levels of activity, and more rapid return to remunerative employment when appropriate. The risks and limitations of exercise rehabilitation relate substantially to the extent of residual ventricular dysfunction and its often slow or limited postoperative improvement, such that problems regarding exercise training are comparable to those for patients with heart failure.

NEEDS FOR FUTURE RESEARCH

Major outcomes assessment needs relate to the expanded scope and methods of delivery of cardiac rehabilitation services. Three categories of needs are addressed in this section. The first category concerns needs for understudied groups: older adult cardiac patients, women with heart disease, cardiac patients from lower socioeconomic strata and ethnic miniorities, and patients with heart failure. The following is a listing of research needed to evaluate effects of cardiac rehabilitation in these targeted groups:

1. Evaluation of the effects of cardiac rehabilitation exercise training, and education, counseling, and behavioral interventions on older adult coronary patients, with specific evaluation of the effects on postponing disability and dependency and on enhancing quality of life

2. Evaluation of the effects of rehabilitative care in women, many of whom are older adult patients; on patients from different ethnic groups; and for those with a less advantageous educational background or at a lower socioeconomic level

3. Evaluation of the safety and efficacy of strength training in higher-risk populations such as older adult patients, women, unfit cardiac patients, and others at moderate-to-high cardiovascular risk

4. Evaluation of the safety and benefit of exercise training of patients with compensated heart failure and ventricular systolic dysfunction, not only in regard to outcome events but also related to changes in ventricular function

The second category targets newer interventions and their relevant outcomes: risk reduction, return to work, adherence to rehabilitative strategies, psychologic functional status, and quality of life. The following listing identifies specific research needs to improve the knowledge about outcomes of these newer interventions:

1. Development and assessment of optimal education and counseling strategies for cost-effective coronary risk reduction. Development of behavioral interventions for lifestyle changes applicable to large populations of patients, with prospective evaluation of gender, age, ethnic, and educational and socioeconomic differences in outcomes.

2. Evaluation of the effects of exercise training and of improved functional capacity, as well as of education, counseling, and behavioral interventions, on return to work. Ascertainment of the effect of a targeted vocational rehabilitation intervention as compared with usual cardiac rehabilitative care on return to work.

3. Identification factors that promote adherence to cardiac rehabilitation services, both to exercise training and to coronary risk reduction in different populations and across the life span.

4. Development and assessment of psychologic measures that may better ascertain improvement in psychologic functioning and status and quality-of-life issues (particularly as they pertain to lessening of disability and dependency) as a result of cardiac rehabilitation care in medically ill patients, rather than in those with psychologic or psychiatric illness.

The final aspect relates to outcomes among patients treated with recently available medical and surgical therapies and to innovative approaches for the delivery of cardiac rehabilitation services, with attention to cost-effectiveness. The following are research needs to improve the knowledge base about outcomes following recently developed therapies and using new approaches for delivery of cardiac rehabilitation services:

1. Evaluation of the outcomes of cardiac rehabilitation services in patients following myocardial infarction treated with contemporary therapies,

including coronary thrombolysis and acute angioplasty, and in patients with valvular heart disease treated with newer therapies, including balloon valvuloplasty and valvular repair procedures.

2. Evaluation of outcomes of exercise rehabilitation with and without supervision and/or ECG monitoring and surveillance of high-risk patients, for example, those with myocardial ischemia, heart failure, serious arrhythmias, complications of cardiovascular disease, and older adult patients.

3. Ascertainment of the outcomes of contemporary multidisciplinary cardiac rehabilitation, where specific components of care are tailored to individual patient needs and preferences.

4. Evaluation of the most cost-effective means of delivery of cardiac rehabilitative care, both exercise training and education, counseling, and behavioral interventions. This should address various models of delivery of cardiac rehabilitation services, including supervised versus unsupervised exercise training and group versus individual versus programmed-type or computer-based education and counseling.

CONCLUSIONS

Cardiac rehabilitation services are an essential component of the contemporary management of patients with multiple presentations of a variety of cardiovascular illnesses. Cardiac rehabilitation services should be integrated into the comprehensive care of cardiac patients.

REFERENCES

Ades, P.A., Waldmann, M.L., & Gillespie, C. (1995). A controlled trial of exercise training in older coronary patients. *Journal of Gerontology, 50A*, M7–11.

Ades, P.A., Waldmann, M.L., Polk, D., & Coflesky, J.T. (1992). Referral patterns and exercise response in the rehabilitation of female coronary patients aged ≥62 years. *American Journal of Cardiology, 69*, 1422–1425.

Agency for Health Care Policy and Research (AHCPR). (1991). *Cardiac rehabilitation programs.* (Health Technology Assessment Report No. 3). Rockville, MD: U.S. Department of Health and Human Services, Public Health Service, Agency for Health Care Policy and Research. (AHCPR Publication No. 92-0015)

American College of Physicians, Health and Policy Committee. (1988). Cardiac rehabilitation services (position paper). *Annals of Internal Medicine, 109*, 671–673.

American College of Sports Medicine, Preventative and Rehabilitative Exercise Committee. (1991). *Guidelines for exercise testing and prescription* (4th ed.). Philadelphia: Lea & Febiger.

Ben-Ari, E., Rothbaum, D.A., Linnemeir, T.J., Landin, R.J., Steinmetz, E.F., Hillis, S.J., Noble, J.R., Hallam, C.C., See, M.R., & Shiner, R. (1989). Benefits of a monitored rehabilitation program versus physician care after emergency percutaneous transluminal coronary angioplasty: Follow-up of risk factors and rate of restenosis. *Journal of Cardiopulmonary Rehabilitation, 7*, 281–285.

Blumenthal, J.A., Rejeski, W.J., Walsh-Riddle, M., Emery, C.F., Miller, H., Roark, S., Ribisl, P.M., Morris, P.B., Brubaker, P., & Williams, R.S. (1988). Comparison of high- and low-intensity exercise training early after acute myocardial infarction. *American Journal of Cardiology, 61,* 26–30.

Cannistra, L.B., Balady, G.J., O'Malley, C.J., Weiner, D.A., & Ryan, T.J. (1992). Comparison of the clinical profile and outcome of women and men in cardiac rehabilitation. *American Journal of Cardiology, 69,* 1274–1279.

DeBusk, R.F., Houston Miller, N., Superko, H.R., Dennis, C. A., Thomas, R.J., Lew, H.T., Berger, W.E., III, Heller, R.S., Rompf, J., Gee, D., Kraemer, H.C., Bandura, A., Ghandour, G., Clark, M., Shah, R.V., Fisher, L., & Taylor, C.B. (1994). A case-management system for coronary risk factor modification after acute myocardial infarction. *Annals of Internal Medicine, 120,* 721–729.

Feigenbaum, E., & Carter, E. (1988). *Cardiac rehabilitation services.* Health technology assessment report, 1987, no. 6. Rockville, MD: U.S. Department of Health and Human Services, Public Health Service, National Center for Health Services Research and Health Care Technology Assessment, (DHHS publication no. PHS 88-3427).

Fuster, V., Badimon, L., Badimon, J.J., & Chesebro, J.H. (1992). The pathogenesis of coronary artery disease and the acute coronary syndromes (2). *New England Journal of Medicine, 326,* 310–318.

Giannuzzi, P., Tavazzi, L., Temporelli, P. L., Corra, U., Imparato, A., Gattone, M., Giordano, A., Sala, L., Schweiger, C., & Malinverni, C. (1993). Long-term physical training and left ventricular remodeling after anterior myocardial infarction: Results of Exercise in Anterior Myocardial Infarction (EAMI) trial. *Journal of the American College of Cardiology, 22,* 1821–1829.

Goble, A.J., Hare, D.L., Macdonald, P.S., Oliver, R.G., Reid, M.A., & Worcester, M.C. (1991). Effect of early programmes of high and low intensity exercise on physical performance after transmural acute myocardial infarction. *British Heart Journal, 65,* 126–131.

Harlan, W.R., III, Sandler, S.A., Lee, K.L., Lam, L.C., & Mark, D.B. (1995). Importance of baseline functional and socioeconomic factors for participation in cardiac rehabilitation. *American Journal of Cardiology, 76,* 36–39.

Haskell, W.L. (1978). Cardiovascular complications during exercise training of cardiac patients. *Circulation, 57,* 920–924.

Haskell, W.L., Alderman, E.L., Fair, J.M., Maron, D.J., Mackey, S.F., Superko, H.R., Williams, P.T., Johnstone, I.M., Champagne, M.E., Krauss, R.M., & Farquhar, J.W. (1994). Effects of intensive multiple risk factor reduction on coronary atherosclerosis and clinical cardiac events in men and women with coronary artery disease: The Stanford Coronary Risk Intervention Project (SCRIP). *Circulation, 89,* 975–990.

Kelemen, M.H. (1989). Resistance training safety and essential guidelines for cardiac and coronary prone patients. *Medicine and Science in Sports and Exercise, 21,* 675–677.

Konstam, M., Dracup, K., Baker, D., Bottorff, M.B., Brooks, N.H., Dacey, R.A., Dunbar, S.B., Jackson, A.B., Jessup, M., Johnson, J.C., Jones, R.H., Luchi, R.J., Massie, B.M., Pitt, B., Rose, E.A., Rubin, L.J., Wright, R.F., & Hadorn, D.C. (1994). *Heart failure: Evaluation and care of patients with left-ventricular systolic dysfunction.* Clinical practice guideline no. 11. Rockville, MD: U.S. DHHS, PHS, Agency for Health Care Policy and Research. (AHCPR Publication No. 94-0612).

Lavie, C.J., Milani, R.V., & Littman, A.B. (1993). Benefits of cardiac rehabilitation and exercise training in secondary coronary prevention in the elderly. *Journal of the American College of Cardiology, 22,* 678–683.

Leon, A.S., Certo, C., Cosmoss, P., Franklin, B.A., Froelicher, V., Haskell, W.L., Hellerstein, H.K., Marley, W.P., Pollock, M.L., Ries, A., Sivarajan, E.F., & Smith, L.K. (1990). Scientific evidence of the value of cardiac rehabilitation services with emphasis on patients following myocardial infarction. Section I: Exercise conditioning component (position paper). *Journal of Cardiopulmonary Rehabilitation, 10,* 79–87.

Mark, D.B., Naylor, C.D., Hlatky, M.A., Califf, R.M., Topol, E.J., Granger, C.B., Knight, J.D., Nelson, C.L., Lee, K.L., Clapp-Channing, N.E., Sutherland, W., Pilote, L., & Armstrong, P.W. (1994). Use of medical resources and quality of life after acute myocardial infarction in Canada and the United States. *New England Journal of Medicine, 331,* 1130–1135.

Meyer, T.R., Casadei, B., Coats, A.J., Davey, P.P., Adamopoulos, S., Radaelli, A., & Conway, J. (1991). Angiotensin-converting enzyme inhibition and physical training in heart failure. *Journal of Internal Medicine, 230,* 407–413.

O'Connor, G.T., Buring, J.E., Yusuf, S., Goldhaber, S.Z., Olmstead, E.M., Paffenbarger, R.S., Jr., & Hennekens, C.H. (1989). An overview of randomized trials of rehabilitation with exercise after myocardial infarction. *Circulation, 80,* 234–244.

Oldridge, N.B., Guyatt, G.H., Fischer, M.E., & Rimm, A.A. (1988). Cardiac rehabilitation after myocardial infarction: Combined experience of randomized clinical trials. *Journal of the American Medical Association, 260,* 945–950.

Oldridge, N.B., Guyatt, G., Jones, N., Crowe, J., Singer, J., Feeny, D., McKelvie, R., Runions, J., Streiner, D., & Torrance, G. (1991). Effects on quality of life with comprehensive rehabilitation after acute myocardial infarction. *American Journal of Cardiology, 67,* 1084–1089.

Parmley, W.W. (1986). Position report on cardiac rehabilitation: Recommendations of the American College of Cardiology on cardiovascular rehabilitation. *Journal of the American College of Cardiology, 7,* 451–453.

Raft, D., McKee, D.C., Popio, K.A., & Haggerty, J.J., Jr. (1985). Life adaptation after percutaneous transluminal coronary angioplasty and coronary artery bypass grafting. *American Journal of Cardiology, 56,* 395–398.

Rechnitzer, P.A., Cunningham, D.A., Andrew, G.M., Buck, C.W., Jones, N.L., Kavanagh, T., Oldridge, N.B., Parker, J.O., Shephard, R.J., Sutton, J.R., & Donner, A.P. (1983). Ontario Exercise-Heart Collaborative Study: Relation of exercise to the recurrence rate of myocardial infarction in men. *American Journal of Cardiology, 51,* 65–69.

Sparling, P.B., Cantwell, J.D., Dolan, C.M., & Niederman, R.K. (1990). Strength training in a cardiac rehabilitation program: A six-month follow-up. *Archives of Physical Medicine and Rehabilitation, 71,* 148–152.

Stevenson, L.W., Steimle, A.E., Fonarow, G., Kermani, M., Kermani, D., Hamilton, M.A., Moriguchi, J.D., Walden, J., Tillisch, J.H., Drinkwater, D.C., & Laks, H. (1995). Improvement in exercise capacity of candidates awaiting heart transplantation. *Journal of the American College of Cardiology, 25,* 163–170.

Stewart, K.J., Mason, M., & Kelemen, M.H. (1988). Three-year participation in circuit weight training improves muscular strength and self-efficacy in cardiac patients. *Journal of Cardiopulmonary Rehabilitation, 8,* 292–296.

Superko, H.R. (1983). Effects of cardiac rehabilitation in permanently paced patients with third-degree heart block. *Journal of Cardiopulmonary Rehabilitation, 3,* 561–568.

Van Camp, S.P., & Peterson, R.A. (1986). Cardiovascular complications of outpatient cardiac rehabilitation programs. *Journal of the American Medical Association, 256,* 1160–1163.

Walter, P.J. (Ed.). (1985). *Return to work after coronary artery bypass surgery: Psychosocial and economic aspects.* Berlin: Springer-Verlag.

Wenger, N.K. (1987). Impairment, disability, and the cardiac patient [editorial]. *Quality of Life and Cardiovascular Care, 3,* 56.

Wenger, N.K., Balady, G.J., Cohn, L.H., Hartley, L.H., King, S.B., III, Miller, H.S., Jr., & Weiner, D.A. (1990). Cardiac rehabilitation services following PTCA and valvular surgery: Guidelines for use. *Cardiology, 19,* 4–5.

Wenger, N.K., et al. (1995). *Cardiac rehabilitation.* Clinical practice guideline no. 17. Rockville, MD: U.S. Department of Health and Human Services, Public Health Service, Agency for Health Care Policy and Research and the National Heart, Lung, and Blood Institute. (AHCPR Publication No. 96-0672)

Wenger, N.K., Haskell, W.L., Kanter, K., Squires, R.W., & Yusuf, S. (1991). Cardiac rehabilitation services after cardiac transplantation: Guidelines for use. *Cardiology, 20,* 4–5.

Wenger, N.K., & Hellerstein, H.K. (Eds). (1992). *Rehabilitation of the coronary patient* (3rd ed.). New York: Churchill Livingstone.

Wilke, N.A., Sheldahl, L.M., Levandoski, S.G., Hoffman, M.D., Dougherty, S.M., & Tristani, F.E. (1991). Transfer effect of upper extremity training to weight carrying in men with ischemic heart disease. *Journal of Cardiopulmonary Rehabilitation, 11,* 365–372.

World Health Organization Expert (WHO) Committee. (1964). *Rehabilitation of patients with cardiovascular diseases.* (Technical report series no. 270). Geneva, Switzerland: Author.

World Health Organization (WHO) Expert Committee. (1993). *Rehabilitation after cardiovascular diseases, with special emphasis on developing countries.* (Technical report series no. 831). Geneva, Switzerland: Author.

CHAPTER 16

Early Development–Related Conditions

Margaret A. Turk

Outcomes research has been limited and particularly difficult in developmental-onset disabilities. The impact of growth and development offers special problems in pediatric-onset disabilities. Function, functional change, community integration, and family and consumer quality-of-life issues are neither well represented in the literature nor well appreciated by health care providers in general. Regarding outcomes from discrete interventions, the reported consequences are often based on morbidity and mortality, laboratory values, and functional measures; follow-up is usually time-limited (Young & Wright, 1995). Developmental milestone inventories have limitations in measurement of outcomes in children with moderate to severe impairments (Haley, Coster, & Ludlow, 1991). The effects of specific types of therapies have been studied, and, through meta-analysis, more quantitative information has become available (Ottenbacher, 1982; Ottenbacher et al., 1986; Ottenbacher & Petersen, 1985a, 1985b). The need for tools to evaluate change due to rehabilitation interventions for a wide range of disabilities has been recognized (Haley, Coster, & Ludlow, 1991; Palisano, Kolobe, Haley, Lowes, & Jones, 1995). Multidimensional health status measures in children and adolescents are being developed with limited application to children with disabilities (Vivier, Bernier, & Starfield, 1994). There is a need for long-term follow-up, longitudinal studies, appropriate development and selection of measurement instruments, broad health status measurement, inclusion of family-related or handicap-level measures, and concern with issues of lifelong disability.

As in adults, disabling conditions in children can be defined in very broad terms. For purposes of this chapter, these conditions are limited to cognitive and physical impairments, with onset early in life. Congenital disorders are those that are present from the time of birth (e.g., spina bifida); they may be further specified as genetically based (e.g., Down syndrome) or caused by an extrinsic factor during gestation (e.g., fetal alcohol syndrome). Acquired disorders are those that occur later and are usually the result of trauma, infection, or other causes. Acquired disorders should not be confused with disorders that manifest later after birth that may be genetically based (e.g., Duchenne muscular dystrophy). The duration of the disabling condition also requires description: Disorders may be transient (e.g., acute inflammatory demyelinating neuropathy), progressive (e.g., juvenile rheumatoid arthritis), or nonprogressive (e.g., cerebral palsy). However, the simultaneous occurrence of growth, development, and disease progression will affect the functional level and disability continuum through a lifetime for a person with a developmental disability.

Throughout this chapter, the term *rehabilitation* is used, rather than *habilitation,* to describe the general services or strategies employed to enhance or facilitate function and community integration. It is recognized that, for children with very early–onset disabilities, there is no loss of skills; rather, there is an acquiring of developmental skills confounded by a disability.

This chapter discusses a sample of outcomes measurement instruments used in pediatrics; two common pediatric disability groups with the typical manifestations, rehabilitation interventions, and outcomes research available for each of these groups; and the general need for future outcomes research.

PEDIATRIC OUTCOMES MEASUREMENT

Health outcomes in children have been measured much as they have been in adults—with morbidity, mortality, clinical, or laboratory measures. As in adults, there is a need for measures that are more comprehensive, functionally directed, and standardized. Choice of outcomes measured and timing of measurement affect evaluative or predictive measures. Functional outcomes measures differ from developmental assessment measures. Functional measures assess independence (not normality), have some sensitivity to functional change, and consider adaptive and contextual issues. This section describes a selection of outcomes measures often used in pediatric research.

General Health Measures

Formal measures of health status for children and adolescents have been developed to discriminate between groups of patients. Maternal perceptions and ratings are often used to determine health status (Stein & Jessop, 1990). Often adult measures are modified for children (Orenstein, Nixon, Ross, & Kaplan, 1989), although concepts underlying health status are different when comparing adults with children and adolescents. Health and illness are separate concepts for youth, not at opposite ends of a continuum as for adults (Natapoff, 1978). Also, perceptions of health and illness are not well established for people with disabilities or for their parents, families, or friends.

Domains of health status for children and adolescents have been explored. Quality of life is a single domain that has been considered separately in adults and children. The Child Health and Illness Profile is a multidimensional health status assessment developed with six domains: activity, comfort, satisfaction, disorders, achievement, and resilience (Starfield et al., 1993). It is a self-administered questionnaire requiring about 45 minutes to complete and is designed to be completed by children age 11–17. Instruments have been adapted (McCormick, Brooks-Gunn, Workman-Daniels, & Peckham, 1993) from the Rand Health Insurance Study (Eisen, Ware, Donald, & Brook, 1979), although the original and modified scales represent parents' report and perception of their children's health status. There are no reports of these instruments being used with children or adolescents with disabilities.

General Functional Measures

Traditionally, clinical measures (e.g., range of motion, change in laboratory values, radiographs) have been used to evaluate interventions or to predict eventual extent of disability or quality of life. The rehabilitation field has been at the forefront in developing more functionally directed measures to better evaluate the effectiveness of programs and intervention strategies. In children, functional outcomes measures determine the level of independence for a given physical or cognitive limitation and for a given developmental level. They are important for monitoring and planning rehabilitation programs and interventions. Contextual and environmental factors are often noted; differentiation between capability (i.e., task completion in an ideal situation) and performance (i.e., task completion in a more typical situation) may be helpful in both education and rehabilitation goal setting (Haley, Coster, & Binda-Sundberg, 1994). Level-of-care provision, use of adaptive equipment, and environmental modifications are often factors documented in these scales. The instruments usually measure disability (*International Classification of Impairments, Disabilities and Handicaps* [World Health Organization, 1993] classification). Often a variety of outcomes measures, developmental assessments, interviews, and clinical examinations or assessments are used to determine a comprehensive functional assessment.

There are a few pediatric tools that have been used nationally or internationally as functional measures. The Functional Independence Measure (FIM) for Children (WeeFIM) builds on the conceptual framework of the FIM but is not meant to replace developmental motor, communicative, or cognitive assessments (see Chapter 5). It comprises 18 items over six domains in children 6 months to 7 years old, rated by a reliable informant, to track outcomes over time (evaluative) and to describe the care provision and resources required (Msall, DiGaudio, & Duffy, 1993). The WeeFIM has been standardized on a normative sample (Msall et al., 1994). The Pediatric Evaluation of Disability Inventory (PEDI) was designed to evaluate function over time and for response to interventions. Care provider assistance and modifications or adaptive equipment required are also recorded. The PEDI is designed to be used with children with ongoing health conditions and disabilities (ages 6 months to 7½ years) over three domains using parent report or structured interview (Feldman, Haley, & Coryell, 1990). By assessing functional skills, care provider assistance, and modifications separately, the instrument measures both capability and performance and allows clinical interpretation of the functional performance (Haley, Coster, & Ludlow, 1991). The Tufts Assessment of Motor Performance was developed to assess motor performance underlying functional abilities. It covers three domains of physical performance using clinician observation for an overall scale that is generally consistent across age groups (ages 6 years and older) (Haley, Ludlow, Gans, Faas, & Inacio, 1991).

These instruments are disability measures, with some description of social, environmental, or burden-of-care levels. The context of the performance measure is also important and may complicate outcomes analyses (Haley et al., 1994). Choice of outcomes measures is determined by purpose of measurement (e.g., predictive, discriminative, descriptive, evaluative) and standardization of the measure (e.g., reliability or validity, normative sample, disability comparison sample, scalability, responsiveness). Consideration should be given to method of administration (e.g., self, parent report, direct observation) and timing of measurement (e.g., time since injury, time since intervention completed). It is necessary to know the purposes, domains measured, method of administration, and standardization of the instruments used to adequately choose and compare outcomes studies reports.

Specific Outcomes Measures

The Gross Motor Function Measure (GMFM) and the Gross Motor Performance Measure (GMPM) were developed to measure change in motor function and performance over time in children with cerebral palsy (CP) and acute brain injury. The GMFM evaluates motor function over five gross motor activities, and the GMPM evaluates aspects of gross motor function over five descriptive motor qualities (Boyce et al., 1992). Both require clinician observation for completion and are reported to be useful in documenting qualitative and function changes.

The field of rheumatology has developed instruments for adults with arthritis to measure health and functional outcomes. Tools also have been developed to measure disability in children with juvenile rheumatoid arthritis (JRA). The Juvenile Arthritis Functional Assessment Scale is a timed performance of 10 activities with clinician observation that discriminates between controls and children with JRA (Lovell et al., 1989). The Juvenile Arthritis Functional Assessment Report for Children and for Parents are interviewer-administered and self-administered questions, respectively, on 23 items of activities with an analogue pain scale (Howe et al., 1991). Age-specific norms are not required. The longitudinal validity of the scale and questionnaires is expected to be assessed. The Childhood Health Assessment Questionnaire has been developed for use with children with JRA and consists of parent or self-report to questions involving eight domains. Validity and reliability data are not available (Timko, Stovel, Moos, & Miller, 1992).

CHILDHOOD DISABLING CONDITIONS

Two common pediatric disabling conditions are presented here. They represent disabilities commonly followed in rehabilitation and developmental centers. CP is the most common cause of paralysis in childhood, and spina bifida (SB) is the most common cause of deformity in childhood (Wenger, Kaye, & LaPlante, 1996). SB is a discrete entity that involves multiple body systems, whereas CP is a more difficult impairment to define and usually includes other associated conditions. Although a wealth of knowledge exists regarding acute management issues and options for rehabilitation and therapy interventions, there is a dearth of information regarding the natural history of the disabling process; the long-term, intermediate, and relatively short-term result of interventions in childhood; and substantiation of recommended practices. No true population-based longitudinal studies regarding natural history exist, because even minimal interventions are not withheld.

Cerebral Palsy

Cerebral palsy (CP) is a constellation of symptoms and conditions defined as a lifelong motor dysfunction resulting from a one-time nonprogressive injury to the immature brain. As a result, central control of muscle function is limited for a lifetime. The prevalence is about 2 per 1,000 individuals with about 500,000 people of all ages in the United States having CP. Incidence is approximately 1 per 1,000 live births. Traditionally, children under the age of 5 who sustain brain injuries from any cause are classified as having CP. CP ranks third among causes of childhood disabilities, and sixth among the middle-aged (LaPlante, 1989).

The types of CP are described by the neurologic pattern and topography of body dysfunction. Typical terms used to describe these dysfunctions are spastic, dyskinetic, mixed, ataxic, and hypotonic. Spastic is the most frequently documented type of CP in the United States and is characterized by increased resting muscle tone and spread or exaggeration of reflex responses. In *spastic hemiparesis*, the affected upper limb is involved more than the lower. *Spastic diplegia* refers to dysfunction in legs more than arms; upper-limb involvement is often subtle. In *spastic quadriplegia*, all four limbs are affected; the term may also imply that trunk, head, and neck control are limited. In this chapter, so-called rigid tone is included in the spastic type.

The dyskinetic type includes a number of movement disorders. The most commonly reported is athetosis (i.e., generalized involuntary and irregular movements of muscle groups, most notably the head, face, and arms), although dystonias (i.e., trunk or limb posturing or tonal changes with function) are also seen. This movement control problem is often noted after the first year of life, following a period of decreased or fluctuating muscle tone. In the mixed type, a combination of spasticity and movement disorders can occur and may be more common than is reported. The least common type is ataxic, which is characterized by unsteadiness and difficulty with rapid or fine movements. It can involve the trunk and the limbs. Low muscle tone is often the prelude to either the spastic or dyskinetic type of CP. Hypotonic CP is rare, and other etiologies, including mental retardation, should be excluded before making this diagnosis. Common etiologies for CP include prematurity, ischemia, hypoxemia, hyperbilirubinemia, and external or internal trauma (Nelson & Ellenberg, 1986; Stanley & Alberman, 1984).

Clinical Manifestations CP is a disabling condition defined by a motor impairment. There are associated conditions that are also a result of the injury or pathology that are linked to the primary condition. These include seizures, mental retardation, learning disabilities, oral motor problems (e.g., drooling, feeding problems, dysarthria), communication problems, and sensory problems (e.g., hearing, vision). These associated conditions may, in some cases, be more disabling than the motor problem and can be classified as impairments. There also are secondary conditions that may occur at any point during a person's life and that are present because of the primary disabling condition. Secondary conditions include osteoporosis, musculoskeletal complaints (e.g., contractures, pain), and pressure sores resulting from an ill-fitting wheelchair or orthotic. Age-related changes may also be noted, sometimes earlier than expected, and may include decreasing endurance and documented osteoarthritis (Turk, Overeynder, & Janicki, 1995). Each of these categories may be impairments and may be a cause of disabilities or handicaps.

Health and medical issues also need to be considered and may be associated or secondary conditions. Children with significant feeding problems may have difficulties with nutrition, esophageal reflux, or aspiration pneumonia. Urinary and bowel incontinence may persist and present as a handicapping condition, limiting community activities or peer acceptance. Neurogenic bladders have been reported in people with CP. Constipation is an often-noted problem for children and adults with CP. Neuroendocrine problems should be considered in people with extensive brain injuries; irregular menstrual cycles may be related to this system.

Although there are no population-based longitudinal studies reporting functional levels of people with CP, there are clinic-based reports and anecdotal experiences (published and unpublished) that give a sense of expected function for each neurologic pattern of presentation (Bleck, 1975; Molnar, 1979). Generally, motor development is delayed; other areas of development also may show delay. During the developmental years, spasticity may change often as a consequence of growth or attainment of skills. Functional achievements are directed as much by cognitive skills as by motor capabilities. Anticipated functional levels for the common neurologic patterns are further described in this section.

Children with *spastic hemiplegia* are usually recognized by 6 months of age, although very mild forms may not be noted until 1 year of age or later. Early gross motor milestones are usually delayed. Despite usually limited function of the hemiparetic hand, most children and adults are independent in adaptive skills. Generally, children become independent in walking by 3 years of age and maintain walking for mobility throughout life. Presence of cognitive or perceptual limitations may interfere with acquisition of these motor functions. Seizures are noted in about 50% of children with hemiparetic CP (Aksu, 1990). Contractures are common in the involved extremities. There may be limited growth and underdevelopment in the involved limbs. Mental retardation is not common (Süssová, Seidl, & Faber, 1990).

Spastic diplegia is the common presentation of CP in children born prematurely. Motor development and functional level vary in this group (Bleck, 1975; Largo, Molinari, & Weber, 1985). Studies have been reported that prognosticate functional outcomes. Molnar and Gordon (1976) reported that sitting by age 2 years was a positive predictive sign for walking, whereas persistent obligatory primitive reflexes beyond age 18 months were associated with a poor prognosis for walking. Watt, Robertson, and Grace (1989) also noted that sitting by age 2 years had a strong correlation with walking, and other variables did not improve the predictive value. Badell-Ribera (1985) noted that sitting by age 1½ years and crawling by age 2½ years predicted the walking potential of children with diplegic CP. The typical early pattern in children is a predominant extensor posturing in the lower limbs (scissoring), which eventually translates into the characteristic crouched positioning for walking. Independent walking may be with or without assistive devices, and some children may require a wheelchair for independent mobility. Adolescents, young adults, and adults may choose a wheelchair as the main means of independent mobility to conserve energy. Hip pathology is common because of muscle imbalance from spastic posturing; surgery may be indicated for hip subluxation or dislocation. The avoidance of a painful dislocated hip is key. Pelvic obliquity and scoliosis are associated with hip pathology. Contractures are often noted at the hips, knees, ankles, and feet. Because the hands are usually minimally affected, adaptive skills are performed independently, sometimes with modifications. Mental retardation and seizures are less common in people with diplegia than in those with quadriplegia. Again, function is affected by cognitive skills.

Spastic quadriplegic CP typically manifests the highest level of severity for function and associated conditions. Commonly, this category implies poor head, neck, and trunk control, or total body involvement. However, in this type, there may exist a wide variation from mild to severe impairment; therefore, a severe level of disability or handicap is not always the case. Gross motor development follows that seen in diplegic CP, although trunk control is usually difficult to attain. Consequently, some children and adults in this group demonstrate a significant disability in motor and adaptive skills, and they may never walk for mobility, may be dependent for any mobility, and are dependent for all self-care. Dependency is more common in this type of CP. Because of the high energy expenditure required, adolescents, young adults, and adults with spastic quadriplegic CP may choose a wheelchair (often powered) as the main means of mobility. Musculoskeletal impairments are more common in this group and are usually more severe, including dislocated hips and scoliosis. Oral motor problems are more common in this group, and feeding, swallowing, drooling, and articulation problems are frequently noted. Dental problems are also seen. Mental retardation is common, and severe deficits are frequently noted. More than half have seizures (Aksu, 1990). The most common *mixed type* is spastic athetoid CP and follows the course for quadriplegic CP. Again, a variety of functional capabilities are noted, although there are usually fewer deformities, owing to the movement component.

The *dyskinetic types* usually present with hypotonia during the first year of life. Athetosis is the most common form, but its frequency has decreased since the advent of RhoGAM and fetal transfusions. Therefore, there are fewer children and a larger adult population with this manifestation. Athetosis represents a generalized involvement, and dystonias may be focal or generalized. It has traditionally been held that most children and adults walk for mobility. Self-care is more difficult because upper limbs are usually more affected. Contractures are rare in athetosis but can be seen in dystonias and often consist of equinovarus foot deformities and scoliosis. Mental retardation is not common. Seizures are also less common than in spastic hemiplegia and quadriplegia. Oral motor problems are more common.

Adults with CP note problems with fatigue, pain, and change in function (T. Seekins, personal communication, May 1995). However, little is understood about the effect of the aging process on a lifelong disabling condition. Many adults report concerns about possible unknown future issues and about changes in function for which they felt unprepared (Overeynder, Turk, & Janicki, 1994; Turk, Overeynder, & Janicki, 1995). Significant deterioration or loss of function should not be anticipated in adults with CP.

Rehabilitation Interventions Rehabilitation interventions and strategies for children with CP use a developmentally based plan to foster the acquisition of skills and to anticipate potential complications. Such a plan involves the family, health care providers (e.g., physicians, therapists, nutritionists, nurses), and other professionals (e.g., case managers, program coordinators, social workers). Realistic expectations are the basis of the success of these plans. Programs and protocols have used developmental assessment tools for evaluation, but there are no published data using standardized outcomes measurements (i.e., impairment, disability, and handicap measures) to determine effectiveness. Pediatric functional outcomes measurement instruments may prove helpful in evaluating traditional programs and focused interventions.

Early intervention programs provide services for infants and toddlers at risk for, or with known, developmental disabilities. Although services began in the 1970s, they were mandated in 1986 by the Education of the Handicapped Act Amendments (PL 99-457). Eligibility is based on physical, linguistic, or cognitive delays, and a multidisciplinary team is focused on a family-centered approach. Service provision may be home- or center-based. The rationale is based on research data that show that the infant–care provider interaction and the infant exploration of the environment have an influence on early development. A range of stimulation and training activities are provided and include family support, counseling, education, and direct therapy or education. The type of program provided is based on the perceived needs of the infant or child and the philosophic orientation of the disciplines involved (Simeonsson, Cooper, & Scheiner,

1982). Experimental evidence is mixed regarding the efficacy of these programs, although recent research techniques (e.g., single-subject design, meta-analysis) suggest the effectiveness of these interventions in promoting developmental progress (Harris, 1991).

The most common management strategy for the motor impairment in CP is developmental (i.e., physical, occupational, speech) therapy. There are many schools of therapy approaches that are promoted, but it is the general belief that the most effective is that which combines the primitive reflex behaviors of children with CP with a basic understanding of motor learning (Gans, 1993). No single approach has been demonstrated to be more effective than another (Bower & McLellan, 1992). The most common approaches include the traditional flexibility and strengthening exercises, neurodevelopmental treatment, and sensory integration. General goals are to promote the development of postural and movement control; to improve fine, gross, and oral motor skills; to enhance communication; to promote age-appropriate self-care; to encourage independent mobility; to support cognitive skills; and to advance a positive self-image. Short-term goals are based on developmental changes, skill attainment, realistic expectations, and focused needs. There is no information available regarding the duration or intensity of therapy related to short-term, long-term, or lifelong function. Home programs are universally thought to be effective to practice or maintain activities. These are also promoted for people with CP. Issues of financial burden and family and child time commitment also must be considered.

Orthotics, adaptive equipment, specific spasticity-reducing regimens, and orthopedic surgery are also part of the intervention options. Orthoses are used to improve function or to prevent deformities. They are most commonly used to improve walking but have been used to decrease tone or improve deformity. Typically, orthotics prescribed to assist with walking are to control tone or position at the ankle and foot; long leg braces are prescribed much less often. There are many types of ankle-foot orthoses and supramalleolar orthotics that may combine different trimlines with tone inhibition. Serial casting may be used to improve a deformity prebracing, and inhibitive casts may be used therapeutically. Casting and orthotics or splints have been used to improve function, improve deformity, or maintain position in the upper limb and hand. Bracing also may be used for scoliosis management. Adaptive equipment is prescribed to improve functional independence in mobility, self-care, communication, environmental control, and school or work activities. There are no definitive studies regarding how to make the best choice among all the options, what the most effective way is to use them, or which options improve function the most and for how long.

Orthopedic surgery plays an important role in the management of those with CP. Typical goals of surgery are to improve posture and function (usually gait, with many fewer upper-limb surgeries), to alleviate or prevent deformity, or to decrease pain from deformity. Published reports of case series usually are a follow-up of 6 months to a number of years. Outcomes are usually based on clinical measures rather than on function. Gait analysis is often used as a measure. Use of physical therapy postoperatively is variable. There are no studies that consider long-term functional outcomes following procedures.

Options for spasticity management have increased since the mid-1980s. Oral medications have been the typical management strategy used, with varying degrees of success having been achieved. Motor point or nerve blocks have been used as a temporizing method. Selective posterior rhizotomy gained popularity in the late 1980s and early 1990s and is promoted with reports of improved function, with up to 10 years of follow-up data available using clinical measures. Postoperative use of physical therapy is not consistent, ranging from inpatient rehabilitation services on a daily basis to home program with limited direct physical therapy service. Baclofen pumps also have been promoted as a means of spasticity management; however, limited follow-up data are available. In the early 1990s, botulinum toxin injection gained popularity, with reports of decreases in spasticity with its use over a limited time. There is no definitive information regarding patient characteristics to determine the best choice of management options.

Psychosocial, educational, and vocational issues are also addressed, often within school programs. Appropriateness of therapy in the classroom or for individual service during the school day continues to be questioned as resources continue to shrink. Systems to address adult needs and services are not as well organized as they are for children, except possibly for adults with CP who have severe cognitive and motor impairments. There is a need for limited direct therapy services for adults with onset of secondary conditions or age-related changes. Generally, young adults and adults do not participate in routine fitness or exercise programs. This is as much a result of the limited knowledge in this area as it is of the attitudes of care providers of, and families of, people with disabilities.

Outcomes and Life Status Studies

As previously noted, outcomes studies are very limited regarding people with CP. Generally accepted treatment or intervention strategies may not be well substantiated in the literature. Surgical interventions and their outcomes are reported in case series, usually using clinical or laboratory measures, and often for only limited epochs. There has been advocacy for use of functional measurement in the orthopedic literature (Young & Wright, 1995). The WeeFIM has been used to measure outcomes following posterior rhizotomy for up to 8 years (D.J. Gaebler-Spira, personal communication, March 1996), and the PEDI has been used as a pre- and postoperative measurement (Bloom & Nazar, 1994). The GMPM showed statistically significant improvements in motor performance in older children (ages 7–12 years) with CP than in younger children over a 4- to 6-month period (Boyce et al., 1992). There are no reports of functional measures used in adults with CP to evaluate interventions or to determine capabilities or changes over a lifetime.

A report of health status in children with developmental disabilities reviewed the data from the 1988 National Health Interview Survey Child Health Supplement (Boyle, Decouflé, & Yeargin-Allsopp, 1994). The overall impact on health and school functioning was greatest for children with CP and epilepsy. There was greater utilization of health care, poorer school performance, and a greater frequency of their parents to rate health as fair to poor for these two groups. However, children with CP lost fewer school days to absences. In a population-based study of adults with CP in a mid-size metropolitan area, people with CP were generally healthy (based on clinical information and self-report), but worried and concerned about their health status (Turk, Weber, Geremski, & Pavin, 1995). Further study regarding the health status of children and adults is warranted.

Mortality statistics over the population are not reported. Children with severe or profound mental retardation have shown an increased risk of dying in a retrospective time-limited population-based study (Kudrjavcev, Schoenberg, Kurland, & Groover, 1985). The most commonly reported cause of death in children and young adults with CP was respiratory in a retrospective review of a British CP registry (Evans & Alberman, 1990). Shortened life expectancy was reported in people with mental retardation and severe motor impairments, particularly those with a feeding disability, as noted in review of a state service registry (Eyman, Grossman, Chaney, & Call, 1990).

Spina Bifida

Spina bifida is a congenital abnormality of the spinal axis resulting in spinal cord dysfunction and therefore encompasses all the typical impairments seen in patients with spinal cord injuries. Along with the neural tube defect, there may also be an associated cephalic anterior neuropore abnormality giving rise to hydrocephalus and possibly resulting in brain dysfunction. The etiology is considered genetic, with both chromosomal and environmental factors contributing to the condition. Nutritional aspects began to be recognized in the early 1990s. The incidence is quite low at 0.5 per 1,000 live births. Prevalence is also low; before the advent of the shunt (pre-1960), mortality was quite high, which may contribute to these prevalence figures. However, this condition represents a multisystem impairment for which there often is an organized management system in health care.

Clinical Manifestations   Spinal cord and brain pathology are the causes for the resulting impairments, which commonly are paraplegia (motor and sensory component), neurogenic bladder and bowel, and cognitive dysfunctions. Early acute care is directed to surgical closure of the lesion and assessment for hydrocephalus and of urinary function. Hydrocephalus occurs in about 90% of cases (Gans, 1993). Secondary conditions are also noted, the most common of which are pressure sores. Age-related changes are also likely present.

Paraplegia with sensory and motor involvement is the typical motor impairment. The level and extent of the lesion determines the function of lower limbs. Activation of major muscle groups is usually apparent in infants without detailed muscle testing to assist with functional determination. There are general anticipated functional activities regarding spinal-level involvement. Cognitive abilities also affect motor function. Asymmetry in function may be present and may modify intervention or outcome.

In *thoracic paraplegia*, legs are flaccid and trunk control may be limited. There may be contractures from in utero position at birth or later occurrence of conforming to a sitting posture. Trunk support may be required for sitting in early development and may continue to be required for routine function for self-care, school, or other activities. Mobility may be aided with orthotics (e.g., hip-knee-ankle-foot orthosis with or without trunk support, parapodium) and walking aids if needed and requires significant energy. Walking is often therapeutic or in-home; thus, wheelchair mobility is often chosen. Hip dislocation is common secondary to poor joint development. Scoliosis is also common.

Children with *high lumbar* or *midlumbar paraplegia* have the highest risk for progressive hip dislocation. Surgical intervention is usually advisable for prevention of hip dislocation. Contractures are noted at joints with unopposed movement patterns and may be asymmetric (e.g., hip flexion, hip adduction, knee extension). Ankle and foot deformities may be arthrogrypotic and difficult to correct. Orthotics and walking aids are usually prescribed and usually require significant energy. Walking may be used in the community, but wheelchair mobility may be chosen to conserve energy.

In *low lumbar paraplegia*, independent walking for community mobility is expected, barring any complications. Ankle-foot orthosis with or without walking aids is usually required. Foot deformities may be problematic. Hip pathology may progress over childhood, with dislocation occurring by adolescence. *Sacral* paralysis presents with foot deformities that may be problematic for pressure sores in late childhood or in adolescence. Often the only limitations to walking are the pressure sores.

Neurogenic bladder dysfunction requires special routines for management and follow-up. Both incontinence and retention can be seen, depending on the type of neurogenic bladder. Poorly managed incontinence is a serious disability and handicap. Retention with dyssynergy of external sphincter and detrusor function can cause upper renal tract pathology, a secondary condition. The objective of management is to prevent renal damage and achieve social continence. Intermittent self-catheterization with the use of medications is a typical management strategy, but it requires a certain cognitive level and perceptual skill level to be accomplished. Surgical interventions may be considered. Neurogenic bowel dysfunction is often a difficult management problem. Social continence with routine evacuation is the goal.

Problems with perceptual skills and low IQ scores have been noted (Friedrich, Lovejoy, Shaffer, Shurtleff, & Beilke, 1991), particularly in people with a history of shunt malfunctions and infections (McClone, Czyzewski, Raimondi, & Sommers, 1982). Pressure sores are a common secondary condition for people with SB because there are areas of the body with no sensation (impairment) secondary to the spinal cord dysfunction. Prevalence rates for pressure sores are about 40%–60% (Farley, Vines, McCluer, Stefans, & Hunter, 1994; Shurtleff, 1986). Preventive strategies should be a part of daily management. Obesity is common in adolescents and more frequent in adults. Osteoporosis (Type III: secondary osteoporosis) is common and may result in fractures. Latex allergy also is common, with the presence of latex antibodies in people with SB reported to be 38% (Tosi, Slater, & Shaer, 1993).

Deterioration of function or skills should not be expected in children or adults with SB. There are two specific conditions that must be considered with changes in functional skills. First, the Arnold Chiari malformation can cause progressive deterioration, particularly in swallowing problems, in both children and adults. Second, a tethered cord must be considered in children or adults who note new or increased spasticity, weakness, progression of deformities, and pain.

Age-related changes should be considered in young adults and adults with SB. People with SB begin to choose wheelchairs as the main means of mobility if energy expenditure is great, usually between the ages of 10 and 20 years (Findley et al., 1987). Adults with SB may show typical musculoskeletal aging changes earlier than their peers without disabilities (Dunne, Gingher, Olsen, & Shurtleff, c. 1984).

Rehabilitation Interventions As for any child with a developmental disability, intervention programs are designed with growth and developmental issues at the forefront. Parents of infants with SB are taught care needs, handling, and positioning in the newborn nursery. A team consisting of family, health care providers, and other professionals work toward common goals. Infants and toddlers with SB participate in early intervention programs. Anecdotal reports of positive response to this organized approach is noted, although there are no studies to substantiate this.

Developmental therapies are the most common intervention strategy. Realistic expectations are to be considered in development of therapy and program goals, along with time and financial constraints. General goals are to promote mobility, promote independent self-care (including neurogenic bladder and bowel management at age-appropriate times), prevent secondary conditions, determine adaptations for educational and vocational issues, and advance a positive self-image. No specific therapy approach has been proved more effective than another. Developmental activities to promote strengthening, flexibility, and range of motion are the typical physical therapy approach.

Use of orthotics is common in children with SB. A variety of orthotics and walking aids may be used and include traditional orthoses and aids, the parapodium, the swivel walker, and reciprocal orthoses. Prescription is defined by level of function first, although regional preferences and professional experiences are a part of the decision. Early supported standing is promoted with use of orthotics; however, no studies exist to support the belief that this enhances skeletal alignment; prevents osteoporosis; or improves urinary, gastrointestinal, or pulmonary function. It has been shown that muscle activity is more important than weight bearing in determining extent or presence of osteoporosis (Rosenstein, Green, Herrington, & Blum, 1987). Orthotics are used for scoliosis management.

Orthopedic surgical intervention is common. General indications are to improve muscle imbalance about joints (particularly hip and ankle); to release soft tissue contractures recalcitrant to stretching, which can produce further deformities; to correct congenital deformities; or to improve function, hygiene, or pain complaints. The need for physical therapy postoperatively has not been substantiated or refuted in the literature. Usually, case series are reported using clinical measures and over relatively short time frames.

Use of adaptive equipment may allow a child or adult to be independent at a task. Wheelchairs, both power and manual, are the most common piece of equipment prescribed. Equipment may also be used to assist with care needs and to enhance educational, vocational, or social pursuits.

Educational and vocational issues are usually addressed in the school system. Psychosocial and independence issues may be supported by the medical system in the area of independence in self-care (management of neurogenic bladder and bowel). Adults with SB may require focused and limited therapy interventions with age-related changes or secondary conditions. Programs of fitness and exercise are not usually part of regular routines of people with SB.

Outcomes and Life Status Studies For the most part, outcomes studies are limited to clinical measures and complications following surgical procedures, usually over a limited time. No studies use standardized measures of function to determine pre- and postoperative abilities. A few studies discuss outcomes at some level in adults and young adults (Charney, Melchionni, & Smith, 1991; Hunt, 1990; Liptak, Shurtleff, Bloss, Baltus-Hebert, & Manitta, 1992).

A report of a survey of young adults and adults for the Spina Bifida Association of America documented issues and concerns of this self-selected group, although no standardized functional measures or health measures were employed (Dunne et al., c. 1984). Unemployment was high, and parents primarily provided needed assistance with care. A 1994 survey of people identified in a state registry as having SB was reported (Farley et al., 1994) in which descriptive and clinical measures were collected (including secondary conditions), with report of education, employment, and independence being used as markers of handicap and quality of life. For these quality-of-life measures, adults with SB had low educational achievement, low employment status, and low social independence. Also of note is a study to determine better prognostication of walking function based on lower extremity muscle strength rather than on level of spinal dysfunction (McDonald, Jaffe, Shurtleff, & Menelaus, 1991). No other reports have used this measure for prognostication.

Reported mortality statistics are limited. Reports from the early 1970s noted survival to adulthood to be 60%–70% of infants referred to regional centers (Shurtleff, Hayden, Chapman, Broy, & Hill, 1975). A 1990 study reported survival of 60% of consecutive cases, treated unselectively, over a 16- to 20-year time frame (Hunt, 1990).

FUTURE OUTCOMES RESEARCH

As this chapter has indicated, there are no population-based longitudinal studies that can give a true picture of the natural history of developmental disabilities. The effects of growth and development clearly confound the assessment of treatment-related functional outcomes of infants and children with disabling conditions. Interventions are based on accepted empirically derived practices, anecdotal experience, and case series or cross-sectional reports. Standardized measures of functional outcomes for evaluation of intervention or characterization of individuals have not been applied routinely to measure outcomes of specific interventions or for life course determination. As of 1994, standard measures applicable for outcomes prognostication have not been developed. The impact of the disabling condition on the family and vice versa has not been demonstrated, and it is not clear how a change in function of a person with a disability over a lifetime affects that interaction. Recommendations for future research are given in this section.

Longitudinal Studies

Children and adults with developmental disabilities and their families often request information regarding natural history and recommended practices for specific disabling conditions to assist with decisions regarding interventions and planning for lifelong needs. Professionals also need this information for treatment or research design. However, what little information is available is based on personal experience, limited descriptive case reports or series, or generalization from other experiences or disability groups. The relative impact of development and early intervention (e.g., therapy, surgery) over a lifetime is not known. Published information on developmental disabilities is often collected from a nonrepresentative population, does not use accepted standardized measures, and often is outdated. These small, cross-sectional studies may not contain sufficient enough variability in the spectrum of the disability, may not offer variability in treatment (e.g., from the same service program), and may have outcomes that are not generalizable. Therefore, longitudinal studies with representative populations should be undertaken. This requires careful identification of cohorts on which to base the studies and development of protocols that address the family and community elements of developmental disabilities, define methods determining the impact of development on interventions and the reverse, and enable collaboration with agencies and organizations serving the population with developmental disabilities.

Measurement Development

There are no measurement systems that address each of the domains of the disability continuum for children or adults with developmental disabilities and none that predict function or evaluate the benefits of a specific intervention over a lifetime. There are some pediatric measures for impairment or for disability and pilot studies for measures for the handicap or quality-of-life domains. Standard developmental assessments exist for typical children, but their use in children with disabilities does not yield a valid evaluation of an intervention, and they do not provide prognostic information over a lifetime. There are no methods by which to discriminate between the effects of development and of interventions in children with developmental disabilities. There are a few instruments available that provide descriptive disability-specific information. General health status instruments have not been standardized for populations with disabilities. Self-report measures are difficult or impossible in younger children and in people with cognitive impairments. Parent or care provider report measures are subject to questions of accuracy and bias, issues that must be acknowledged and addressed where proxy information is used. Assessment using a combination of questionnaires, structured interviews, and clinical judgment is less time-consuming than a complete, direct observation. Although this type of assessment may contain some factual errors, it can provide a more accurate, contextually valid response.

Those standardized measures that exist have been poorly used in studies. Using an existing outcomes measurement instrument for a study requires both recognizing that its use does not carry an extension of validity developed for other purposes and ensuring that the measure provides sufficient applicable data to reach a conclusion. Instruments designed for evaluation of rehabilitation intervention must be distinguished from those that prognosticate future function or define burden of care. Qualitative or minimal changes are often difficult to determine with some existing instruments and within differing contexts. In trauma, prognostic scales (as limited as they are) have been standardized for adults, but not for children. Most important, these instruments usually define status and change in status between measurements. They do not inherently relate to cause of change. They may have validity in statistically significant samples, but applying these general relationships to small samples or individuals is usually not valid.

Outcomes measurement protocols are increasingly being used in a variety of contexts. Program evaluation, quality assurance, patient outcomes, and reimbursement issues have been bound together by service organizations, managed care organizations, government agencies, and policy makers. Care must be taken in review of outcomes measurement methods to define their purposes, measurement properties, scoring and interpretation, and statistical power to validate these tools for use in each new area of application.

Therefore, a research agenda must strengthen or further develop existing measurement systems, accurately describe and validate the purposes of each, develop valid and reliable quality-of-life measures, and develop transition issues and lifelong function measures. Issues of development (e.g., cognitive, adaptive, physical function) and environmental and social context (e.g., gender, culture) must be addressed. Although outcomes measurement development in children is quite complex, collaboration of researchers and clinicians can provide an effective framework.

Service Delivery Models

There are many models of service delivery for people with developmental disabilities and their families. Traditionally, these models provide medical and/or educational services. Services may be home-based or center-based. Services may be provided directly by professionals, as a professional consultation on a single or periodic basis, in group settings, and by trained nonprofessionals. There are varying intensities and a variety of time courses. Description of interventions are imprecise and may have different meanings to different providers or consumers. Services may be direct intervention, evaluation or assessment, didactic in nature, or supportive. Goals span maintenance of function to specific attainment of function. The effectiveness of each model, including cost-effectiveness, is unknown. The generalization of certain models to or applicability of models in various cultures and environments is also unknown. There are usually simultaneous or sequential multiple interventions that often lack communication between medical and educational disciplines in formulating a care plan or individual educational plan. This may further complicate ongoing plans and adjustments by children with disabilities and their families.

Interventions and outcomes measures must be gender-sensitive and culturally and environmentally sensitive. To be sustainable they should be compatible with both health and education delivery systems, separately and in combination. This requires collaboration and dissemination of these protocols among service providers at both the system and individual levels. The ultimate goal of these protocols is to identify the best coordination, continuity, and mix of service for people with developmental disabilities over a lifetime.

A research agenda must include evaluation and comparison of various systems of care delivery. This implies that the definitions of intervention and measures must be clear and precise to better delineate the black box of rehabilitation. Cost analysis through a true economic model must be a part of any comparative study of service models. Traditional and nontraditional approaches should be evaluated by using education-based measures and/or medical-based measures where appropriate to determine how each service system relates to outcomes.

Transition Issues

Transition from dependent to independent living is a particularly important event for people with developmental disabilities, whatever their chronologic age. Minimal information exists regarding these transitions and interventions that may assist or enable them. Specific information available may not be generalizable to other disability groups or settings, or it may be too general for application. Transition concerns often deal less with the person with the disability than with perceived or anticipated problems. Providers and professionals assisting in these transitions may draw on personal experiences or maternal or paternal instincts rather than directly assisting with the priorities of the individual. Support system strategies also may deal more with perceived concerns than with actual concerns and may seek a system-directed rather than an individual-directed effectiveness. Therefore, effective interventions should be established to ease transitions or key changes occurring during development.

The research agenda must identify and measure stages involved in key transition issues. For example, these stages may include issues involved with transitions from school to work or with issues of sexuality and positive body image during adolescence. Normative and comparative sampling could determine differences in stages in those with developmental disabilities compared with their peers without disabilities and among disability groups. Once issues are identified, effectiveness of interventions for transitions could be evaluated by using established outcomes measurement protocols.

Effectiveness of Assistive Technology over a Lifetime

Assistive technology has become more accessible to children with disabilities since the mid-1980s. Light- as well as high-technology measures have been promoted to enhance the function of individuals with a variety of impairments, and many of these have been shown to be effective. Cost, parent or consumer preference, knowledge of the provider, and environment limit the application of technology. Young adults and adults with developmental disabilities may be offered technology but may find it of limited use because other long-used strategies have proved effective, because long-held beliefs and attitudes prohibit its use, or because change is difficult for those with a disability or for their support system. The risk of musculoskeletal secondary conditions may warrant consideration or reevaluation of use of assistive technology for some motor tasks as a prevention strategy (e.g., use of power mobility to conserve energy) or as a cause (e.g., use of a manual wheelchair for long distances causing shoulder impingement syndromes) for secondary conditions. It is a generally held belief that assistive technology can improve the functional performance of an individual with impairments. However, there is no information to substantiate the benefit of using that technology over a lifetime or when best to change (or upgrade) technology based on developmental and transition issues.

In addition to longitudinal studies, the research agenda must consider lifelong use of assistive technology, documenting effectiveness of that technology as an intervention, identifying stages for reconsideration of its use, and defining environmental and social considerations. Outcomes measurement instruments in the realms of disability, handicap, and quality of life, particularly those that are sensitive enough to document change, would prove beneficial in this endeavor.

Impact of the Child and Disability Continuum on the Family

Parent and family issues are entwined with those of a child or adult with a developmental disability. It has long been recognized that families play an important role in the functional performance and health of a child with a disability. Some existing measurement instruments include information from parent or care provider and attempt to weight these elements along with observed components to provide a total assessment. There are existing descriptive studies of family coping strategies and interactive styles. Maintaining a cohesive family unit has proved difficult for some. Rehabilitation interventions include family involvement by providing education and support to families and having families provide direct service with training. These added responsibilities and activities may have both positive and negative effects. However, long-term impact, stages for change in family involvement, successful coping strategies, and effective service interventions considering gender, social, and cultural issues have not been described using outcomes measures.

Therefore, research in the area of family dynamics related to the child or adult with a developmental disability, at different stages and over a lifetime, is imperative. Equally important is the correlation of the individual's functional status with his or her family's support and coping strategies.

Impact of the Environment on the Child with a Disability

The environmental, social, and cultural framework is an important factor in any child's life, and this is also the case for a child with a disability. A child's performance is tied to the surroundings and supports, including physical environment, the social context, and the participation of other people. Achievement of independence may be enhanced by physical environmental accessibility as well as by the contributions of people and systems that facilitate and enable independent behaviors and goals. For a child with a disability, an inherent developmental process may be modified by impairments that limit specific activities and by personal experiences. The child's intrinsic functional capacity can be further adjusted to a more functional performance by a change in the environment through modification of the setting, conditions of the task, social supports, and the degree of adult direction. Outcomes measurement must take into account the environmental variables as a contribution to functional performance. Specific environmental barriers or enhancements to functional performance must be identified, including effective modifications to the environment.

Training for Research and Clinical Professionals

Outcomes measurement development and use has become an acknowledged priority in research and practice in pediatric care and rehabilitation.

There has been an increasing demand for documentation and accountability. However, clinical pediatric practice use of these instruments has been limited. The majority of research has been in standardization and validation of instruments. No single measure has been embraced by clinicians, and outcomes issues remain throughout the framework of the development and the disability continuum. Although outcomes measurement development and use have been recognized as important, application of that principle has been less notable. Although standardized measurement protocols are often used for routine documentation in adult rehabilitation, there has been less interest in their use in pediatrics.

Consequently, training of clinicians in the role of outcomes measures should be undertaken. Clinicians should be aware of the protocols, their purposes, the practicality of each, the scoring and interpretation, and, most important, their limitiations for clinical use. Researchers should be encouraged to use the protocols within large populations and validate them for specific or multiple purposes. Researchers and clinicians should collaborate on outcomes measures and promote their use for research and application.

CONCLUSIONS

Outcomes measurement in childhood-onset disabilities is moving slowly from a development stage to an implementation phase. Clinicians are beginning to recognize the importance of measuring outcomes from an interventional perspective, as well as from a lifelong functional perspective. Although developmental assessment instruments have been utilized, true measures to assess independence and response to treatment interventions have been used in a limited fashion. Choices of outcomes measures must be determined by the purpose of the measurement and standardization of the measure. The clinician must also be aware of the methods of administration and the timing of measurement to use the information appropriately.

Outcomes measurement of pediatric disabling conditions is a necessity to identify descriptive, evaluative, and predictive information. Promotion of traditional and new interventions must be based on functional measures. The issues of lifelong disabilities must be better identified. This therefore requires continued development and standardization of functional measures. Issues specific to the pediatric population must be recognized and addressed, and professionals must be educated in appropriate use of these measures.

REFERENCES
Aksu, F. (1990). Nature and prognosis of seizures in patients with cerebral palsy. *Developmental Medicine and Child Neurology, 31*, 287–292.

Badell-Ribera, A. (1985). Cerebral palsy: Postural-locomotor prognosis in spastic diplegia. *Archives of Physical Medicine and Rehabilitation, 66,* 614–619.

Bleck, E.E. (1975). Locomotor prognosis in cerebral palsy. *Developmental Medicine and Child Neurology, 17,* 18–23.

Bloom, K.K., & Nazar, G.B. (1994). Functional assessment following selective posterior rhizotomy in spastic cerebral palsy. *Children's Nervous System, 10,* 84–86.

Bower, E., & McLellan, D.L. (1992). Effects of increased exposure to physiotherapy on skill acquisition of children with cerebral palsy. *Developmental Medicine and Child Neurology, 34,* 25–39.

Boyce, W., Gowland, C., Rosenbaum, P., Lane, M., Plews, N., Goldsmith, C., Russell, D., Wright, V., Zdrobov, S., & Harding, D. (1992). Gross motor performance measure for children with cerebral palsy: Study design and preliminary findings. *Revue Canadienne de Santé Publique, 83,* S34–S40.

Boyle, C.A., Decouflé P., & Yeargin-Allsopp, M. (1994). Prevalence and health impact of developmental disabilities in U.S. children. *Pediatrics, 93,* 399–403.

Charney, E.B., Melchionni, J.B., & Smith, D.R. (1991). Community ambulation by children with myelomeningocele and high-level paralysis. *Journal of Pediatric Orthopaedics, 11,* 579–582.

Dunne, K.B., Gingher, N., Olsen, L.M., & Shurtleff, D.B. (c. 1984). *A survey of the medical and functional status of members of the adult network of the Spina Bifida Association of America.* Unpublished manuscript, Spina Bifida Association of America, Washington, DC.

Education of the Handicapped Act Amendments of 1986, PL 99-457, 20 U.S.C. §§ 1400 *et seq.*

Eisen, M., Ware, J.E., Donald, C.A., & Brook, R.H. (1979). Measuring components of children's health status. *Medical Care, 17,* 902–921.

Evans, P.M., & Alberman, E. (1990). Certified cause of death in children and young adults with cerebral palsy. *Archives of Disease in Childhood, 66,* 325–329.

Eyman, R.K., Grossman, H.J., Chaney, R.H., & Call, T.L. (1990). The life expectancy of profoundly handicapped people with mental retardation. *New England Journal of Medicine, 323,* 584–589.

Farley, T., Vines, C., McCluer, S., Stefans, V., & Hunter, J. (1994). Secondary disabilities in Arkansans with spina bifida (abstract). *European Journal of Pediatric Surgery, 4*(Suppl.), 39–40.

Feldman, A.B., Haley, S.M., & Coryell, J. (1990). Concurrent and construct validity of the Pediatric Evaluation of Disability Inventory. *Physical Therapy, 70,* 981–993.

Findley, T.W., Agre, J.C., Habeck, R.V., Schmalz, R., Birkebak, R.R., & McNally M.C. (1987). Ambulation in the adolescent with myelomeningocele I: Early childhood predictors. *Archives of Physical Medicine and Rehabilitation, 68,* 518–522.

Friedrich, W.N., Lovejoy, M.C., Shaffer, J., Shurtleff, D.B., & Beilke, R.L. (1991). Cognitive abilities and achievement status of children with myelomeningocele: A contemporary sample. *Journal of Pediatric Psychology, 16,* 423–428.

Gans, B.M. (1993). Rehabilitation of the pediatric patient. In J.A. DeLisa (Ed.), *Rehabilitation medicine: Principles and practice* (2nd ed., pp. 623–641). Philadelphia: J.B. Lippincott.

Haley, S.M., Coster, W.J., & Binda-Sundberg, K. (1994). Measuring physical disablement: The contextual challenge. *Physical Therapy, 74,* 443–451.

Haley, S.M., Coster, W.J., & Ludlow, L.H. (1991). Pediatric functional outcomes measures. In K.M. Jaffe (Ed.), *Physical medicine and rehabilitation clinics of*

North America: Pediatric rehabilitation (pp. 689–723). Philadelphia: W.B. Saunders.

Haley, S.M., Ludlow, L.H., Gans, B.M., Faas, R.M., & Inacio, C.A. (1991). Tufts Assessment of Motor Performance: An empirical approach to identifying motor performance categories. *Archives of Physical Medicine and Rehabilitation, 72,* 359–366.

Harris, S.R. (1991). Efficacy of early intervention in pediatric rehabilitation: A decade of evaluation and review. In K.M. Jaffe (Ed.), *Physical medicine and rehabilitation clinics of North America: Pediatric rehabilitation* (pp. 725–742). Philadelphia: W.B. Saunders.

Howe, S., Levinson, J., Shear, E., Hartner, S., McGirr, G., Schulte, M., & Lovell, D. (1991). Development of a disability measurement tool for juvenile rheumatoid arthritis. *Arthritis and Rheumatism, 34,* 873–880.

Hunt, G.M. (1990). Open spina bifida: Outcome for a complete cohort treated unselectively and followed into adulthood. *Developmental Medicine and Child Neurology, 32,* 108–118.

Kudrjavcev, T., Schoenberg, B.S., Kurland, L.T., & Groover, R.V. (1985). Cerebral palsy: Survival rates, associated handicaps, and distribution by clinical subtype (Rochester, MN, 1950-1976). *Neurology, 35,* 900–903.

LaPlante, M.P. (1989). *Disability risks of chronic illness and impairments.* San Francisco: Disability Statistics Program.

Largo, R.H., Molinari, L., Weber, M., Comenale Pinto, L., & Duc, G. (1985). Early development of locomotion: Significance of prematurity, cerebral palsy and sex. *Developmental Medicine and Child Neurology, 27,* 183–191.

Liptak, G.S., Shurtleff, D.B., Bloss, J.W., Baltus-Hebert, E., & Manitta, P. (1992). Mobility aids for children with high-level myelomeningocele: Parapodium versus wheelchair. *Developmental Medicine and Child Neurology, 34,* 787–796.

Lovell, D.J., Howe, S., Shear, E., Hartner, S., McGirr, G., Schulte, M., & Levinson, J. (1989). Development of a disability measurement tool for juvenile rheumatoid arthritis: The Juvenile Arthritis Functional Assessment Scale. *Arthritis and Rheumatism, 32,* 1390–1395.

McClone, D.G., Czyzewski, D., Raimondi, A.J., & Sommers, R.C. (1982). Central nervous system infections as a limiting factor in the intelligence of children with myelomeningocele. *Pediatrics, 70,* 338–342.

McCormick, M.C., Brooks-Gunn, J., Workman-Daniels, K., & Peckham, G.J. (1993). Maternal rating of child health at school age: Does the vulnerable child syndrome persist? *Pediatrics, 92,* 380–388.

McDonald, C.M., Jaffe, K.M., Shurtleff, D.B., & Menelaus, M.B. (1991). Modifications to the traditional description of neurosegmental innervation in myelomeningocele. *Developmental Medicine and Child Neurology, 33,* 473–481.

Molnar, G. (1979). Cerebral palsy: Prognosis and how to judge it. *Pediatric Annals, 8,* 43–56.

Molnar, G.E., & Gordon, S.U. (1976). Predictive value of selected clinical signs for early prognostication of motor function. *Archives of Physical Medicine and Rehabilitation, 57,* 153–158.

Msall, M.E., DiGaudio, K.M., & Duffy, L.C. (1993). Use of functional assessment in children with developmental disabilities. In C.V. Granger & G.E. Gresham (Eds.), *Physical medicine and rehabilitation clinics of North America: New developments in functional assessment* (pp. 517–527). Philadelphia: W.B. Saunders.

Msall, M.E., DiGaudio, K., Duffy, L.C., LaForest, S., Braun, S., & Granger, C.V. (1994). WeeFIM: Normative sample of an instrument for tracking functional independence in children. *Clinical Pediatrics,* 431–438.

Natapoff, J. (1978). Children's views of health: A developmental study. *American Journal of Public Health, 68,* 995–1000.

Nelson, K.B., & Ellenberg, J.H. (1986). Antecedents of cerebral palsy. *New England Journal of Medicine, 315,* 81–86.

Orenstein, D.M., Nixon, P.A., Ross, E.A., & Kaplan, R.M. (1989). The quality of well-being in cystic fibrosis. *Chest, 95,* 344–347.

Ottenbacher, K. (1982). Sensory integration therapy: Affect or effect. *American Journal of Occupational Therapy, 36,* 571–578.

Ottenbacher, K.J., Biocca, Z., DeCremer, G., Gevelinger, M., Jedlovec, K.B., & Johnson, M.B. (1986). Quantitative analysis of the effectiveness of pediatric therapy. *Physical Therapy, 66,* 1095–1101.

Ottenbacher, K.J., & Petersen, P. (1985a). A meta-analysis of applied vestibular stimulation research. *Physical and Occupational Therapy in Pediatrics, 5*(2/3), 119–134.

Ottenbacher, K., & Petersen, P. (1985b). The efficacy of early intervention programs for children with organic impairment: A quantitative review. *Evaluation and Program Planning, 8,* 135–146.

Overeynder, J., Turk, M.A., & Janicki, M.P. (1994). *Aging and cerebral palsy— pathways to successful aging: A national action plan.* Albany, NY: State Developmental Disabilities Planning Council.

Palisano, R.J., Kolobe, T.H., Haley, S.M., Lowes, L.P., & Jones, S.L. (1995). Validity of the Peabody Developmental Gross Motor Scale as an evaluative measure of infants receiving physical therapy. *Physical Therapy, 75,* 939–948.

Rosenstein, B.D., Green, W.B., Herrington, R.T., & Blum, A.S. (1987). Bone density in myelomeningocele: The effects of ambulatory status and other factors. *Developmental Medicine and Child Neurology, 29,* 486–494.

Shurtleff, D.B. (1986). Decubitus formation and skin breakdown. In D.B. Shurtleff (Ed.), *Myelodysplasia and exstrophies: Significance, prevention, and treatment* (pp. 299–311). New York: Grune and Stratton.

Shurtleff, D.B., Hayden, P.W., Chapman, W.H., Broy, A.B., & Hill, M.L. (1975). Myelodysplasia. Problems of long-term survival and social function. *Western Journal of Medicine, 122,* 199–205.

Simeonsson, R.J., Cooper, D.H., & Scheiner, A.P. (1982). A review and analysis of the effectiveness of early intervention programs. *Pediatrics, 69,* 635–641.

Stanley, F., & Alberman, E. (Eds.). (1984). *The epidemiology of the cerebral palsies.* Philadelphia: J.B. Lippincott.

Starfield, B., Bergner, M., Ensminger, M., Riley, A., Ryan, S., Green, B., McGauhey, P., & Skinner, A. (1993). Adolescent health status measurement: Development of the child health and illness profile. *Pediatrics, 91,* 430–435.

Stein, R.E.K., & Jessop, D.J. (1990). Functional status II (R): A measure of child health status. *Medical Care, 28,* 1041–1055.

Süssová, J., Seidl, Z., & Faber, J. (1990). Hemiparetic forms of cerebral palsy in relation to epilepsy and mental retardation. *Developmental Medicine and Child Neurology, 32,* 792–795.

Timko, C., Stovel, K.W., Moos, R.H., & Miller, J.J., III. (1992). Adaptation to juvenile rheumatic disease: A controlled evaluation of functional disability with a one-year followup. *Health Psychology, 11,* 67–76.

Tosi, L.L., Slater, J.E., & Shaer, C. (1993). Latex allergy in pediatric spina bifida patients: Incidence and implications [Abstract]. *Developmental Medicine and Child Neurology, 69,* 17.

Turk, M.A., Overeynder, J.C., & Janicki, M.P. (Eds.). (1995). *Uncertain future— aging and cerebral palsy: Clinical concerns.* Albany, NY: State Developmental Disabilities Planning Council.

Turk, M.A., Weber, R.J., Geremski, C.A., & Pavin, M. (1995). Medical secondary conditions among adults with cerebral palsy (abstract). *Archives of Physical Medicine and Rehabilitation, 76,* 1055.

Vivier, P.M., Bernier, J.A., & Starfield, B. (1994). Current approaches to measuring health outcomes in pediatric research. *Current Opinion in Pediatrics, 6,* 530–537.

Watt, J.M., Robertson, C.M.T., & Grace, M.G.A. (1989). Early prognosis for ambulation of neonatal intensive care survivors with cerebral palsy. *Developmental Medicine and Child Neurology, 31,* 766–773.

Wenger, B.L., Kaye, H.S., & LaPlante, M.P. (1996). Disabilities among children. *Disability Statistics Abstract* (No. 15). Bethesda, MD: U.S. Department of Education, National Institute on Disability and Rehabilitation Research.

World Health Organization (WHO). (1993). *International classification of impairments, disabilities, and handicaps: A manual of classification relating to the consequences of disease.* Geneva, Switzerland: Author.

Young, N.L., & Wright, J.G. (1995). Measuring pediatric physical function. *Journal of Pediatric Orthopedics, 15,* 244–253.

CHAPTER 17

Aging-Related Conditions

Bryan Kemp and Laura Mosqueda

There is a dramatic increase in both the prevalence and the incidence of ongoing disabilities as people age. The percentage of people with a disability increases from 8% for people in the 18 and younger age group to more than 50% for the over-75 age group (Pope & Tarlov, 1991). Most of this increase is due to the large number of people who acquire a disability late in life. However, part of this increase is due to people who had a disability earlier in life and now are aging. This chapter touches on both populations, although the former is the primary focus. Although becoming disabled early in life is relatively rare (about 11% of people under age 30; National Center for Health Statistics, 1989), acquiring a disability late in life is practically a normative life event. More than half of the population over age 65 acquire a significant disability before death (Pope & Tarlov, 1991). Some people (Ferrini & Ferrini, 1992) believe that disability among the older population is one of the most serious public health problems and long-term care issues facing the United States today. The baby boom generation (those born between 1946 and 1964) will soon swell the ranks of people with disability and bring even more attention to the need for geriatric rehabilitation. Conditions such as stroke, hip fracture, amputations, Alzheimer's disease, vision loss, Parkinson's disease, respiratory illnesses, and heart disease will challenge the health and rehabilitation systems.

THE OLDER DISABLED POPULATION

The older adult population has a disproportionate amount of disability. Although they compose about one eighth of the U.S. population, they account for more than one third of the total disabled population. Of the approximately 35 million people in the United States with some degree of

This chapter was supported in part by Grants H133B30004 and H133B30029 from the National Institute on Disability and Rehabilitation Research.

disability, 8% are under age 18, 57% are in the 18–64 age range, and 35% are over age 65 (see Figure 1). Severity of disability also increases with age. Data from the Survey of Income and Program Participation (SIPP) (U.S. Department of Health and Human Services, 1989) indicate that 20% of people with a disability ages 18–64 need help with instrumental activities of daily living (IADL; i.e., skills needed to live in the community) and one third of them need additional help with activities of daily living (ADL; i.e., skills needed to live at home), reflecting a higher degree of disability. However, about 50% of people with a disability over age 65 need help with IADL, and half of those people need additional help with ADL (Ficke, 1992). Thus, both the prevalence of disability and its severity increase with age.

AGING WITH A DISABILITY

Those who acquired a disability early in life, including people with a history of polio, spinal cord injury, cerebral palsy, mental retardation, childhood arthritis, brain injury, low vision, schizophrenia, and other conditions, are, for the first time in history, aging into late life in large numbers. For example, it is established that people with spinal cord injury (SCI) have a life expectancy that is 85% of that of the population without disabilities (Sasma, Patrick, & Ferusser, 1993). In the 1950s, people with SCI had a life expectancy of only 5 years postinjury. People with these and other impairments are not aging typically, however. As they age, the majority of them appear to be experiencing new and unexpected medical and functional problems that impair their health, threaten their independence, stress their support systems, and challenge them psychologically. Individuals with polio, for example, have an 80%–90% probability of developing secondary conditions in middle or late life (Halstead, 1991). People experiencing changes as they age with a disability are estimated to range from 3 to 5

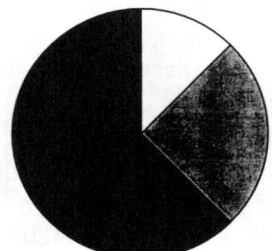
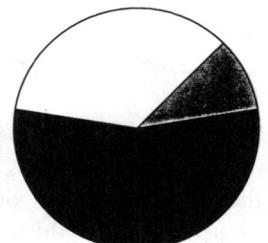

Age Distribution of U.S. Population   Age Distribution of U.S. Population
                                                       with a Disability

Figure 1. Percentages of total U.S. population by age and percentage with disability. (□ < 18 years, ■ = 18-64 years, ■ > 65 years.) (Adapted from Pope and Tarlov (1991).)

million people (Campbell, Kemp, & Brummel-Smith, 1994). For both groups, older adults and those aging with disability, the short-term and long-term benefits of rehabilitation are important if independence and quality of life are to be maintained. This chapter discusses the nature of disability in both groups, the unique problems each face, the outcomes of rehabilitation, and the needed research to further improve understanding of these outcomes.

REHABILITATION TERMS

The disablement process was conceptualized by the World Health Organization in its *International Classification of Impairments, Disabilities and Handicaps* (1980) as a process ranging from the cellular to the social levels. In this scheme, several terms are essential and are commonly used. Earlier chapters in this book review these terms (see Chapter 2); this chapter provides only a brief overview to aid further sections.

Pathology refers to dysfunction at the cellular level. It can be due to a variety of causes, including injury, genetic defects, toxins, viral infections, or other mechanisms. A particular pathology can be temporary (a fracture) or permanent (a stroke). *Impairment* refers to dysfunction at the organ-system level; it reflects the organ's inability to carry out its principal functions. Thus, muscle impairment (organ) manifests as weakness (function). Not all pathologic changes produce significant impairment. The brain can (and normally does) lose millions of cells before thinking is impaired. Osteoporosis exists long before it causes an impairment. This is because these organ systems have a high degree of reserve capacity. A dysfunction at the level of task performance (a series of sequenced and planned actions) is termed a *disability*. A person may have a locomotion disability, a learning disability, or a work disability. Just as not all pathology causes impairment, not all impairment causes disability. Hypertension rarely causes disability, for instance. Also, disabilities are not absolute limitations. Viewed in relative terms, a disability occurs because the person's capabilities are out of balance with the demands of the task. A disability can be improved by changing the environment as well as changing the person. A *handicap* is a dysfunction at the level of social integration. People are handicapped to the extent that society does not make accommodations for them through social acceptance, environmental accessibility, job opportunities, recreational involvement, and so forth. A person with a disability is more often handicapped by the attitudes and practices of others rather than by his or her own disabilities.

Using this typology, the goals and objectives of rehabilitation can be defined either broadly or narrowly. When defined broadly, the goals of rehabilitation are to reduce impairment, improve functioning, promote personal independence, reduce handicap, promote self-determination, and increase life satisfaction for people with disabilities. When defined narrowly, rehabilitation's goal is to improve functioning of specific abilities, such as walking. The particular philosophy adopted by an organization determines the kinds of outcomes measured and the most likely way to measure them. How well rehabilitation can achieve any of these goals will determine its importance as health care funding becomes even more competitive.

A SEQUENTIAL-STAGE THEORY OF GERIATRIC REHABILITATION

To effectively measure rehabilitation outcomes, it is important to understand the rehabilitation process, that is, the necessary ingredients in rehabilitation. Only after determining these necessary ingredients is it possible to understand how outcomes are achieved, influenced, and therefore measured. Additionally, a theory of rehabilitation process and outcomes can help guide selection of measurement variables as well as define how they relate to each other. Geriatric rehabilitation (if not all rehabilitation) can be thought of as a multistage process (Kemp, Brummel-Smith, & Ramsdell, 1990). To some degree, rehabilitation progresses sequentially through these stages. These stages are as follows:

1. Stabilization of the underlying impairments and pathology
2. Prevention and treatment of secondary impairments
3. Evaluation and correction of any psychological factors affecting rehabilitation
4. Evaluation of functional deficits and provision of function-improving therapies
5. Modification of the home and community environments
6. Education and support of significant others
7. Societal integration and long-term care

The tenets of this theory are as follows. First, the stages of rehabilitation can be arranged somewhat sequentially because some outcomes must be achieved before others can be addressed. For example, a patient who is not medically stable cannot participate in rehabilitation, and a patient who is severely depressed cannot gain significantly in rehabilitation therapy. Second, several stages of rehabilitation may be addressed at the same time, even if one takes precedence over the other. Third, when rehabilitation is successful in the broad sense, it is because all stages have been accomplished. Fourth, success and failure in rehabilitation can occur for a variety of reasons, but it is proposed here that inability to solve problems in the first three stages keeps people from participating in rehabilitation in the first place, whereas the adequate provision of services in the last four stages accounts for success. Fifth, any given stage of the rehabilitation process is strongly influenced by adjacent stages; therefore, it cannot be properly treated and outcomes cannot be properly measured without some knowledge of those adjacent stages. Thus, to understand how well a person ultimately does in improving functional abilities, the home environment in which those skills will be practiced has to be looked at as well as the person's psychological motivation and learning ability to practice those skills. Sixth, the mechanisms that determine success vary from stage to stage but are believed to relate to both the proficiency of the practitioners who are responsible for that stage as well as characteristics of the patient. Seventh, progress between stages requires communication, coordination, and involvement of the team, patient, and significant others. This model is described in Figure 2.

This model has important implications for the measurement of rehabilitation outcomes. For narrowly focused models of rehabilitation, outcomes at the disability level, such as ADL and IADL, would be suitable. For more broadly conceived programs, measures at each of the different stages would be appropriate. The best measure at each stage would be an outcome reflecting that stage's goals. A program that chooses to focus only on improvement of functional disabilities should not be evaluated by how well it prevents secondary complications or promotes social integration. However, a national or state program of rehabilitation should probably be evaluated by how well it meets all those goals.

HOW AGING AFFECTS REHABILITATION

When the aging process is added to this model, the rehabilitation process is complicated in many ways because older individuals have several unique problems or characteristics, including: 1) typically having multiple, coexisting impairments; 2) being highly susceptible to secondary conditions (e.g., deconditioning, incontinence, pressure sores, infection); 3) having a higher rate of coexisting psychological problems, especially depression; 4) progressing more slowly in therapy because of age differences and medical limitations; 5) having a support system that often lacks in resources; 6) having less familiarity with technology that could be useful at home; and 7) lacking meaningful roles and social acceptance as an older person with a disability in the community. Individuals who are aging with a disability also have unique problems, including 1) a relatively rapid decline in functioning and health after a long period of stability, 2) the onset of new medical problems of unknown etiology, 3) a need to renegotiate or enlist support from others, 4) a lack of understanding of their problems by professionals, and 5) few services available to help them. This chapter now briefly describes the most common kinds of impairments affecting older and aging people with disability.

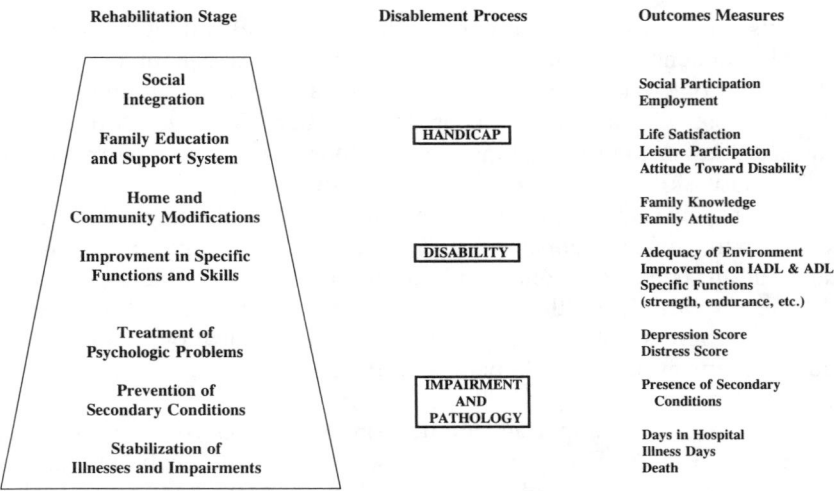

Rehabilitation Stage	Disablement Process	Outcomes Measures

Figure 2. A multistage theory of rehabilitation processes and outcomes.

Impairments Causing Disability in Older People and Those Aging with Disability

It is important to distinguish purely health problems from disability problems in late life. Hypertension, minor arthritis, osteoporosis, heart disease, bronchitis, intestinal disorders, and sensory problems, for instance, are responsible for the majority of doctor visits, prescriptions, and hospitalizations but do not account for much disability (Ferrini & Ferrini, 1993). Stroke, hip fractures, heart failure, Alzheimer's disease, amputations, severe osteoporosis and arthritis, pulmonary diseases, Parkinson's disease, severe diabetes, and heart diseases are the most common impairments causing disability in late life. Once a disability occurs, it puts the older person at great risk of loss of independence and even institutionalization. When an older person cannot sufficiently perform critical ADL, his or her chances of entering a skilled nursing facility within the next year increase dramatically (Manton, 1989). This may be because about 30% of older people with a disability live alone and about 30% live below the poverty line (Ferrini & Ferrini, 1993). There is also a 50% chance that the spouse's health is impaired or shortly will be. Furthermore, patterns of referral show that primary care physicians do not frequently refer older people to rehabilitation services, often out of negative expectations or lack of knowledge (American Medical Association, 1990).

Stroke There are more than 500,000 new cases of stroke each year, and the incidence of stroke increases with age. The majority of strokes are related to hypertension, atherosclerosis, and diabetes. African Americans have a higher rate, and Mexican Americans have a lower rate, than the Caucasian population. Using the model of rehabilitation previously described, stabilization of this illness requires medically managing risk factors by reducing blood pressure, changing diet, losing weight, eliminating smoking, and reducing stress. Common preventable or treatable secondary conditions in people with stroke include contractures, incontinence, shoulder pain, pressure sores, and urinary infections. Functionally, stroke typically produces hemiplegia, sensory loss, cognitive impairment, language disturbance (aphasia), and perceptual dysfunction (e.g., neglect). Consequently, the person has great difficulty with most ADL and IADL tasks. Mobility, transfers, bathing, dressing, and toileting are especially affected. Depression is the most common psychological reaction and may approach an incidence of 50% among stroke survivors (Robinson, Starr, & Price, 1984). Caregiving and support by the family are paramount to being able to function at home and remain in the community. The spouse, however, is also usually older, and other family members, usually the daughters or daughters-in-law, must assist, which creates stresses on them as well. As many as 70% of caregivers experience excess stress. Rehabilitation following stroke occurs in a variety of settings, including a rehabilitation center, a rehabilitation section of a general hospital, a skilled nursing facility, or at home.

Hip Fracture   There are more than 250,000 new hip fractures in the United States every year, with the vast majority occurring to older people (Kane, Ouslander, & Abrass, 1993). Fractures of the hip, femoral neck, and femur are major causes of disability. Frequently, the older person has other major illnesses coexisting that may even have played a role in the fracture, such as osteoporosis, poor vision, or Parkinson's disease. Unless well managed, 30%–40% of older people with hip fracture will either be in a nursing facility or die within 1 year from secondary complications (Kane et al., 1993). Hip fractures are treated surgically; the type of surgery and the nature of any prosthesis depend on the site of the fracture. Subcapital fractures disrupt blood supply to the femoral head and have a higher rate of necrosis of the femoral head. A prosthesis is often installed. Intertrochanteric and subtrochanteric require fixation by pinning and side plates. The most common secondary complications are coexisting medical conditions (e.g., heart failure, anemia, infection) and deconditioning secondary to dysmobility. Rehabilitation programs stress mobility as soon as medically tolerated, to increase conditioning and range of motion. The most common psychological complications are anxiety, especially the fear of falling ("fallaphobia"), and depression. People who have fallen, been injured, and been left unassisted on the ground for even an hour can develop excess fear that inhibits their functioning later. Many people receive rehabilitation in a skilled nursing facility after surgery, particularly since the advent of the prospective payment system. If rehabilitation is provided, most older people do well after a hip fracture.

Heart Disease Diseases of the heart, including coronary artery disease, arrhythmias, and congestive heart failure, are not typically primary causes of disability unless they are severe. They are, however, the leading causes of death in people over age 65, and they add to the level of disability in people with other chronic illnesses, such as stroke. Patients with severe heart disease benefit from a rehabilitation program that reestablishes functional independence and restores confidence. A graduated walking program, diet control, and managing other risk factors such as smoking are important. Most cardiac rehabilitation can be accomplished in an outpatient setting or at home after acute care is provided in the hospital. Fear and anxiety are often as disabling as the cardiac condition and must be addressed as part of rehabilitation. A return to normal or near-normal avocational, leisure, sexual, and family activities are important goals. (For more detailed discussion of cardiac rehabilitation, see Chapter 15 of this book.)

Arthritis Arthritic conditions affect millions of people over the age of 65. It is the most frequent impairment in people over age 70, even more common than hypertension (Kane et al., 1993). The most common forms of arthritis are osteoarthritis and rheumatoid arthritis. When severe, arthritic conditions can cause major disability because of pain, limited joint mobility, and limb deformation. Surgical correction of limb deformity or joint replacements is common. Rehabilitation may be required for people with disabling arthritis. Rehabilitation focuses on pain relief, joint protection, alternative ways of accomplishing ADL, and preventing other injuries. Home modification and the use of simple assistive devices (e.g., jar opener, rocker knife) are especially important in arthritis rehabilitation. Except for those people needing surgical correction, most rehabilitation for arthritis is done on an outpatient basis. Depression is quite common in arthritis, especially in women, when associated with loss of valued home activities and with exacerbations (flare-ups) associated with the illness or triggered by psychosocial stress.

Alzheimer's Disease Because it is a progressive, ultimately fatal disease, most people do not think of Alzheimer's disease (AD) as suitable for a rehabilitation model. However, such a model does work quite well for people with AD. Preventing secondary complications (e.g., delirium, incontinence, injury), promoting function, supporting the family, and addressing psychiatric complications (e.g., hallucinations, agitation) are reasonable and achievable goals. The principal effect of AD (loss of new memory and learning) is the greatest disadvantage for rehabilitation purposes. However, people with AD can use long-term memory for a long time after onset and, with the assistance of others, remain at home and engage in leisure, family, and social activities. The growing number of people with AD (4 million in 1996 but projected to grow to 14 million by 2030) and the tremendous cost to society of AD (estimated at $30 billion–$50 billion annually) make it imperative that better care be provided for these people.

Parkinson's Disease   Parkinson's disease results from progressive degeneration of the basal ganglia. This disease's prevalence is about 16 per 100,000 people, with the rate increasing from the fifth to the eighth decade (Shults, 1990). Parkinson's disease (PD) typically produces motor dysfunction, autonomic pathology, and, in many cases, cognitive impairment. The pathologic elements are the presence of Lewy bodies, a concentric hyaline ectoplasmic inclusion, in multiple neuronal centers and the loss of cells in the substantia nigra. The functional losses resulting from PD include loss of motor control (e.g., tremor, bradykinesia, rigidity), characteristic cognitive change (i.e., impaired recall, difficulty organizing thoughts and memory, slowness), and autonomic dysregulation (e.g., drooling, blurred vision, skin changes). The most common secondary risks are falling and injury. Functionally, the most common disabilities are impaired mobility, difficulties in managing money (secondary to cognitive change), and work performance if tremor or slowness interferes. Eventually, other IADL and ADL become affected as the disease worsens. Depression is the most common psychological disorder of PD. Primary treatment of PD is aimed at trying to restore the dopamine deficiency by drugs such as levadopa. Rehabilitation is usually done on an outpatient basis or at home. Modifications of the home, the use of assistive devices (e.g., weighted eating utensils), and family education have been shown to be effective (Beattie & Caind, 1980).

Aging Changes in People with a Disability

Although most geriatric rehabilitation is still concerned with people who sustain a disability late in life, a new group requiring further rehabilitation attention cannot be overlooked. People who sustained a disability in early life are now becoming older in significant numbers, and it is expected that this trend will increase. This has occurred because of improved medical care and the prevention of secondary complications, resulting in increases in life expectancy.

As they age, people with SCI, polio, cerebral palsy, rheumatoid arthritis, Down syndrome, and other conditions are experiencing new and unexpected changes in their health and functioning, often at alarming rates. People with SCI, for example, have been shown to have high rates of atherosclerotic cardiovascular changes, insulin-resistant diabetes, osteoporosis, shoulder pain, bowel and bladder changes, fatigue, weakness, needs for assistance, and job loss (e.g., Gerhart, Bergstrom, Charlifue, Menter, & Whiteneck, 1993). People with polio have been experiencing fatigue, pain, weakness, and loss of function (postpolio syndrome). People with cerebral palsy are having trouble with ambulation, joint dislocations, and arthritic changes. People with Down syndrome are developing Alzheimer's-type dementia. All of these people are facing major support problems as their conditions change and deteriorate. Many have been out of contact with rehabilitation programs for years and have few professional supports in the community. It is clear that the previous notion that these conditions represent stable, unchanging impairments is obsolete. Rehabilitation programs now face the task of adapting a life-span perspective in their programs instead of focusing only on outcomes that can be achieved within months.

Research has begun to investigate the causes of these changes. At least four possible factors may be involved:

1. *Undetected medical illnesses.* The high rate of early onset atherosclerotic heart changes among people aging with SCI fits in this category.
2. *Overuse or misuse of the body.* The use of the arms to propel a wheelchair for decades eventuates in shoulder pain for many people.
3. *The era in which the person became disabled and matured.* Many of the changes people are experiencing may reflect the treatment they received during their rehabilitation. Such treatments have changed and improved. Harrington rod surgery to stabilize the spine is no longer used, but people who did receive it often develop complications in later life that will probably not occur in future patients.
4. *Normal aging.* Both by itself and in combination with these other factors, the normal aging process affects people with disabilities.

Any problem a person experiences in later life after an impairment earlier in life can be due to any one or more of these factors. These long-term outcomes are just as important to understand as the more immediate outcomes of rehabilitation. The growing recognition of these late-life changes may even require an alteration in rehabilitation practices.

REHABILITATION OUTCOMES FOR OLDER PEOPLE

There is considerable literature regarding the outcomes of rehabilitation for older people who acquire disability. In selecting representative studies, only those that controlled for natural recovery; those that specified the nature of the intervention provided; and those with sound methodologic controls, preferably with matched control designs (e.g., control over subject assignment to different treatment groups), were included. It seems reasonable to divide outcomes studies into the kind of outcomes achieved within the rehabilitation definitions of *impairment, disability,* and *handicap,* because different studies have had clearly different goals.

Impairments, Primary and Secondary

Rubenstein and Ouslander (1987) conducted a randomized control study of specialized geriatric assessment of older individuals to determine if assessment of their problems by trained geriatricians would result in a greater number of health impairments being found as compared with assessments by nongeriatricians. At issue here was the point that medical problems can be treated only if they are detected, and many problems are often overlooked in older patients by physicians who are not geriatrically trained. If an impairment is not identified, it most certainly can interfere with rehabilitation. Older patients in a veterans' hospital were randomly assigned to an assessment, through either internal medicine or family medicine, or they were assigned to a geriatric evaluation unit, where they were seen by a geriatrician and other specialists. All of the participants also had some degree of functional limitation. In the group seen by the geriatric evaluation unit, an average of 4 new problems were identified per patient, as opposed to 1.5 problems in the control group. Because undetected medical problems among geriatric patients are a major contributor to their functional problems, this study is of great importance.

Several other studies of geriatric evaluation programs have been conducted, all leading to the same general finding. Rubenstein et al. (1984) randomly assigned geriatric patients with a high probability of nursing facility placement to either a geriatric unit or a regular acute care ward. Each group had an average of 4.5 medical problems. Only one third of each group could walk one block, climb stairs, or function independently at home. The average length of stay was 43 days. Treatment focused primarily on improving their health, reducing impairment, and recommending interventions to improve functioning. At follow-up, the experimental group had lower morbidity (23% versus 48%), fewer hospitalizations, and was less likely to have spent time in a nursing facility. Dumas, Brahan, and Haywood (1993) assessed the effect of geriatric assessment on 120 inpatients over the age of 70. All received comprehensive medical, functional, and psychosocial assessment and recommendations but no rehabilitation therapy. At 6-month follow-up, 21% of the control subjects had died, as opposed to 6% of the geriatric assessment patients. At 1-year follow-up, the control group had significantly more rehospitalizations and twice the death rate but showed no differences on ADL throughout the study. Rubenstein (1994) summarized the results of studies on geriatric evaluation units and concluded that these programs are effective in discovering and treating previously unknown problems, but that, in and of themselves, they are not sufficient to lead to functional improvement.

Improvement or prevention of secondary impairments is also espe-cially important in geriatrics because of their high frequency, their tendency to interfere with rehabilitation, and their high treatability. Secondary im-pairments such as deconditioning, contractures, incontinence, confusion, and dehydration are quite common in older patients. Brummel-Smith (1985) described the unique characteristics of older people that favor the development of these secondary problems and the approach to care that is needed. Deconditioning, the physical consequences of underactivity that result in impaired endurance, strength, and coordination, is quite common in older people. Moreover, older people are faster to become deconditioned with bed rest or underactivity, and they are slower to recover. Decondi-tioning can then lead to complications such as falls, fractures, pulmonary infections, emboli, and depression. If the older person already has a disa-bility, the problem is exacerbated because he or she is probably less active than an older person without disability. Morey et al. (1991) provided ex-ercise programs to older individuals on an outpatient basis to improve conditioning. They found that specific exercise had a beneficial effect last-ing up to 2 years and that advanced age or ongoing health condition did not necessarily interfere. Many studies have shown the beneficial effects of exercise in older people without disabilities (e.g., DeVries, 1979).

These results suggest that programs that specifically target impair-ments for intervention can produce improvements over nonspecialized pro-grams. However, improvements in impairment do not necessarily mean that gains in functional performance will occur. A study by Silliman, Mc-Garvey, Raymond, and Fretwell (1990) supported this caveat. They ran-domly assigned older individuals (mean age, 75) who were acutely hospitalized ($n = 142$) to a comprehensive geriatric assessment program or to a regular admission. Under the comprehensive assessment, patients were seen by a nurse coordinator, physical therapist, social worker, dieti-tian, pharmacist, and geriatrician. Their recommendations were then given to the primary care physician, but treatment was not provided by the ger-iatric team. Follow-up telephone calls postdischarge were made weekly to the participants. The intervention did not have any effect on functioning in terms of ADL or IADL. However, the intervention did produce better coping in caregivers and better self-reported health. Care in the hospital also was improved for the patients. Thus, improvements in the patient's functional capacities probably require direct intervention at that level.

Functional Improvement and Reduction in Disability

Not all of the evidence concerning improvements in functional capacity and disability within the geriatric arena is in a rehabilitation context. Many studies, both of specific functional skills (e.g., strength) and of more gen-eral abilities such as ADL or IADL, are carried out by geriatricians and gerontologists who do not necessarily identify themselves with rehabilitation. Their interest in functional outcomes stems from the concern that geriatricians have because older individuals have such high rates of ongoing conditions.

One fact that is clear from both function-specific studies and more general outcomes studies is that age is no deterrent to ultimate improvement, although older people typically require more time to achieve the same goal (Banes & Dunovan, 1987). DeVries (1979) found no differences in improvement from exercise in community-dwelling older people, regardless of their age. He included people 55–88 years of age who were not acutely ill. A 1991 study showed that residents of a nursing facility could improve muscular strength by weight training up to age 90 and that this led to improved activity (Fisher, Pendergast, & Calkins, 1991). Kemp (1985) reviewed existing geriatric rehabilitation outcomes studies and found that there was little evidence that age makes a difference in achieving success in rehabilitation.

Numerous studies have shown the beneficial effects of rehabilitation for older individuals. So many studies have shown the clear benefits of rehabilitation for older people that it can hardly be considered an experimental question any more. Instead, research is faced with detailing the specific mechanisms of improvement in older people. Many studies have used a matched control group design (Applegate et al., 1990; Garroway, Alchtar, Prescott, & Hockey, 1980; Kennie, Reid, Richardson, Kiamari, & Kelt, 1988; Sivenius, Pyorala, Heinonen, Salonen, & Rickkinen, 1985; Smith et al., 1981) or other rigorous designs (Lehmann et al., 1975a, 1975b). Sivenius et al., (1985) compared the effect of different intensities of rehabilitation in 95 individuals with stroke. Individuals in the control group received normal physical therapy in a conventional medical ward. The intensive therapy consisted of admission to a rehabilitation unit with the goal of rehabilitation. Therapy on the rehabilitation unit continued as long as functional improvement could be attained or until the person became independent. Both groups remained in the hospital for the same length of time. The intensive group received 10 more rehabilitation days of treatment during the first 3 months. In the analysis of outcomes, the intensive treatment group was 28% better on ADL scores at follow-up and also had significantly better motor scores. The differences in ADL persisted at 6 months but fell slightly short of significance.

Lehmann et al. (1975a) also studied functional improvements in older people with stroke. To control for spontaneous recovery, patients were accepted an average of 10 months postonset. They had been treated at other acute hospitals but had shown little functional gain. Comprehensive rehabilitation, including physical therapy, occupational therapy, speech therapy, psychology, social work, and recreation therapy, was provided. There was no separate control group. Significant improvements in several ADL measures were achieved during rehabilitation, and these were retained at follow-up 24 months later. Because most spontaneous recovery occurs within 6 months of a stroke's onset, it is hard to argue that the rehabilitation was not the responsible agent of change. That the gains persisted so long is encouraging. Of the population, 25% were living in a nursing facility at follow-up. This did not increase from the time of discharge and is a positive indication of long-term success. The presence of severe medical illness was the main factor predicting nonsuccess. Family involvement was another key factor in determining final disposition. Patients with more family involvement were more likely to return home after discharge. In a large-scale study, Hamilton and Granger (1994) assessed more than 27,000 rehabilitation cases of stroke using the Functional Independence Measure (FIM) (State University of New York at Buffalo, 1993). The mean age was 71, and patients had an average of 28 days of rehabilitation. Seventy-four percent were discharged to their homes, and the majority improved in rehabilitation. The largest gains were in memory, problem solving, and mobility.

Not all interventions designed to improve functioning are successful. Mulrow et al. (1994) conducted a randomized control trial with 194 elderly residents of nursing facilities to determine if regular physical therapy was better for mobility than "friendly visiting." Therapy was not much more effective compared with the control condition, even though there were fewer subsequent falls in the treatment group (suggesting better strength) and patients were less likely to use a wheelchair at the conclusion of treatment. It must be pointed out, however, that these participants had severe disabilities and had several medical comorbidities that were not addressed in the study. This finding does lend support to the proposed model of rehabilitation presented earlier in that medical conditions were not treated and could have interfered with therapy gains.

Kennie et al. (1988) examined the effects of having a geriatrician as part of the rehabilitation team for older individuals with hip fractures. Using a randomized assignment procedure, the control group remained in the orthopedic ward and the experimental group was moved to an equivalent nearby hospital. The average age was 82. Both groups received physical therapy and other services. The primary difference in treatment, therefore, was the presence of a geriatric specialist working in collaboration with the rehabilitation team. The experimental group produced significantly more independent people, a shorter stay, and more discharges to independent living. These results are similar to Rubenstein et al. (1984), who found not only improved health and less impairment among geriatric patients treated on a specialized geriatric assessment unit but also improved functional outcomes for those receiving rehabilitation services. Thus, the added expertise of a geriatrician seemingly helped these older adult patients significantly. Possible reasons for this are better detection of medical complications, better guidance of rehabilitation therapy, maintaining more of a functional perspective, and patient education. Smith et al. (1981) also demonstrated the benefits of outpatient rehabilitation compared with a control group for older individuals with less severe disabilities. Three levels of therapy intensity were used: 1) 4 days a week, 2) 3 half-days a week, and 3) no routine rehabilitation (home health visiting and encouraging the patient to exercise at home). At follow-up, there were significant differences between all three groups with the degree of benefit being proportional to the intensity of the treatment.

It seems conclusive that improvement of older individuals in rehabilitation is not only possible but commonly achieved. The keys to such improvements appear to be careful assessment of the older person, the provision of rehabilitation services, and the possible addition of a geriatric specialist for the oldest of patients. In addition, several studies suggest that family support is especially important to the success of older people (see Becker & Kaufman, 1988). Providing emotional support to families is important because they play a large role in supporting their elders (D'Afflite & Wertz, 1977). Research shows that the family also plays a large role in maintaining rehabilitation goals after discharge (Garroway, Alchtar, Hockey, & Prescott, 1980).

As changes in health care financing and delivery occur, epitomized by the move toward managed care and prospective payment, there is concern whether older people will get the rehabilitation they need, especially because it seems they may need even longer rehabilitation care than younger persons. Fitzgerald, Moore, and Pittus (1988) compared differences in the quality of care and in the outcomes of rehabilitation in elderly people with hip fracture before and after the implementation of the prospective payment system (PPS). A total of 338 people was compared, about half before and half after the advent of PPS. Those treated post-PPS had shorter acute hospitalizations (22 versus 13 days) and fewer physical therapy sessions (7.6 versus 6.3). Of the pre-PPS group, 46% could ambulate at discharge as opposed to 40% for the post-PPS group. At 1-year follow-up, 9% of the pre-PPS group were residing in a nursing facility, as opposed to 33% for the post-PPS group. These results strongly suggest that the method of payment can have a major effect on outcomes.

Improvements in Handicap

Few studies have attempted to directly measure improvements in handicap among older people with a disability. This may be because handicap is so difficult to measure. Because handicap is a dysfunction at the level of societal integration, it involves the individual's disability, attitudes, socioeconomic status, and degree of social involvement as well as the community's resources and accessibility. The following studies have measured the impact of programs on some of these aspects of handicap.

Evans, Werkhoven, and Fox (1982) provided group telephone psychotherapy to elderly, isolated individuals who had been blind for several years. Eight 1-hour sessions were provided. Before treatment, these individuals engaged in virtually no outside social activities. After treatment, loneliness scores and household activities improved, as did social activities for the experimental group, although short of significance. These results were supported by Amaral and Ringering (1988). In another study involving individuals with poor vision, volunteers assisted older individuals to become better integrated into senior citizen centers by accompanying them to the centers, working with center staff to help integrate the person with poor vision into the activities of the center, and staying with the person with visual impairment for several days during a transition period. Only by performing these extra services was the older person able to become integrated into the center (Michaelson, 1990).

CONCLUSIONS

Rehabilitation can be effective in improving the functioning and independence of older people with ongoing disabilities. Support for this conclusion comes from both the rehabilitation literature and the geriatrics literature. Although both fields have much in common, they are not well integrated. The fact that older people can improve in rehabilitation to such a high degree runs counter to what is often believed about older people. This fact, together with the growing number of older people, further highlights that geriatrics will probably occupy a larger role in rehabilitation, certainly as the percentage of older people increases with its high rates of disabling conditions. This chapter outlined a multistage theory of geriatric rehabilitation in which successful outcomes at the successive levels of impairment, disability, and handicap require different processes to be addressed. A new problem emerging in rehabilitation is the number of people who acquired a disability early in life and are now aging. These people are experiencing new and problematic medical, functional, and support changes that require additional research and care.

The following listing contains some areas needing more research attention:

- Evaluation of a multistage model of rehabilitation as presented in this chapter
- Improved understanding of the specific mechanisms of rehabilitation treatments that make them effective with older people
- Cost-effectiveness studies on providing geriatric rehabilitation
- Studies on gaining access to rehabilitation services for older people

- Additional studies on reducing handicap in older people with a disability
- How to better intervene with people aging with a disability to preserve their health and functioning
- The impact of managed care on rehabilitation

REFERENCES

Amaral, P., & Ringering, L. (1988). Enhancing low vision rehabilitation through peer telephone counseling. *Journal of Vision Rehabilitation, 2,* 61–68.

American Medical Association. (1990). White paper on elderly health. *Archives of Internal Medicine, 150,* 2359–2471.

Applegate, W.B., Miller, S.T., Graney, M.S., Elan, J.T., Burns, R., & Akins, D.E. (1990). A randomized, controlled trial of a geriatric assessment unit in a community rehabilitation hospital. *New England Journal of Medicine, 32,* 1571–1575.

Banes, B., & Dunovan, K. (1987). Functional outcomes after hip fracture. *Physical Therapy, 67,* 1675–1679.

Beattie, A., & Caind, F.I. (1980). The occupational therapist and the patient with Parkinson's disease. *British Medical Journal, 280,* 1354–1357.

Becker, G., & Kaufman, S. (1988). Old age, rehabilitation and research: A review of the issues. *Gerontologist, 28,* 459–468.

Berman, A., & Blass, G. (Eds.). (1985). *Principles of geriatric medicine and gerontology.* New York: McGraw-Hill.

Brummel-Smith, K. (1985). Rehabilitation of the geriatric patient. In W.R. Hazard, R. Andres, E.L. Bierman, & J.P. Blass (Eds.), *Principles of geriatric medicine and gerontology* (2nd ed., pp. 319–330). New York: McGraw-Hill Information Services Co.

Campbell, M., Kemp, B.J., & Brummel-Smith, K. (1994). *Later life effects of early life disability: Comparisons of age-matched controls on indicators of physical, psychological and social status.* Downey, CA: Rehabilitation Research and Training Center on Aging and Disability, Rancho Los Amigos Medical Center.

D'Afflite, J., & Wertz, G.W. (1977). Rehabilitating the stroke patient through patient-family groups. *International Journal of Group Psychotherapy, 24,* 323–332.

DeVries, H.A. (1979). Physiological effects of an exercise training regimen upon men aged 52 to 88. *Journal of Gerontology, 25,* 335–341.

Dumas, D.R., Brahan, R., & Haywood, B.P. (1993). Inpatient community-based geriatric assessment reduces subsequent mortality. *Journal of the American Geriatric Society, 41,* 101–104.

Evans, R.L., Werkhoven, W., & Fox, H.R. (1982). Treatment of social isolation and loneliness in a sample of visually impaired elderly persons. *Psychological Reports, 51,* 103–108.

Ferrini, A.F., & Ferrini, R.L. (1993). *Health in the later years* (2nd ed.). Dubuque, IA: Brown and Benchmark.

Ficke, R. (1992). *Digest of data on persons with disabilities.* Washington, DC: National Institute on Disability and Rehabilitation Research.

Fisher, N.M., Pendergast, D.R., & Calkins, E. (1991). Muscle rehabilitation in impaired elderly nursing home residents. *Archives of Physical Medicine and Rehabilitation, 72,* 181–185.

Fitzgerald, J.F., Moore, P.S., & Pittus, R.S. (1988). The care of elderly patients with hip fractures: Changes since implementation of the prospective payment system. *New England Journal of Medicine, 319,* 1392–1397.

Garroway, W.M., Alchtar, A.J., Hockey, L., & Prescott, R.J. (1980). Management of acute stroke in the elderly: Follow-up of a controlled trial. *British Medical Journal, 281,* 827–829.

Garroway, W.M., Alchtar, A.J., Prescott, R.J., & Hockey, L. (1980). Management of acute stroke in the elderly: Preliminary results of a controlled trial. *British Medical Journal, 281,* 1040–1044.

Gerhart, K.A., Bergstrom, E., Charlifue, S.W., Menter, R.R., & Whiteneck, G.G. (1993). Long term spinal cord injury: Functional changes over time. *Archives of Physical Medicine and Rehabilitation, 74,* 1030–1034.

Halstead, L. (1991). Assessment and differential diagnosis for post-polio syndrome. *Orthopaedics, 14,* 1209–1217.

Hamilton, B.B., & Granger, C.V. (1994). Disability outcomes following inpatient rehabilitation for stroke. *Physical Therapy, 74,* 494–503.

Kane, R.L., Ouslander, G., & Abrass, I.B. (1993). *Essentials of clinical geriatrics* (3rd ed.). New York: McGraw-Hill.

Kemp, W. (1985). Rehabilitation and the older adult. In J.E. Birren & K.W. Schaie (Eds.), *Handbook of the psychology of aging* (2nd ed., pp. 619–627). New York: Van Nostrand Reinhold.

Kemp, B., Brummel-Smith, K., & Ramsdell, J.W. (1990). *Geriatric rehabilitation.* Austin, TX: PRO-ED.

Kennie, D.C., Reid, J., Richardson, I.R., Kiamari, A., & Kelt, C. (1988). Effectiveness of geriatric rehabilitative care after fracture of the proximal femur in elderly women: A randomized clinical trial. *British Medical Journal, 267,* 1083–1086.

Lehmann, J.F., DeLateur, B.J., Fowler, R.S., Warren, C.G., Arnhold, R., Schertzer, G., Hurka, R., Whitmore, S.S., Masock, A.J., & Chambers, K.H. (1975a). Stroke: Does rehabilitation affect outcome? *Archives of Physical Medicine and Rehabilitation, 56,* 375–382.

Lehmann, J.F., DeLateur, B.J., Fowler, R.S., Warren, C.G., Arnhold, R., Schertzer, G., Hurka, R., Whitmore, S.S., Masock, A.J., & Chambers, K.H. (1975b). Stroke rehabilitation outcome and prediction. *Archives of Physical Medicine and Rehabilitation, 56,* 383–389.

Manton, K.G. (1989). Epidemiological, demographic, and social correlates of disability among the elderly. *Milbank Memorial Fund Quarterly, 67* (Suppl. 2, Pt.1), 13–58.

Michaelson, S. (1990). *Integrating visually impaired older people into senior centers.* New York: The Lighthouse.

Morey, M.C., Cowper, P.A., Feussner, J.R., Di Pasquale, Z.C., Crowley, G.M., & Sullivan, R.J. (1991). Two-year trends in physical performance following supervised exercise among community-dwelling older veterans. *Journal of the American Geriatric Society, 39,* 549–554.

Mulrow, C.D., Gerety, M.D., Kanten, D., Cornell, J.E., DeNino, L.A., Chiodo, L., Aguilar, C., O'Neil, M.S., Rosenberg, J., & Solis, R.M. (1994). A randomized trial of physical rehabilitation for very frail nursing home residents. *Journal of the American Medical Association, 271,* 519–524.

National Center for Health Statistics. (1989). *Current estimates from the National Health Interview Survey, 1988.* Vital and Health Statistics, Series 10, No. 1972. Washington, DC: U.S. Government Printing Office. (DHHS Publication No. (PHS) 89-150)

Pope, A.M., & Tarlov, A.R. (Eds.). (1991). *Disability in America: Toward a national agenda for prevention.* Washington, DC: National Academy Press.

Robinson, R.G., Starr, L.B., & Price, T.R. (1984). A ten-year longitudinal study of mood disorder following stroke: Prevalence and duration at six months follow-up. *British Journal of Psychiatry, 144,* 256–262.

Rubenstein, L.Z. (1994). *Geriatric assessment units: A review.* Paper presented at the American Geriatric Society meeting, Los Angeles, CA.

Rubenstein, L.Z., Josephson, K.R., Wieland, G.D., English, P.A., Sayre, J., & Kane, R.L. (1984). Effectiveness of a geriatric evaluation unit; A randomized clinical trial. *New England Journal of Medicine, 311,* 1664–1670.

Rubenstein, L.Z., & Ouslander, J. (1987). Geriatric assessment on a subacute hospital ward. *Clinical Internal Geriatric Medicine, 3*(2), 1–17.

Sasma, G.P., Patrick, C.H., & Ferusser, J.R. (1993). Long-term survival of veterans with traumatic spinal cord injury. *Archives of Neurology, 50,* 909–914.

Shults, C.W. (1990). Parkinson's disease: New developments in understanding and treatment. In B.J. Kemp, K. Brummel-Smith, & J. Ramsdell (Eds.), *Geriatric rehabilitation* (pp. 121–136). Austin, TX: PRO-ED.

Silliman, R.A., McGarvey, S.T., Raymond, P.M., & Fretwell, M.D. (1990). Does inpatient interdisciplinary geriatric assessment help the family caregivers of acutely ill older persons? *Journal of the American Geriatric Society, 38,* 461–466.

Sivenius, J., Pyorala, K., Heinonen, V.P., Salonen, J.T., & Rickkinen, P. (1985). The significance of intensity of rehabilitation of stroke: A controlled trial. *Stroke, 16,* 928–931.

Smith, D.S., Goldenberg, E., Ashburn, G., Kinsella, G., Sheilch, K., Brennan, P.J., Meade, T.W., Zutshi, D.W., Perry, J.D., & Reback, J.S. (1981). Remedial therapy after stroke: A randomized controlled trial. *British Medical Journal, 282,* 517–522.

U.S. Department of Health and Human Services. (1989). *Population profile on disability.* Washington, DC: Mathematica Policy Research Co.

World Health Organization. (1980). *International classification of impairments, disabilities, and handicaps.* Geneva, Switzerland: Author.

CHAPTER 18

Musculoskeletal Conditions

Jacquelin Perry

Rehabilitation for musculoskeletal conditions relates to all three stages of the World Health Organization's (1980) classification of disablement because the pathologies involved are so diverse in their nature and severity. The need is for functionally oriented programs designed to reduce the impairment, disability, and handicap that are likely to follow either protracted or permanent pathology if only acute, curative care is provided. Yet documenting outcomes is difficult because this category is so broad.

The musculoskeletal system includes all of the body's bones, joints, and muscles from head to toe. These structures determine the person's capacity for physical function. They also can be impaired by any of the major forms of pathology (i.e., trauma; infection; congenital and developmental defects; immune reactions; degenerative, vascular, and metabolic diseases). In the United States, there are approximately 12 million people limited by ongoing or permanent musculoskeletal impairment, making this the most common cause of dysfunction (Holbrook, Grazier, Kelsey, & Stauffer, 1984). In addition, this is the class of impairment that most commonly disrupts patients' ability to work. Hence, a significant handicap is not uncommon.

Musculoskeletal pathology causes reduced joint mobility, pain, muscle weakness, deformity, and possibly loss of limbs. These impairments are the common focus of most medical evaluations. The disability resulting from these impairments includes limitations in patients' ability to walk; climb stairs; carry a load; or manipulate a keyboard, dials, or tools. Criteria for assessing these functions remain in flux. A societal handicap that most frequently follows musculoskeletal impairment is the inability to return to work. Only severe multilimb involvement limits the patients' activities of daily living (ADL) or their ability to live independently.

A categorical list of major musculoskeletal pathology includes arthritis, low back and cervical pain syndromes, limb trauma, amputations, burns, tumors, immune disorders, myopathies, and the postpolio syndrome. Any age group can be involved. This review, however, focuses on the course of young and middle-age adults because other chapters of this book are concerned with early development (see Chapter 16) and aging-related conditions (see Chapter 17).

The accountability for providing musculoskeletal rehabilitation is difficult to identify. Many of the conditions are managed within standard medical environments, that is, private offices and outpatient clinics. This complicates data gathering. The severity and scope of the initial impairment also vary widely. Many levels of musculoskeletal impairment have a good potential for complete healing. Some respond well to standard care, whereas others show the benefits of specialized expertise. Advancement from the obviously curable impairment to a high probability for permanent impairment is often subtle. This can obscure timely recognition of adverse progression into a major disability or handicap, making the indications for musculoskeletal rehabilitation vague.

The first phase of outcomes assessment, impairment management, begins with the clinician's criteria that characterize the levels of pathology. The basic subclassifications are the scope of the impairment (i.e., single or multilimb involvement) and the degree of dysfunction (i.e., mild, moderate, severe). Other variables are the common course of the impairment and the secondary factors that interfere with full physical recovery. These can include contractures, disuse weakness, loss of tissue, and associated medical problems.

For the second phase, assessing the disability resulting from the impairment, clinicians have developed descriptive scales. For the lower extremities, these scales grade ability to walk, climb stairs, limitations in lifting, and so forth. An alternate approach is the use of objective measurements such as walking velocity and repetitious lifts. Upper-extremity function is more difficult to quantify because it involves so many tasks.

Assessing the resulting social handicap is the third phase. Subtle variables are level of lifestyle, degree of independence, recreational capability, and effect on family. To demonstrate the character of outcomes assessment for musculoskeletal conditions, five major musculoskeletal categories are reviewed:

1. Trauma
2. Arthritis
3. Amputations
4. Tumors
5. Low back pain

TRAUMA

Although the broad category of trauma includes all types of musculoskeletal injury, the two most significant types of pathology relative to outcomes analysis are fractures and sports injuries. Both of these modes of dysfunction can involve the upper or lower extremities and can occur across the full spectrum of ages.

Fractures

Fractures are so diverse in their anatomy and severity that both the optimum restoration of function and outcomes analysis are vigorous challenges. A fracture can involve any bone, and the damage may vary from a simple, undisplaced, transverse, midshaft break to one that is significantly angulated, is in several fragments (comminuted), and involves the intricate anatomy of the joint. Other significant variables are the extent of the soft tissue damage and bone penetration of the skin (compounding) (Helfet & Schmeling, 1993). Each of these factors correspondingly threatens alignment stability, joint mobility, healing time, and functional quality. The orthopedist's choice of fracture reduction, stabilization, and mobilization procedures represents a balance between the physiology of bone and fibrous tissue healing and the mechanics of motion relative to adverse determinants.

Nonoperative procedures avoid the potential for infection from penetrating the skin barrier and add no further soft tissue trauma. Contradicting these advantages is the limited ability to restore and maintain precise alignment throughout the healing process. There also is less opportunity to use early mobilization to prevent contracture formation. Surgery facilitates fixation and early mobilization, but it necessitates choosing the device from among the numerous types of screws, plates, and external fixators that are most comparable with the patient's bone quality. The rehabilitation program to preserve and restore joint mobility cannot begin until the fracture is considered sufficiently stable (Aitken & Rorabeck, 1986).

Outcomes evaluations of orthopedic fracture management primarily consider impairment factors (e.g., quality of healing, range of motion, pain). Less frequently, investigators also assess the functional outcomes (disability). That the entire fracture management process, including rehabilitation, customarily is handled within the acute care milieu also makes it difficult to amass a significant number of like cases for discriminating outcomes analysis.

Most follow-up studies compare the effectiveness of new techniques or areas of continuing difficulty. Outcome is related to the anatomical area involved and the extent of the fragmentation. The pronounced variability in the type and magnitude of bone and joint injuries has led to continual changes in the classification criteria, making comparisons between studies difficult.

Outcomes grading criteria also vary. Although the four-level scale of excellent, good, fair, and poor is most common, other investigators merely score the outcome as satisfactory or unsatisfactory. Each rating step also often has differing criteria. For example, in the assessment of elbow fracture management, joint motion is the critical factor. Aitken and Rorabeck (1986) graded their results excellent if the elbow could flex at least 110°. Gabel, Hanson, Bennett, Noble, and Tullos (1987) and Helfet and Schmeling (1993) required 130° flexion for an excellent result; Gabel et al. accepted a 30° flexion contracture, whereas Helfet and Schmeling limited it to 15°. Reflected in these differences is the progress that has been made in the orthopedic surgical management of the severely injured elbow and improved joint mobilization skills from physical therapists' growing experience with sports injuries. These factors demonstrate that the establishment of outcomes criteria must remain timely and be current with the therapeutic potential of modern orthopedists. Each joint—shoulder, hip, knee, foot—presents similar difficulties in classification of the fracture pattern and subsequent outcomes analysis (Benirschke & Sangeorzan, 1993; Ruesch, Holdener, Ciaramitaro, & Mast, 1994; Segal, Mallik, Wetzler, Franchi, & Whitelaw, 1993; Szyszkowitz, Segal, Schliefer, & Cundy, 1993).

When functional use of the extremity is included as an outcomes criterion, the standards also can vary markedly. For example, elbow function has been rated as unlimited, ADL-capable, or just serving as a prop (Aitken & Rorabeck, 1986). For lower-extremity injuries, the patient's ability to resume his or her customary lifestyle may be the standard (Segal et al., 1993). A more discriminating outcome is the ability to return to work (Bednar & Ali, 1993). In an assessment of primary intramedullary fixation for isolated femoral shaft fractures, 85% of patients returned to work within 4 months postinjury, with 90% having full-time employment. These investigators carefully limited their cases to the 47 with one type of fracture from a total population of 136 femoral shaft fractures. More complicated fractures and those involving the knee joint were excluded so that management effectiveness could be accurately evaluated.

In patients with severe limb injury and predictable permanent disability, the value of a protracted treatment course versus early amputation is a common question (Caudle & Stern, 1987). A comparative study showed that the impairment scores for the successfully managed severe (Type III) tibial fractures ranged from 7% to 19%, whereas the impairment levels of the through-knee and above-knee amputees were 36% and 28%, respectively. It was concluded that protracted fracture care that preserved a functional limb led to a better outcome.

Most outcomes studies of fracture management include follow-up intervals of fewer than 2 years. This time period covers the secondary management of a complication, contracture reduction efforts, progressive activity, and the opportunity to resume the customary lifestyle (Gabel et al., 1987; Kemp, Van Niekerk, & Van Meurs, 1993). Beyond this time frame, further restoration of function is unlikely to occur unless an entirely new program can be instituted.

Hip fracture outcome following a fall by older adults commonly is complicated by the vicissitudes of inactivity. This introduces the question of survival as well as function. The ability to return home is the functional measure. A 10-year follow-up study of 103 patients with an average age of 75 who were treated with early surgical fixation and immediate weight bearing showed that an increasing percentage returned home, though survival significantly decreased (Thorngren, Ceder, & Svensson, 1993). At 3 weeks, 54% were home, with only one death having occurred. The 10-year mark showed that most of the survivors were at home, but mortality had increased to 66%.

Sports Injuries

Sports injuries fall into a specific clinical group because soft tissues (i.e., ligament, capsule, tendons) are the usual site of injury, and an athletic activity is the cause. The injury may represent either a single event or accumulative recurrent strain. Most vulnerable to sports injuries are the shoulder, elbow, and knee. Outcome is judged by the individual's ability to return to sports (Mizuno, Nabeshima, & Hirohata, 1993; Rowe, Patel, & Southmayd, 1978). This standard, however, can be compromised by the recreational athlete who chooses not to undergo the rigor of an intense therapeutic program or the potential for reinjury. The second outcomes criterion is return to work (Daniel et al., 1994). Levels of residual disability such as limited range of motion and pain are lesser criteria.

ARTHRITIS

Numerous modes of joint pathology fall within the arthritis category, but rheumatoid arthritis and osteoarthritis are the dominant diagnoses. The course of the other immune diseases can be coupled with rheumatoid arthritis, and the late effects of joint trauma and sepsis present clinical pictures compatible with osteoarthritis.

Rheumatoid Arthritis

Rheumatoid arthritis is potentially the most disabling joint disease. Its dominant pathology of persistent synovial membrane inflammation causes swelling and pain that inhibit function. Secondary effects are joint cartilage destruction and bone erosion, which cause permanent losses of function (Cush & Lipsky, 1991). In addition, this immune system disease includes systemic manifestations of weakness, malaise, and weight loss (Cooke & Scudamore, 1984). Symptoms may start at any age and then burn out at an early stage, have an intermittent course of exacerbations and remissions, or continue to progress in an unrelenting fashion. The involvement can vary from a single joint (e.g., one knee, hand) to include all four limbs and the spine. Even the head's only joint, the jaw, is not immune. Approximately 29% of patients have multiple-joint onset. A benign self-limiting course was found in 25% of the patients requiring hospitalization, even when there were several exacerbations. Symptomatic courses that continued for 10 or more years had a high incidence of unrelenting progression of joint destruction, deformity, and loss of function.

Medical care employs nonsteroidal anti-inflammatory drugs (NSAIDs) to limit synovial inflammation (Paulus, 1991). For the more protracted situations, disease-modifying agents such as gold and selective steroids are added. None offer a specific cure, though the intensity of the symptoms can be significantly lessened (Weinblatt & Maier, 1991). Medicinal effectiveness in rheumatoid arthritis is judged by the reduction in joint tenderness and swelling, more normal laboratory blood levels, and minimization of complications such as gastric irritation (Tilley et al., 1995).

Physical and occupational therapy seek to preserve mobility, strength, and function. They are most effective when considered part of an ongoing program throughout the course of the patient's care (Suteji & Hadler, 1991). Additional rehabilitation efforts include lifestyle management and adaptive devices to enable patients with more disabilities to cope with their limitations (Rodrigo & Gershwin, 1993).

Surgical reconstruction of the damaged joint with metallic or plastic replacements is a common procedure to relieve deformity and restore function. This entire course generally occurs within the standard acute care environment. Referrals to an inpatient rehabilitation center are reserved for patients more disabled by rheumatoid arthritis with multilimb impairment (Classes III and IV dysfunction). Outcome studies have been inconclusive regarding the benefits of such a program (Shope, Barnwell, Jette, Kulik, & Edwards, 1983; Suteji & Hadler, 1991). The inclusion of reconstructive surgery increased the benefit of inpatient rehabilitation (Conaty & Nickel, 1971).

Osteoarthritis

Osteoarthritis, described by Mankin (1984) as the most common "affliction of the joints" (p. 215), represents a progressive degeneration of articular cartilage. Secondary changes are osteophyte formation (bone spurs), capsular thickening, and joint destruction. Most commonly, this pathology arises in the hands and major weight-bearing joints of middle-age and older adults. No single etiology has been identified, but selected populations show strong evidence of genetic errors, repetitive trauma, and mechanical derangements, as well as hormonal and chemical imbalance. Medical management includes NSAIDs and physical and occupational therapy to reduce symptoms and preserve mobility.

Surgical Joint Reconstruction

Surgical reconstruction of joints damaged by arthritis using metallic or plastic replacements is a common procedure to relieve deformity and restore function. The indications are intolerable pain, significant loss of function, and medical fitness for surgery (Moreland, 1993). Outcome of surgical joint replacement most commonly is judged with a descriptive scale that combines impairment signs and function.

Several descriptive scales have been developed by the major orthopedic centers for joint replacement. Based on earlier systems to rate pain relief, joint mobility, and function after hip surgery, Harris (1969) developed a 100-point scale that focused on ability. Pain relief (44 points) and function (47 points related to ADL and gait) have almost equal emphasis. Only 9 points relate to passive mobility. The patient's total scores then are summarized as excellent (90+), good (80+), fair (70+), and poor (less than 70 points). For total knee replacement, the Hospital for Special Surgery (HSS) 100-point scale is preferred (Insall, Ranawat, Aglietti, & Shine, 1976). This assigns less for pain (30 points) and function (22 points) and emphasizes the reduction of impairment (48 points divided among deformity, mobility, muscle strength, and stability). Total scores are similarly described as excellent (85+), good (70+), fair (60+), and failure (60−). An example is the 15-year follow-up of the first 85 patients (112 knees) to have a Total Condylar knee, which showed that 92% of those still alive had a good to excellent result (Ranawat, Flynn, Saddler, Hansraj, & Maynard, 1993). The outcome was poor in 6.5% (under 60 points). The differences in the Harris and HSS rating systems reflect the complex list of variables that determine the final outcome of a major surgical reconstruction such as total joint replacement. Choosing among them has relied on subjective weighting by experienced experts.

Prosthetic survivorship analysis to indicate the reliability of the procedure was added to outcomes assessment in 1993. In the Ranawat et al. (1993) Total Condylar knee study, there was a 100% 7-year survival rate, and, at 15 years, the survival rate was 94%. The results for rheumatoid arthritis (95%) were slightly better than for osteoarthritis (91%). Female survival (93%) was longer than that for males (83%). Body weight proved to be a determinant, with those weighing less than 80 kg having a 96% clinical and roentgenograms survival rate. For the heavier group, clinical survival rate was 89%. These results were not replicated in a survivorship study of 9,200 knee prostheses involving nine different styles and several clinical variables (Rand & Ilstrup, 1991). At 15 years, the overall survival rate was 69%. Four factors were identified that lowered the risk of failure:

1. The absence of prior knee surgery
2. A diagnosis of rheumatoid arthritis (versus osteoarthritis)

3. Age over 60 years
4. A metal-backed tibial component

With all four positive factors present, the 10-year predicted survival rate was 97%.

Formal gait analysis to assess outcome following knee replacement surgery has demonstrated only moderate gains in walking ability. Gait velocity showed a 13% improvement at 3 months, which paralleled the reduction in pain (Steiner, Simon, & Pisciotta, 1989). The gain was related to a significantly longer stride length. This in turn reflected improved joint mobility and weight-bearing tolerance. Cadence registered little change, because keeping a relatively normal step rate had been the patients' mode of compensation. By 18 months, there was a 40% increase in gait velocity (Berman, Zarro, Bosacco, & Israelite, 1987). Gait measurements were limited by difficulties in getting the patients to the gait laboratory (Steiner et al., 1989). Berman et al. (1987) reduced this obstacle by having a gait mat in the physical therapy department, yet his study group still was not large ($N = 28$).

AMPUTATIONS

The three major causes of amputation in 1995 were peripheral vascular disease (including diabetes), tumors, and trauma. Each presents unique characteristics for outcomes evaluation. The basic criteria of therapeutic effectiveness are primary wound healing, ambulation quality, and functional outcome.

Traumatic Amputations

Traumatic amputations have the best potential for long-term function if the cause of the amputation was a single self-limiting episode. Although the healing period may include early complications or associated injuries, the etiology presents no lingering threats to the individual's health. Thus, the traumatic amputee has a normal potential to recover strength, mobility, and function compatible with his or her age group and rehabilitation program. Outcomes criteria can focus on the level of amputation, type of prosthesis, age, and functional level attained (Walker, Ingram, Hullin, & McCreath, 1994).

Dysvascular Amputations

Dysvascular amputations are the consequence of limb pathology secondary to peripheral vascular disease or diabetes. These underlying pathologies are systemic diseases that compromise the patient's basic health. In addition, many have other chronic impairments such as coronary artery disease. The associated physiologic imbalance impairs amputees' ability to generate the strength and energy required to accommodate the added demands of prosthetic gait. Patients' life spans are also threatened by both their disease and their advanced age.

In outcomes assessments for dysvascular amputees, the basic question is the value of prescribing a prosthesis. Both the device and rehabilitation program are expensive. Countering this are the physiologic and psychologic values of being able to walk. The cost–benefit ratio is implied but is approached indirectly. The purpose of prosthetic fitting is to enable the amputee to walk.

A 1993 retrospective review of a six-hospital nationwide sampling of the Veterans Administration (VA) assessed the survival and preservation of ambulation (Pinzur et al., 1993) for patients with transtibial (TT) amputations registered in a Special Teams for Amputation Mobility Prosthetics-Orthotics Program (STAMP). This program had been instituted to upgrade VA amputee care, which appeared to have slipped from its intense post–World War II development. Follow-up was undertaken after a minimum of 1 year. During the 3-year study, 37% died. Of the 299 surviving amputees, 64% were diabetic. Ambulatory ability was judged by a simplified Hoffer descriptive scale that differentiates among unable, household, and community ambulation (Hoffer, Feiwell, Perry, Perry, & Bonnett, 1973). Preamputation status proved to be a major determinant. Of the 56% who had been community ambulators before surgery, 87% retained their independence in the community following amputation. Among the 31% who were household ambulators, a similar proportion remained so postamputation. The percentage of nonambulators increased by only 7%. Study limitations identified by the authors included the lack of standardized criteria among the hospitals for patient selection, treatment protocols, or follow-up evaluation. Despite these limitations, the demographic data, death rate, and functional outcome proved to be similar among the six institutions. There also was general agreement on surgical technique and postoperative care.

Moore et al. (1989) reviewed a mixture of transfemoral (TF) and TT amputations in a wide range of adult ages. Their purpose was to determine exclusion criteria to avoid providing prostheses to amputees who lacked a reasonable potential to walk. The 157 amputees were divided into three groups: 1) noncandidates (28, mean age 72), 2) prosthetic failures (41, mean age 66), and 3) functional prosthetic users (88, mean age 57). The authors indirectly showed that the major determinants of prosthetic gait capability were amputation level, etiology, age, and coronary artery disease, although none was an absolute indicator. Only 46% of the TF amputees were successful walkers; of this group, 65% were young and trauma was the etiology. Only 7% had coronary artery disease. Bilateral amputation and coronary artery disease led to 81% failure, even when performed at the TT level. Among the unilateral TT amputees, coronary artery disease was not a specific determinant, yet only 66% were successful walkers.

Holden and Fernie (1987) found the mean walking endurance for TF amputees at the time of discharge from rehabilitation barely approximated the 600 steps per day required in a small home, and they made little subsequent improvement. In contrast, the TT amputees exceeded the initial threshold by 28% and continued to increase their endurance. The poor potential of TT amputees with the added debilitation of coronary artery disease, a dysvascular etiology, and aging relates to the significantly higher energy demand of walking with an TF prosthesis. That demand is 187% of normal for the TF amputee versus 133% for the TT amputee (Waters, 1992).

The Functional Independence Measure (FIM) (State University of New York at Buffalo, 1993), a rehabilitation assessment tool, was used to determine amputees' potential for prosthetic management. Among 68 amputees between the ages of 50 and 80, a comparison of the patients in the highest (fourth) quartile and the lowest (first) quartile showed a strong correlation between their admission and discharge scores ($r = .84$) and their ambulatory gains (Muecke, Shekar, Dwyer, Israel, & Flynn, 1992). More fourth-quartile patients used crutches (77% vs. 18%) and had a permanent prosthesis (65% vs. 18%), whereas the first-quartile patients generally used a wheelchair (82% vs. 29%). The gait-training program of the fourth-quartile patients, however, required a longer period of rehabilitation hospitalization (110 days vs. 53 days). The need to omit the middle half of the amputee population to obtain meaningful indicators implied significant imprecision in the classification criteria.

There are no precise criteria for effective prosthesis use. One approach used hours per day of prosthesis wearing (Reyes, Leahey, & Leahey, 1977). Among the three stages chosen, 6–8 hours, 2–4 hours, and none, the latter two identified primary wheelchair dependency. A second standard was level of ambulatory function, that is, "able to get out of house" and "use of stairs." Other criteria of ambulatory effectiveness were management of irregular terrain (90% could) and ambulatory aid requirements (i.e., none, cane, crutches, walker). The relative significance of these criteria has not been determined.

The social outcome (handicap) of amputation in the older adults population is less often explored. By adding the ESCROW scale to the Pulses evaluation (Moskowitz & McCann, 1957), a need for social and financial support was identified (O'Toole, Goldberg, & Ryan, 1985). (ESCROW is an acronym for the assessment of the housing environment, personal support, family cluster, financial resources, outlook, and work or school status. Pulses documents the patient's upper and lower extremity, sensory and excretory function, and social support.) Among a group of older amputees with an average age of 64 years, 27% returned to work, but half at a lighter job. Return to work was not related to the availability of realistic work opportunities. Thirty percent regained their ability to drive or to use public transportation.

TUMORS

Both life and limb survival are threatened by malignant tumors. Because the patients generally are teenagers or young adults, all regain the ability to walk. Thus, outcomes measures focus on the ability to preserve life and limb.

Primary tumors of the musculoskeletal system are sarcomas involving the fibrous tissue, cartilage, bone, or muscle (Sim, McDonald, & Wold, 1988). Most often they occur in the lower extremity about the knee or hip. Tumor excision by amputation was the customary method of management (Johnston, 1988). Advances in chemotherapy and the development of internal prostheses to replace the excised bone now allow limb preservation (Horowitz, Glasser, Lane, & Healey, 1993). The residual functional disability relates to the amount of muscle and other soft tissues that also must be removed to create a tumor-free environment. The common practice of concentrating orthopedic tumor management in specialized centers has resulted in valid outcomes data for significantly large groups of patients.

Both tumor location and method of management influence survival. In a 10-year follow-up of 108 patients having limb salvage procedures, life survival was best for patients with proximal tibia tumors (93%) and significantly shorter for those with either a distal (67%) or proximal femur tumor (45%) (Horowitz et al., 1993). A comparison of tumor eradication procedures showed hip disarticulation to offer the best tumor control (0 in 39 cases). The less disabling amputation (TF) allowed an 8% recurrence in 115 patients, and the incidence among 73 limb salvage procedures was 11%.

The residual disability and quality of life following limb salvage procedures and amputation have been compared. The amputees had greater difficulty with stairs and needed more assistance (Nicholson, Mulvihill, & Byrne, 1992; Rougraff, Simon, Kneisi, Greenberg, & Manakin, 1994). Employment status and annual income were similar: 68% worked full-time and 28% had an income of more than $30,000. There were few adverse psychological outcomes, with an average quality-of-life rating of 7/10 and 34% having a rating of 10/10.

LOW BACK PAIN

Low back pain generally starts as an acute episode precipitated by a twist, a fall, or a lifting episode. Most patients recover in a few days or a few weeks; but, in 5%–10% of cases, the disabling symptoms continue for more than 3 months (Nachemson, 1992). Persistent pain, disruption of daily routine, and lack of gainful employment add psychological trauma. The frequency of these episodes makes low back pain the leading cause (52%) of musculoskeletal disability in the working-age group (18–64 years) (Holbrook et al., 1984). For those who fail to recover in a timely fashion, the penalty is the societal handicap of unemployment induced by ill-defined pain mechanisms.

Persistence of the category *low back pain* attests to the complexity of the problem. Despite diagnostic capabilities in the 1990s, precise pathology often cannot be identified, nor can severity be delineated, except by the duration of symptoms as acute, subacute, or ongoing. Although there is the classic, clear-cut herniated disc that responds well to surgical excision, the majority of disc lesions do not (Spengler, 1993). This also is true for spine instability and the arthritic joint (Kane, 1993). These inconsistencies in diagnosis, pathology, and surgical response have made conservative therapy the dominant form of management.

The problem lies in the multifaceted character of back function and the complex anatomy of the lower spine. The low lumbar and lumbosacral joints serve as a critical junction between the lifting and reaching body unit (trunk and arms) and the locomotor supporting unit (lower extremities and pelvis). This functional junction experiences repetitious compressive, stretching, and torsional forces during work, recreation, and ADL. Each intervertebral interval includes a specialized disc for load distribution and two facet joints to guide motion that rely on a multilayered system of short and long muscles for control and protection. Passing through this anatomical complex are nerves that exit from the spinal cord to the legs. All of these tissues have varying tolerances for the stresses they experience and differing capacity to recover from strain. Conservative management includes a variety of physical therapy programs to relieve pain, recover mobility, and strengthen the back muscles, and to establish back protection habits, psychological training in pain management, and orthoses for mechanical protection. The controversy revolves on which procedures are most successful in returning the patient to work.

Outcomes analyses, however, have been sufficiently different in scope and format to make program comparisons difficult. Often the exact therapeutic procedures are not defined. Patient populations differ in chronicity, activity pattern, and physical capability. The therapeutic regimens include different components.

Measurements of impairment are used to ascertain the effectiveness of the individual therapeutic techniques. These include pain, spine mobility, and trunk muscle strength. Return to work, however, is the primary outcome criterion for all low back pain treatment programs. Some consider the percentage of patients who remain employed for least 1 year, and a few programs evaluate longer work histories.

A major area of dispute is the relative value of different physical therapy procedures. One study related the type of exercise to patient characteristics in a comparison of three 4-week protocols randomly applied to 150 patients with subacute or ongoing low back pain. Relief of pain was the outcomes measure. Intense dynamic back muscle exercise was most effective for women and sedentary workers. Conventional physical therapy modalities (e.g., heat, ultrasound, ice) and isometric exercise proved to be more effective for men and individuals with moderate-to-hard physical jobs (Hansen et al., 1993). Two short-term (1-month) programs confirmed the value of dynamic extension exercise for pain relief and the return to work (Gill, Sanford, Binkley, Stratford, & Finch, 1994; Spratt, Weinstein, Lehmann, Woody, & Sayre, 1993). A similar short-term physically intense program that included work hardening (i.e., job-specific tasks) and psychologic testing for 54 nonworking patients was successful in returning 55% to work. Follow-up was undertaken after 1 year (Edwards, Zusman, Hardcastle, Twomey, O'Sullivan, & McLean, 1992).

Quite different was the inconclusive outcome of an intense physical training program for more ongoing low back pain. Physical gains were found not to be indicative of a good rehabilitation outcome (Mellin, Harkeapeaea, Hurri, & Jarvinkowski, 1990). When a group of patients still working (101) was compared with a group on sick leave (79), both showed gains in physical measures; but work potential was inconsistent. Only 28% of those on leave returned to work; 14% of the patients went on sick leave. The only physical change that correlated with return to work was increased spinal mobility in the women. A Swedish study of injury-related low back pain found factors adverse to recovery were lump-sum compensation, psychological disturbances, time off from work, and age. Nonsignificant factors were the type and severity of the injury or associated neurologic deficits (Greenough, 1993). Compensation availability delayed early recovery, but there was no difference after 6 months (Tollison, 1993). A multifaceted program for patients with ongoing low back pain demonstrated a reversal of psychological abnormalities (e.g., hysteria, depression, hypochondria) (Barnes, Gatchel, Mayer, & Barnett, 1990). Merely adding psychological intervention to a standard 3-week inpatient rehabilitation back program, however, made no difference in outcome (Altmaier, Lehmann, Russell, Weinstein, & Kao, 1992).

Prevention of low back injury in heavy demand occupations is another outcomes concern. The use of specific programs to teach the patient how to overcome the limitations of chronic back pain and a lumbosacral corset resulted in less loss of work time compared with untreated controls or with groups in which the orthosis or training program was omitted. Strength and accident rates did not differ among the groups.

CONCLUSIONS

Outcomes analysis of rehabilitation for the multitude of musculoskeletal conditions has followed two major directions. First is classification of the condition by etiology and severity, because these are the underlying determinants of the patients' potential to recover normal function. The second level of analysis has been the effectiveness of the therapeutic procedures employed.

Fractures, sports injuries, and traumatic amputations offer the best rehabilitation potential because they are single, self-limiting events in fundamentally healthy people, though the loss of tissue may not be totally recoverable or replaceable. For these conditions, outcomes assessment has tended to focus on the reduction of impairment. The reports, however, have usually focused on the effectiveness of a particular procedure instead of providing a comparison of therapeutic approaches. The individual studies still could be related, except for the continual refinement of criteria by each sequential investigator, both to classify the initial pathology and to define outcomes. It is time for the experts in these clinical areas to establish a consensus on the significant diagnostic determinants for each of the major areas of trauma. Another need is to consistently extend the analysis to include disability. Return to work or active sport participation is the ultimate goal for this population. More specific definitions of these accomplishments are needed, however, such as duration and level of demand.

Hip fractures in the older adults and malignant tumors include the added variable of survival, but otherwise they are fairly discrete conditions. This diagnostic stability has resulted in outcomes reports that could be related to each other. The other major musculoskeletal conditions have much less predictable courses. Consequently, outcomes analysis has been correspondingly more difficult.

Despite the difficulties in defining the pathology of low back pain, the classifications of acute, subacute, and ongoing have proved useful. Further agreement, however, is needed to define the discriminating time intervals. It also is important to determine why the patient's course continued into the later stages. Does this represent failure to profit from optimum acute care or its unavailability?

Therapeutic programs for low back pain can be grouped into three major areas: physical therapy, work hardening, and psychologic guidance; and each area includes numerous variables. In the desire for brevity, the exact procedures often have not been detailed. As a result, the reasons for differences in outcomes remain obscure. An example of the value of such detail is the Hansen et al. (1993) study, which found that the activity level of the patients significantly influenced the specific type of physical therapy that was effective.

The unpredictability of most arthritic conditions limits the opportunity for meaningful outcomes assessments of nonoperative management programs. As a result, the majority of outcomes studies on arthritis relate to surgical joint replacement. The pathology has been excised so that the duration of success can be considered as an indication of technical effectiveness, unless there is an identifiable flare-up in a new joint. The development of major rating scales, such as the Harris hip and HSS knee systems, has allowed good comparisons between individual studies, though these scales are not used by all surgeons, nor are there similar protocols for all of the other joints. Another significant limitation is the imprecision of the surgical indications. Although a preoperative rating documents the level of disability, no correlations with the need for surgery have been presented.

For dysvascular amputees, the major indecision in clinical management is the appropriateness of providing prostheses because of the patients' medical fragility and age. Attempts to make this determination through outcomes studies have been inconclusive. Most studies have merely considered the patient's postamputation state. These identified adverse situations that reduced the amputee's ability to walk, but they were not sufficiently conclusive to serve as predictive criteria. In contrast, the TT amputee study, which considered the patient's preamputation ambulatory status (i.e., community, household, unable), identified a strong outcomes indicator, with only a 7% error. A similar analysis is needed for TF amputees.

Walking requires both cardiopulmonary energy productivity and limb muscle strength. Outcomes assessment that documents the incidence of coronary disease and multiple complications indirectly considers the patient's energetics, but the data have not been developed into firm criteria. The relationship between the amputee's muscle strength and walking ability has yet to be developed.

Gait analysis offers an objective means of defining the patient's walking ability. This would appear to be a good outcomes assessment instrument, yet it rarely is used for several reasons. First is the inconvenience of getting the patient to the gait laboratory, unless the critical stride measurement system is in the gait-training (i.e., physical therapy) area as was done by Berman et al. (1987). Second, for the arthritic patients, the mean gains in walking speed closely paralleled the reduction in pain. Hence, a simple clinical tool was equally informative. For amputee patients, the use of gait analysis also has been reserved as a research instrument. In both situations, the significance of individual variations has not been identified. In energy cost measurement, the minimal 5-minute test failed to reflect the endurance factor of community ambulation, whereas a 20-minute test showed good correlation. Consequently, informative gait analysis involves a time commitment. Objective gait analysis, however, could become a significant outcomes measure once closer correlations are developed with the individual patient's clinical picture.

REFERENCES

Aitken, G.T., & Rorabeck, C.H. (1986). Distal humeral fractures in the adult. *Clinical Orthopaedics and Related Research, 207,* 191–197.

Altmaier, R.M., Lehmann, T.R., Russell, D.W., Weinstein, J.N., & Kao, C.F. (1992). The effectiveness of psychological intervention for the rehabilitation of low back pain. *Pain, 49,* 329–335.

Barnes, D., Gatchel, R.J., Mayer, T.G., & Barnett, J. (1990). Changes in MMPI profile levels of chronic low back pain patients following successful treatment. *Journal of Spine Disorders, 3,* 353–355.

Bednar, D.A., & Ali, P. (1993). Intramedullary nailing of femoral shaft fractures: Reoperation and return to work. *Canadian Journal of Surgery, 36,* 464–466.

Benirschke, S.K., & Sangeorzan, B.J. (1993). Extensive intra-articular fractures of the foot. *Clinical Orthopaedics and Related Research, 292,* 128–134.

Berman, A.T., Zarro, V.J., Bosacco, S.J., & Israelite, C. (1987). Quantitative gait analysis after unilateral or bilateral total knee replacement. *Journal of Bone and Joint Surgery, 69*(9), 1340–1345.

Caudle, R.J., & Stern, P.J. (1987). Severe open fractures of the tibia. *Journal of Bone and Joint Surgery, 69A,* 801–807.

Conaty, J.P., & Nickel, V.L. (1971). Functional incapacitation in rheumatoid arthritis: A rehabilitation challenge. *Journal of Bone and Joint Surgery, 53A,* 624–637.

Cooke, T.D.V., & Scudamore, R.A. (1984). Rheumatoid arthritis and allied conditions. In R.L. Cruess & W.R. Rennie (Eds.), *Adult orthopaedics* (pp. 271–359). New York: Churchill Livingstone.

Cush, J.J., & Lipsky, P.P. (1991). Cellular basis for rheumatoid inflammation. *Clinical Orthopaedics and Related Research, 265,* 9–22.

Daniel, D.M., Stone, M.L., Dobson, B.E., Fithian, D.C., Rossman, D.J., & Kaufman, K.R. (1994). Fate of the ACL-injured patient. A prospective outcome study. *American Journal of Sports Medicine, 22,* 632–644.

Edwards, B.C., Zusman, M., Hardcastle, P., Twomey, L., O'Sullivan, P., & McLean, N. (1992). A physical approach to the rehabilitation of patients disabled by chronic low back pain. *Medical Journal of Australia, 156,* 167–172.

Gabel, G.T., Hanson, G., Bennett, J.B., Noble, P.C., & Tullos, H.S. (1987). Intra-articular fractures of the distal humerus in adults. *Clinical Orthopaedics and Related Research, 216,* 99–108.

Gill, C., Sanford, J., Binkley, J., Stratford, P., & Finch, E. (1994). Low back pain: Program description and outcome in a case series. *Journal of Orthopedic Sports Physical Therapy, 20,* 11–16.

Greenough, C.G. (1993). Recovery from low back pain. 1–5 year follow-up of 287 injury-related cases. *Acta Orthopaedica Scandinavica, 254*(Suppl.), 1–34.

Hansen, F.R., Bendix, T., Skov, P., Jensen, C.V., Kristensen, J.H., Krohn, L., & Schioler, H. (1993). Intensive, dynamic back-muscle exercises, conventional physiotherapy or placebo-control of low back pain: A randomized, observer blind trial. *Spine, 18,* 98–108.

Harris, W.H. (1969). Traumatic arthritis of the hip after dislocation and acetabular fractures: Treatment by mold arthroplasty. *Journal of Bone and Joint Surgery, 51A*(4), 737–755.

Helfet, D., & Schmeling, G.J. (1993). Bicondylar intraarticular fractures of the distal humerus in adults. *Clinical Orthopaedics and Related Research, 292,* 26–36.

Hoffer, M.M., Feiwell, E., Perry, R., Perry, J., & Bonnett, C. (1973). Functional ambulation in patients with myelomeningocele. *Journal of Bone and Joint Surgery, 55A*(1), 137–148.

Holbrook, T.L., Grazier, K., Kelsey, J.L., & Stauffer, R.N. (1984). *The frequency of occurence, impact and cost of selected musculoskeletal conditions in the United States.* Chicago: Academy of Orthopaedic Surgeons.

Holden, J.M., & Fernie, G.R. (1987). Extent of artificial limb use following rehabilitation. *Journal of Orthopedic Research, 5,* 562–568.

Horowitz, S.M., Glasser, D.B., Lane, J.M., & Healey, J.H. (1993). Prosthetic and extremity survivorship after limb salvage for sarcoma. *Clinical Orthopaedics and Related Research, 293,* 280–286.

Insall, J.H., Ranawat, C.S., Aglietti, P., & Shine, J. (1976). A comparison of four models of total knee replacement prostheses. *Journal of Bone and Joint Surgery, 58A,* 754–765.

Johnston, J.O. (1993). Principles of limb salvage surgery. In M.W. Chapman & M. Madison (Eds.), *Operative orthopaedics* (2nd ed., pp. 2495–2512). Philadelphia: J.B. Lippincott.

Kane, W.J. (1993). Posterior arthrodesis of the thoracolumbosacral spine. In M.W. Chapman & M. Madison (Eds.), *Operative orthopaedics* (2nd ed., pp. 2765–2772). Philadelphia: J.B. Lippincott.

Kemp, A.G., Van Niekerk, J.L., & Van Meurs, P.A. (1993). Impairment score of type III open tibial fractures. *Injury, 24,* 161–162.

Mankin, H. (1984). The articular cartilages, cartilage healing and osteoarthritis. In R.L. Cruess & W.R. Rennie (Eds.), *Adult orthopaedics* (pp. 163–270). New York: Churchill Livingstone.

Mellin, G., Harkeapeaea, K., Hurri, H., & Jarvinkowski, A. (1990). A controlled study on the outcome of inpatient and outpatient treatment of low back pain: Part IV. Long term effects on physical measurements. *Scandinavian Journal of Rehabilitation Medicine, 22,* 189–194.

Mizuno, K., Nabeshima, Y., & Hirohata, K. (1993). Analysis of Bankhart lesion in the recurrent dislocation or subluxation of the shoulder. *Clinical Orthopaedics and Related Research, 288,* 158–165.

Moore, T.J., Barron, J., Forney, H.I., Golden, C., Ellis, C., & Humphries, D. (1989). Prosthetic usage following major lower extremity amputations. *Clinical Orthopaedics and Related Research, 238,* 219–234.

Moreland, J.R. (1993). Primary total hip arthroplasty. In M.W. Chapman & M. Madison (Eds.), *Operative orthopaedics* (2nd ed., pp. 1873–1887). Philadelphia: J.B. Lippincott.

Moskowitz, E., & McCann, C.B. (1957). Classification of disability in the chronically ill and aging. *Journal of Chronic Disease, 5,* 342–346.

Muecke, L., Shekar, S., Dwyer, D., Israel, E., & Flynn, J.P. (1992). Functional screening of lower-limb amputees, a role in predicting rehabilitation outcome. *Archives of Physical Medicine and Rehabilitation, 73,* 851–858.

Nachemson, A. (1992). Newest knowledge of low back pain: A critical look. *Clinical Orthopaedics and Related Research, 279,* 8–20.

Nicholson, H.S., Mulvihill, J.J., & Byrne, J. (1992). Late effects of therapy in adult survivors of osteogenic sarcoma and Ewings sarcoma. *Medical and Pediatric Oncology, 20,* 6–12.

O'Toole, D.M., Goldberg, R.M., & Ryan, B. (1985). Functional changes in vascular amputee patients: Evaluation by Barthel Index, PULSES profile, ESCROW scale. *Archives of Physical Medicine and Rehabilitation, 66,* 508–511.

Paulus, H.E. (1991). Current medicinal approaches to the treatment of rheumatoid arthritis. *Clinical Orthopaedics and Related Research, 265,* 96–102.

Pinzur, M.S., Gottschalk, F., Smith, D., Shanfield, S., DeAndrade, R., Osterman, H., & Roberts, J.R. (1993). Functional outcome of below-knee amputations in peripheral vascular insufficiency. *Clinical Orthopaedics and Related Research, 286,* 247–249.

Ranawat, C.S., Flynn, W.F., Saddler, S., Hansraj, W.W., & Maynard, M.J. (1993). Long-term results of the total condylar knee arthroplasty. *Clinical Orthopaedics and Related Research, 286,* 94–102.

Rand, J.A., & Ilstrup, D.M. (1991). Survivorship analysis of total knee arthroplasty, cumulative rates of survival of 9200 total knee arthroplasties. *Journal of Bone and Joint Surgery, 73A,* 397–409.

Reyes, R.L., Leahey, E.B., & Leahey, E.B.J. (1977). Elderly patients with lower extremity amputations: Three year study in a rehabilitation setting. *Archives of Physical Medicine and Rehabilitation, 58,* 116–123.

Rodrigo, J.J., & Gershwin, M.E. (1993). Management of the arthritic joint. In M.W. Chapman & M. Madison (Eds.), *Operative orthopaedics* (2nd ed., pp. 1795–1809). Philadelphia: J.B. Lippincott.

Rougraff, B.T., Simon, M.A., Kneisi, J.S., Greenberg, D.B., & Manakin, H.J. (1994). Limb salvage compared with amputation for osteosarcoma of the distal end of the femur, a long-term oncological, functional and quality of life study. *Journal of Bone and Joint Surgery, 76A,* 649–656.

Rowe, C.R., Patel, D., & Southmayd, W.W. (1978). The Bankhart procedure. *Journal of Bone and Joint Surgery, 60A,* 1–16.

Ruesch, P.D., Holdener, H., Ciaramitaro, M., & Mast, J.W. (1994). A prospective study of surgically treated acetabular fractures. *Clinical Orthopaedics and Related Research, 305,* 38–46.

Segal, D., Mallik, A.R., Wetzler, M.J., Franchi, A.V., & Whitelaw, G.P. (1993). Early weight bearing of lateral tibial plateau fractures. *Clinical Orthopaedics and Related Research, 294,* 232–237.

Shope, J.T., Barnwell, B.A., Jette, A.M., Kulik, C.L., & Edwards, A.L. (1983, November/December). Functional status outcome after treatment of rheumatoid arthritis. *Rheumatological Practice,* 243–248.

Sim, F.H., McDonald, D.J., & Wold, L.E. (1993). Malignant bone tumors. In M.W. Chapman & M. Madison (Eds.), *Operative orthopaedics* (2nd ed., pp. 2535–2553). Philadelphia: J.B. Lippincott.

Spengler, D.M. (1993). Lumbar disc herniation. In M.W. Chapman & M. Madison (Eds.), *Operative orthopaedics* (2nd ed., pp. 2735–2744). Philadelphia: J.B. Lippincott.

Spratt, K.F., Weinstein, J.N., Lehmann, T.R., Woody, J., & Sayre, H. (1993). Efficacy of flexion and extension treatments incorporating braces for low back pain patients with retrodisplacement, spondylolisthesis or normal sagittal translation. *Spine, 18,* 1839–1849.

State University of New York at Buffalo. (1993). *Guide for the Uniform Data Set for Medical Rehabilitation (Adult FIM), version 4.0.* Buffalo, NY: Author.

Steiner, M.E., Simon, S.R., & Pisciotta, J.C. (1989). Early changes in gait and maximum knee torque following knee arthroplasty. *Clinical Orthopaedics and Related Research, 238,* 174–182.

Suteji, P.G., & Hadler, N.M. (1991). Current principles of rehabilitation for patients with rheumatoid arthritis. *Clinical Orthopaedics and Related Research, 265,* 116–124.

Szyszkowitz, R., Segal, W., Schliefer, P., & Cundy, P.J. (1993). Proximal humeral fractures. *Clinical Orthopaedics and Related Research, 292,* 13–25.

Thorngren, K.G., Ceder, L., & Svensson, K. (1993). Predicting results of rehabilitation after hip fracture. A ten year follow-up study. *Clinical Orthopaedics and Related Research, 287,* 76–81.

Tilley, B.C., Alarcon, G.S., Heyse, S.P., Trentham, D.E., Deuner, R., Kaplan, D.A., Clegg, D.O., Leisen, J.C., Buckley, L., & Cooper, S.M. (1995). Minocycline in rheumatoid arthritis. An 8 week double-blind placebo-controlled trial. MIRA trial group. *Annals of Internal Medicine, 122,* 81–89.

Tollison, C.B. (1993). Compensation status as a predictor of outcome in nonsurgically treated low back injury. *Southern Medical Journal, 86,* 1206–1209.

Walker, C.R., Ingram, R.R., Hullin, M.G., & McCreath, S.W. (1994). Lower limb amputation following injury, a survey of long term functional outcome. *INJURY, 25,* 387–392.

Waters, R.L. (1992). Energy expenditure. In J. Perry (Ed.), *Gait analysis: Normal and pathological function* (pp. 443–489). Thorofare, NJ: Slack.

Weinblatt, M.E., & Maier, A.I. (1991). Disease-modifying agents and experimental treatment in rheumatoid arthritis. *Clinical Orthopaedics and Related Research, 265,* 103–115.

World Health Organization. (1980). *International classification of impairments, disabilities, and handicaps.* Geneva, Switzerland: Author.

CHAPTER 19

Postscript and Commentary

Marcus J. Fuhrer

The preceding chapters form an intricate tapestry portraying the present status and future promise of outcomes research relevant to medical rehabilitation. This chapter is not designed to be a summarizing miniature into which the larger work is compressed. Instead, its purpose is simply to supply some reinforcing strands and to tie up a few loose ends. The following topics are particularly highlighted:

1. The domains in which medical rehabilitation outcomes are found
2. The various value-laden perspectives in terms of which outcomes can be viewed
3. The distinction between outcomes research that is rehabilitation science–oriented and program management–oriented
4. The significance of continuing outcomes research for fostering the evidence-based practice of rehabilitation medicine

DOMAINS OF MEDICAL REHABILITATION OUTCOMES

Considerable progress has been made since the mid-1980s in achieving consensus about the principal domains of human functioning that rehabilitation practices affect. Attaining that consensus is of pivotal importance for outcomes research for several reasons. The development and refinement of relevant outcomes measures will be encouraged, study planners will have a stronger rationale for selecting particular outcomes criteria and their related measures, and published findings can more readily be compared because similar variables and measures will have been used. That accord also will facilitate the cumulative development of a body of theory to explain why particular interventions achieve the outcomes attributed to them.

Foundational to this emerging consensus are the domains of human functioning distinguished originally by Nagi (1976) and then adopted in modified form by Wood and colleagues in their development of the *International Classification of Impairments, Disabilities, and Handicaps* (ICIDH; World Health Organization, 1980). Indeed, the influence of the ICIDH-specified domains of impairment, disability, and handicap is so great that few contemporary outcomes investigators ignore these concepts and the related measures in designing their studies or interpreting their findings.

Notwithstanding agreement about the utility of the ICIDH-related concepts, these concepts must not be allowed to become an orthodoxy that stifles continuing analysis and conceptualization. Consistent with that goal, the concepts themselves, subsumed collectively under the rubric of *disablement*, continue to undergo an internationally coordinated process of review and revision. Among the impetuses of that effort is the conviction that influences of the physical, attitudinal, and social policy environments in limiting social role functioning (handicap) are not accounted for adequately by the original conceptualization of disablement (see Chapters 4 and 6). Reflecting an individual effort to strengthen and expand the conception of disablement, Peters (1995, in press) elaborated on the implications of impairments, disabilities, and handicaps from the perspective of people's subjective experience.

Acknowledging the relevance of the ICIDH-related concepts to describing the likely consequences of chronic physical impairments is one thing; agreeing that they are sufficient by themselves to describe the domains of functioning that medical rehabilitation practices affect is quite another. Illustrating the insufficiency of those concepts, Dijkers (Chapter 7) shows how the construct of quality of life is useful for identifying many other areas of people's lives that may be touched by the cascading effects of disabling impairments and that may be influenced by rehabilitation services. Other analysts feel that entirely new concepts are needed. For instance, Fiedler and Granger (Chapter 5) advance the innovative concept of quality of daily living and an associated conceptual model that emphasize the balance between people's opportunities for functioning and the demands for functioning that are made of them.

The health problems for which people with disabilities are at elevated risk exemplify another outcomes domain that is not readily accommodated by the concepts subsumed within disablement. Some of those problems, frequently designated as secondary conditions, have an etiology that can be traced directly to features of an individual's primary disabling condition.

For example, that is the nature of the urinary tract infections and pressure ulcers to which people with spinal cord injury are prone. Other health problems may be determined more complexly, for example, the nutritional deficits, injuries associated with falls, and cardiopulmonary deconditioning incurred by some people recovering from stroke. All of these conditions have a potential for compromising people's functioning at the levels of disability or handicap. Some commentators propose that this diversity of health problems be conceptualized under the rubric of *secondary impairments* and that their implications be considered in terms of secondary disability and secondary handicap (see Chapter 4). However, many of these problems, especially the ones that are more episodic in nature, are more akin to acute illness than to impairments, with their implied chronicity. Consequently, a more cogent alternative may be to consider them in terms of the separate constructs of health status (see Chapter 8) or morbidity.

Continuing efforts to clarify the principal domains of functioning affected by rehabilitation practices need to be paralleled by initiatives to conceptualize, classify, and quantify the principal components of which rehabilitation practices are composed (see Chapters 1, 11, and 13). The challenge for theory is to build upon that classification system to identify processes that link designated components of practices to designated changes in specific domains of people's functioning.

MULTIPLE PERSPECTIVES
CONSIDERATION OF MEDICAL REHABILITATION OUTCOMES

As much as any other area of human services, the character of medical rehabilitation practice is shaped by the people involved: patients, service providers, and payers, among others. The values, treatment goals, and information needs of these and other stakeholders in the rehabilitation process must be considered in deciding on the relative importance of the outcomes being assessed.

A more complete listing of the major interest groups with a stake in medical rehabilitation would include

- Service recipients, both individually and as a group
- Service recipients' family members and other people significant in their lives
- Rehabilitation practitioners
- Facility administrators
- Payers, both public and private

DeJong (Chapter 3) discusses some of the differences and generally unrecognized similarities in perspective that characterize several of these groups. His discussion makes clear how little systematic investigation has been devoted to verifying such comparisons.

Many of the questions that need to be addressed by research were identified in a conference organized by the National Center for Medical Rehabilitation Research (NCMRR; Fuhrer, 1995). Which rehabilitation outcomes are most cherished by each interest group? For example, is achieving independence in activities of daily living (ADL) or mobility within the community similarly valued by service recipients, family members, and sponsors? How different are the groups in the trade-offs they are willing to make among different outcomes? To what degree are the groups heterogeneous in their preferences, and to what extent do variables such as gender, age, and income account for that heterogeneity? Medical rehabilitation outcomes research will grow substantially in utility when speculative commentary about the perceptions and expectations of these groups is replaced by solid empirical data. Flexible approaches must be found as well to weighting the findings of multidimensional outcomes studies to make allowance for the groups' values and preferences.

The comparative questions that have been raised have counterparts in questions applicable to each interest group considered separately. The following discussion focuses on research approaches to better understanding the perspectives of service recipients.

Patients' Perspectives on Rehabilitation Outcomes

Respect for patients' values, perceptions, and preferences has long been integral to the ideology of medical rehabilitation practice. Because the long-term success of rehabilitation depends so much upon the sustained initiative of patients, no other approach has seemed to be reasonable. Anomalously, however, the perspective of patients, whether considered as individuals or as a group, is missing from most medical rehabilitation outcomes studies. Briefly cited below are three exceptions in the research literature that exemplify the needed correctives. They are the use of goal attainment scaling techniques, means of weighting various dimensions of disability or handicap to take into account individual patients' preferences, and measures of subjective well-being.

Goal Attainment Scaling

Goal attainment scaling techniques were developed during the heyday of evaluation research that focused on the social and mental health programs associated with the Great Society initiatives of the Johnson administration (Kiresuk & Sherman, 1968). Goal attainment scaling makes expressed provision for considering the individual patient's goals and expectations in assessing the outcomes of rehabilitation. This approach calls for formulating a number of concrete, measurable goals for each rehabilitee that, in the aggregate, will be used to evaluate the success of rehabilitation. Patients and family members participate fully in formulating the goals. Ratings of the extent of goal attainment obtained periodically during rehabilitation and at its completion can be used to monitor the patient's progress and outcomes. Methods exist as well for combining goal attainment data of a group of patients to assess overall program performance.

A study by Malec, Smigielski, and DePompolo (1991) is one of only a handful of applications of goal attainment scaling to evaluating the outcomes of medical rehabilitation practices. They applied the method to assessing outcomes for 16 patients with brain injuries who had participated in a comprehensive, postacute rehabilitation program. They found the method to be feasible and to generate information that importantly augmented findings based on more conventional measures reflecting outcomes criteria applied uniformly to all participants.

The criticisms that have been leveled at goal attainment scaling through the years do not seem to be consequential enough to discourage its more widespread use in rehabilitation outcomes research. It can be an especially demanding research procedure unless the process of goal setting and the monitoring of goal attainment are made integral parts of clinical practices in the particular setting. That is not at all unrealistic, because individualized goal setting is frequently a routine, albeit unsystematized, aspect of rehabilitation care.

Individual Weighting of the Dimensions of Disability or Handicap

Weighting the dimensions of disability from the rehabilitee's standpoint is another underexploited approach to taking into account individual patients' values and lifestyle preferences. Conventional scales for quantifying patients' abilities to perform ADL assess everyone on the same array of activities. Many take an objective viewpoint by determining the amount of assistance required to perform each activity. For reasons of feasibility, the source of that information may be the individual being assessed, especially when a telephone interview or mailed questionnaire must be relied on to reach people who have resumed their lives in the community. Nevertheless, the approach remains a fundamentally objective one because, at least in principle, the kind of information being sought can be obtained by external observers.

An approach to weighting various disability-related activities in terms of the importance that individual patients assign to them in their lives is exemplified by the study of Laman and Lankhorst (1994). For 39 items reflecting various impairments, disabilities, and handicaps, respondents rated their level of performance as well as how important that performance was for them in their overall quality of life. The scoring algorithm called for multiplying the two ratings for each activity. Thus, little or no disability was reflected by activities that were performed poorly but were of little or no importance to the individual. The scale is designed primarily to monitor changes in functional status over the course of rehabilitation. Additional research is required to determine whether subjective weighting of this kind makes a difference in assessing the impacts of specific interventions on groups of patients.

Measures of Patients' Subjective Well-Being

Subjective quality of life or its synonym, *subjective well-being,* refer to the degree to which people have positive thoughts and feelings about their lives considered as a whole. Expressed less precisely but more evocatively, this dimension is concerned with how happy people are with their lives overall. Considering impacts on subjective well-being as a rehabilitation outcome is to suggest that in the final analysis, after experiencing all the rigors and expense of rehabilitation, patients ought to be happier with their lives than if opportunities for rehabilitation were forgone.

Measures of subjective well-being have been used only rarely to assess the outcomes of medical rehabilitation interventions. However, their use is likely to increase markedly. Helping people to think and feel more positively about their lives overall is an acknowledged, albeit frequently implicit, goal of many different kinds of rehabilitation services. It is appropriate, therefore, to evaluate the outcomes of those services in terms of enhancements of subjective well-being. The second reason relates to the frequently (almost euphemistically) stated intent of most rehabilitation providers to enhance their patients' quality of life. Writers such as Gill and Feinstein (1994) emphasize that if quality of life is to be a measurable construct distinct from other constructs such as functional status, it must be approached from a subjective point of view. In a similar vein, Andrews and Withey (1976) and Campbell, Converse, and Rodgers (1976) have pointed out that, to be meaningful, estimations of people's quality of life should be theirs alone to make.

Outcomes researchers will find that subjective well-being has been operationalized in a number of ways that facilitate its quantitative assessment. Greater subjective well-being is attributed to people who experience a larger number of positive thoughts and feelings about their lives as a whole. The construct is construed as consisting of four components:

1. A cognitive appraisal of the satisfactoriness of life overall
2. Cognitive appraisals of the satisfactoriness of separate domains into which life may be divided (e.g., work, leisure, health)
3. The relative presence of positive affective experience
4. The relative absence of negative affective experience (Diener, 1994)

Although the affective components are integral to the notion of subjective well-being, the most widely used instruments focus only on respondents' cognitive appraisal of their satisfaction with life as a whole. That practice is justified in part by the finding that, when assessed concurrently, the cognitive and affective components covary to a substantial degree (Frisch, 1992).

Dijkers (Chapter 7) cites the writing of Calman (1984) and others who point out that people's level of subjective well-being is influenced by how large the gap is between their expectations of life and their actual achievements. This expectancy-congruence concept of subjective quality of life is consistent with the general philosophy that people can attain happiness either by mustering accomplishments to meet their aspirations or by reducing their aspirations to the level of their actual accomplishments. Applied to rehabilitation, this principle suggests that patients' subjective well-being can be enhanced in several ways. One is to help them increase their level of functioning (e.g., their independence in ADL) so that it is more in line with their expectations. Another is to encourage them to reduce their expectations to conform more with their actual functional capabilities.

This expectancy-congruence conception of subjective well-being makes even greater psychological sense if patients' self-assessed achievements are taken into account in relation to their expectations. The distinction between people's perceived (i.e., subjectively assessed) achievements and their actual (i.e., objectively assessed) achievements simply acknowledges the common observation that the two may sometimes be at variance. For example, people with disabilities may perceive their degree of independence quite differently from that portrayed by an objective assessment. Some patients who, following rehabilitation, are dependent on others' assistance in only a few areas of daily life may nonetheless assess their independence as being severely compromised.

The distinctions between service recipients' expectations, actual achievements, and self-assessed achievements have implications for both medical rehabilitation outcomes research and practice, especially if increasing patients' subjective well-being is taken seriously as an outcomes criterion. The implication for research is that methodologically sound methods of operationalizing the three concepts need to be introduced into outcomes studies so that more can be learned about how various interventions affect patients' subjective well-being. The implication for practice is the reminder that options for increasing patients' subjective quality of life go beyond conventional efforts of helping patients make objective gains in areas such as their strength, mobility, or independence in ADL. Improved subjective well-being may be achieved as well by helping patients alter the way they assess their functioning or by helping them moderate their aspirations associated with that functioning. Although it is likely that many clinicians use all of these strategies in daily practice, their implications and interrelationships are discussed remarkably little in the literature of the rehabilitation professions. This reticence is probably due in part to discomfort about the ethical justification of attempting directly to manipulate patients' perceptions and expectations, especially when little more is being done to elevate their actual level of useful functioning. These are issues that warrant continuing consideration by clinicians and rehabilitation outcomes researchers alike.

TWO APPROACHES TO OUTCOMES RESEARCH: PROGRAM MANAGEMENT AND REHABILITATION SCIENCE

As emphasized in this chapter and in previous chapters, medical rehabilitation outcomes research is subject to diverse expectations from a variety of standpoints. Practitioners want more of it to help guide their treatment decisions; payers are increasingly requiring it as a basis for deciding which services will be reimbursed; and rehabilitation scientists view it as a means of validating theories of how rehabilitation practices work. A multiplicity of research principles, strategies, and methods can be called upon to meet these diverse information demands. Some components of this armamentarium are more appropriate than others for meeting particular information needs. In appraising both prospective and completed studies, it is useful to have in mind the distinction between outcomes research that is rehabilitation science–oriented and the research that is program management–oriented. Their distinguishing features are summarized in Table 1 and are discussed below.

Aims

The expressed purposes of the two kinds of studies distinguish them most sharply. Rehabilitation science–oriented studies are part and parcel of the process of accruing a body of testable theories, scientifically verified principles, and validated interventions upon which to base medical rehabilitation practices. As discussed by Wilkerson and Johnston (Chapter 12) under the rubric of clinical program monitoring systems, program management–oriented studies are a kind of operations research conducted by particular rehabilitation facilities or units in order to assess the value of one of their service programs or practices. The intent is to generate information that justifies continuation of the program or that can be used to improve it.

Regardless of which motivation an outcomes study has, the interpretability of the findings depends upon the clarity and appropriateness with which the goals of the intervention are stated. Several contributors to this book, Whyte (Chapter 2) most explicitly among them, plead for clear distinctions between the more immediate impacts of an intervention and the longer-term effects that may result from achieving it.

Table 1.   Comparative features of program management-oriented and rehabilitation science-oriented outcomes research

Feature	Program management-oriented research	Rehabilitation science-oriented research
Expressed aims	Generating practical information immediately applicable to the provision or sponsorship of services provided by the local rehabilitation program	Accruing generalizable knowledge relevant to developing or confirming theories and principles of rehabilitation practices; demonstrating the efficacy or effectiveness of designated types of interventions in efforts to improve them
Principal audiences	Local administrators and practitioners, and, selectively, payers, accreditors, and potential patients	Researchers, practitioners, administrators, payers, and patients
Bases for outcomes criteria	Expressed goals of the local program	Hypothesized impacts of the intervention, as well as impacts relevant to theory or specific research issues
Role of treatment theory	Frequently left implicit	Characteristically made explicit in planning a study and reporting its findings
Internal validity concerns	Frequently of interest, but seldom addressed adequately	Frequently a key standard for evaluating the soundness of investigations
External validity concerns	Focused on the influence of future changes in the local service setting or in the staff providing the intervention	Focused on all such interventions, wherever conducted
Investigative strategies	Effectiveness studies of local rehabilitation programs and, less frequently, of their component practices	Effectiveness and efficacy studies of types of programs and types of component practices, including decomposition studies
Integration of cost data	Intervention costs frequently considered, either formally or informally	Cost data only infrequently incorporated into analyses
Principal sources of sponsorship for studies	The local rehabilitation facility	Federal agencies supporting medical rehabilitation research
Dissemination of findings	Often limited by administrative policy to local administrators and providers and, selectively, to payers and accreditors	Widespread within limits imposed by publication standards of journals and other media

Audiences

Studies' different purposes dictate differences in the audiences to which their findings are directed. The results of studies conducted for the purpose of program management tend to be made available solely on a need-to-know basis. Results are shared generally with the facility's clinical staff and administrators and selectively with representatives of payer or accrediting organizations. The proprietary nature of the information results in it characteristically being withheld from publication in the professional literature. In marked contrast, the imperatives of science dictate that the findings of rehabilitation science–oriented studies be widely disseminated, with peer-reviewed professional journals being the venue of choice to reach clinicians and researchers.

Outcomes Criteria

Outcomes variables for program management–oriented studies are carefully chosen to reflect the professed goals of the intervention being evaluated. Studies conducted from a rehabilitation science perspective are also likely to include variables reflecting an intervention's putative goals, but other variables may be added as well that are prominent in previous studies or relevant theories.

Treatment Theory

All clinical practices have associated with them one or more theories, varying in explicitness, that attempt to account for their observed or presumed effects. Program management–oriented researchers may make little or no effort to state the theoretical bases of the intervention they are assessing. Their concern is with the degree to which the program works and much less so with why it works. However, rehabilitation science–oriented researchers characteristically take pains to document the presumed theoretical bases of the intervention being evaluated. As explained by Keith (Chapter 11), that explication is important for achieving several goals, including

1. Generalizing the findings of a study to a larger universe
2. Making explicit otherwise hidden assumptions underlying the intervention's use
3. Providing a means of accumulating knowledge across successive studies
4. Guiding the planning of future studies by identifying variables that warrant being manipulated, controlled, or assessed

Internal Validity

As discussed by Ottenbacher (Chapter 10), the findings of an outcomes study have internal validity to the extent that it can be concluded that the intervention studied was responsible for the effects observed. The issue is therefore one of inferring the existence of a causal relationship between the study's independent variables (i.e., the practices being assessed) and its dependent variables (e.g., measured changes in patients' performance). Findings characterized by weak internal validity are those that can be reasonably attributed to influences other than those associated with the intervention studied. Those influences may relate to natural recovery processes, features of the care setting, nonspecific aspects of the intervention such as emotional support afforded by the treatment staff, or characteristics of service recipients affecting their receptivity to the intervention. The design of choice for ruling out such competing explanations is the randomized control design, in which the people to be studied are assigned on a random basis to intervention and control groups. Randomization is unrivaled as a procedure for assuring that observed effects are attributable to the intervention and not to preexisting differences between the intervention and control groups.

Research designs that accord high internal validity to findings are esteemed from the standpoint of rehabilitation science, but they are generally infeasible for outcomes studies conducted under the aegis of program management. Constraints emanating from payers, family members, or patients themselves often rule out the use of control groups or of comparative interventions that do not promise the benefits associated with the intervention being evaluated. The only feasible design is often one in which measures of patients' status are obtained before and after they are exposed to an intervention. These "pre–post" designs yield findings that are susceptible to a variety of competing explanations about the causal factors that were operating. As such, they have low internal validity. However, clinicians and program administrators may have other legitimate concerns for which the pre–post design is of unassailable value. For example, administrators may simply want to know if an intervention is achieving the patient benefits that were documented at an earlier time or that are expected by sponsors. Alternatively, clinicians may be concerned with identifying at admission the patients who are most likely to benefit from an intervention. Changes in patients' status that are revealed by a pre–post design lend themselves nicely to such predictive analyses.

External Validity

The information yield of individual outcomes studies may be powerfully constrained by distinctive features of the treatment environment in which they are conducted, regardless of steps taken to assure the internal validity of their findings. Those features may entail 1) the manner in which various treatments (including the one being studied) are organized and delivered; 2) the training and skill levels of the people who provide them; or

3) characteristics of the patients admitted to the particular facility, including their sponsorship. Factors like these can materially influence how the technical features of any intervention affect patients. The question arises, therefore, whether the intervention would yield similar results if conducted in other treatment environments having their own particularities. That question pertains to the external validity of the findings, that is, the likelihood that they can be generalized to other treatment settings.

The degree of concern with external validity sharply differentiates outcomes studies that are rehabilitation science–oriented from those that are program management–oriented. The latter are intended to yield information required by the facility that commissioned them. If generalization is an expressed concern at all, it is usually one of generalizing across time from when the study was conducted to later times, when changes, large or small, have occurred in the treatment environment. However, the generalizability of findings is a first-order concern of rehabilitation science–oriented studies, apropos of the intent of science to move beyond concrete observations to more general characterizations of the world.

A desire to maximize the external validity of findings poses its own design requirements on studies. For instance, a deliberate effort may be made to maximize individual differences among people within a study sample in order to be able to generalize the findings to a more broadly delineated population. However, that tactic may well be employed at the expense of the study's internal validity, which is generally enhanced by minimizing individual differences within the study sample. Trade-offs of this kind abound in the design of outcomes studies and are the reason why important issues require a family of different but related research efforts for their resolution.

Notwithstanding efforts to strengthen the external validity of findings from individual studies, there is no substitute for launching studies in other settings in an attempt to confirm the generalizability of earlier results. Facilitating such efforts ought to become the objective of national (and possibly international) consortia of rehabilitation facilities concerned with upgrading the demonstrated effectiveness of their services. Such consortia could be enormously helpful in the following ways:

1. Developing treatment guidelines to assist in standardizing practices, which in turn become more feasible subjects of outcomes studies
2. Promoting consensus on measurement standards for outcomes research to facilitate the selection of specific measures and indices
3. Providing technical assistance for the design and conduct of outcomes studies
4. Attracting funding from sources (e.g., federal agencies or managed care organizations) that might be reluctant to fund research proposed by individual facilities

5. Encouraging the dissemination and transfer into practice of information yielded by outcomes studies

Similar possibilities are envisioned by Wilkerson and Johnston (Chapter 12).

Strategies

Textbook discussions of how to design outcomes studies typically consider a planned investigation as an isolated abstraction unrelated to projects that have preceded it or to others that may follow. In actuality, individual studies are almost always components in an interlocking array of investigations, some already completed and others merely envisioned (see Chapters 2 and 10). The projection of future studies is a natural byproduct of the many trade-offs that are entailed in arriving at the structure and procedures of a particular study. Individual studies thus represent components in an investigative strategy, often not spelled out, that is aimed at answering a significant question or confirming an important hypothesis.

Early studies in a strategy may be based on single-subject or pre–post designs and may emanate from management-oriented research. These studies are important for demonstrating an association between the intervention of interest and outcomes that are valued. The question of a causal relationship between the intervention and observed changes in patients' statuses cannot be answered by such studies; but, if the association is found to be reasonably strong, the findings can lend importance to resolving that question. Rehabilitation science–oriented investigators are especially likely to undertake supplying an answer if the intervention is significant from the standpoint of the principles and theories of medical rehabilitation. Their studies may be conducted as pristine efficacy trials or, less likely, as effectiveness studies under conditions of ordinary service provision. Positive findings of studies with randomized control or strong quasi-experimental designs may well be succeeded by studies attempting to confirm the replicability of those findings and their generalizability. Decomposition studies may follow in which particular components of a complex intervention are evaluated individually in an attempt to confirm their hypothesized contribution to observed outcomes. Other, later studies may involve longitudinal designs with multiple waves of data collection in order to confirm the long-term stability of the intervention's impacts. Meanwhile, program management–oriented studies may be called for once again to verify that the intervention continues to yield the benefits documented in earlier studies, despite interim changes in criteria for admitting patients, the composition of treatment staffs, or payers' guidelines for reimbursement.

Consideration of Costs

The literature of medical rehabilitation outcomes research is marked by a conspicuous dearth of studies in which observed outcomes are gauged against the costs of producing them. The failure to inject an economic perspective into outcomes studies is anomalous from a historical standpoint and surely foolhardy from the standpoint of the contemporary health care scene. From its very inception during World War II, medical rehabilitation was touted by its advocates as making compelling economic sense. It was claimed that the costs of services would be returned many times over by recipients' enhanced independence and productivity, often in the form of their being remuneratively employed. However, few relevant studies were conducted to confirm that assertion, and those that were suffered from serious methodologic weaknesses (Johnston & Keith, 1983). Meanwhile, payers began to press increasingly for justifications of rehabilitation costs as part of the growing national debate over health care expenditures. Still, the relevant studies were not forthcoming. That resistance is unlikely to continue, however, in the face of prospects that the reimbursement of rehabilitation services will depend increasingly on convincing evidence that their costs are justified by the benefits conferred on recipients.

Erickson (Chapter 9) describes three analytic strategies—cost–benefit, cost-effectiveness, and cost–utility—for linking medical rehabilitation costs to service outcomes. Cost-effectiveness analysis is likely to be the most widely used of the three. Outcomes need not be translated into monetizable units, as is the case with cost–benefit analysis, and prior studies are not required to establish a basis for estimating years of healthy life or quality-adjusted years, as is the case with cost–utility analysis. Cost-effectiveness analysis simply entails the comparison of two or more interventions that share similar outcomes goals—a situation that abounds in many areas of medical rehabilitation practice.

Researchers conducting program monitoring–oriented studies often gain access to their facility's cost data and relate that information to observed outcomes for particular programs or practices. However, those studies are quite limited for answering questions about the cost-effectiveness of those interventions. That applies especially to questions that implicitly or explicitly allude to their causal impacts. The cost-effectiveness studies needed to answer those questions must be based upon randomized or quasi-experimental designs that confer high internal validity to the findings. As explained above, those designs are generally unfeasible for program monitoring–oriented studies. That makes it particularly incumbent on rehabilitation science–oriented studies to include an economic perspective in order to fill this knowledge gap.

Sources of Sponsorship

Financing the needed investigative effort requires that appropriate priority be given to outcomes research by all of the principal funding sources —federal agencies that sponsor research, the medical rehabilitation industry, payers of services, private foundations, and voluntary health agencies.

Federal Sponsors of Research The agencies that finance medical rehabilitation research can be expected to assign priority to three kinds of outcomes studies, all rehabilitation science–oriented in nature. They are 1) methodologic innovations of significance for outcomes research, 2) hypothesis-testing investigations relevant to theory development, and 3) efficacy studies connected with the development of new interventions.

Encouraging advances in the methodology of outcomes research is a distinctly appropriate mission for agencies like NCMRR and the National Institute on Disability and Rehabilitation Research. Particularly worthy of priority are methodologic innovations with applicability across different kinds of interventions and disabling conditions. Improvements in techniques for measuring outcomes and the factors that affect them are a case in point. Particularly underdeveloped are means of quantifying features of people's environment that have the potential of modulating their longer-term responses to rehabilitation (see Chapter 4). Those features range from individuals' immediate circumstances to personally relevant aspects of the societal environment. Development and application of those measures will yield knowledge that enables rehabilitation providers to do the following:

1. Take environmental influences into account in predicting the likely impacts of rehabilitation
2. Individualize treatments to accommodate known features of patients' environments
3. Account for variability among patients in their responses to particular practices
4. Offer services, typically in collaboration with community-based providers, to favorably modify those influences so that better, more durable rehabilitation outcomes are obtained

Federal agencies will also be disposed to supporting outcomes studies that contribute to the development of theory, both treatment theory and theory bearing on the nature and development of impairments, disability, and handicap. In their design and conduct, these studies may be indistinguishable from garden-variety outcomes studies that are application-oriented. Their distinctiveness will derive from their potentiality to verify one or more hypotheses that have a strong logical relationship to theoretical formulations important for medical rehabilitation.

The most prominent federal agency role will be to finance the development of new rehabilitation interventions that draw upon the enormous reservoir of scientific knowledge that has arisen from basic research and from innumerable areas of clinical research germane to rehabilitation. The capstone of that developmental process is the efficacy study, which seeks to demonstrate that the desired clinical outcomes are yielded by the new intervention. Such studies are conducted with the utmost rigor, with their hallmarks being explicit eligibility criteria for admitting patients into the study, a strong research design that often involves the randomized assignment of participants to study groups, and well-trained administrators of the intervention investigated.

Medical Rehabilitation Industry   The pristine nature of efficacy trials is the basis for delineating the most important sponsorship role for the medical rehabilitation industry: supporting the conduct of effectiveness studies to determine treatment outcomes under ordinary clinical conditions. This is not likely to be accomplished by simply collating retrospectively the findings of program management–oriented studies conducted by individual facilities. Uncontrolled variation in how specific interventions were administered and differences in the outcomes measures used would probably defeat such an effort. Of considerably greater promise are initiatives by consortia of facilities that would develop study protocols on a prospective basis, maintain databases, and analyze and report findings. In addition to modest subscription fees from participating facilities, these consortia could anticipate support from payers, both private and governmental, and from voluntary health organizations and foundations with interests in improving services for people with particular disabling conditions. Federal agencies that support research are not strong candidates to finance effectiveness research of this kind, because limitations on the design and implementation of the research probably would prevent the findings from having much internal validity.

Dissemination

Disseminating the results of outcomes studies conducted for program-monitoring purposes is relatively straightforward because of the restricted audiences being targeted. Most of the relevant individuals belong to the organization that conducted the study, whereas others, such as payer representatives, are known on an individual basis to members of the organization's staff. Effective means of disseminating findings from management-oriented studies are more problematic, though less so for some audiences than for others. Least equivocal are means of reaching members of the research community interested in the intervention or disability group that was studied. Familiarity with the journals and national meetings that focus on particular research topics is the stock-in-trade knowledge of outcomes researchers.

Dissemination to clinicians is much more of a challenge. A repeated lesson is that simply communicating study findings at national meetings and in journals is not sufficient to effect changes in most clinicians' practices, regardless of how incisive the findings are. This is especially true for service areas like medical rehabilitation, whose heritage does not include a strong clinical research literature upon which to base clinical decision making. A transition from relying on clinicians' individual experience or guidance from ostensible authorities to an evidence-based mode of practice inevitably occurs gradually as practitioners become aware of a body of research that is relevant to everyday clinical issues. That awareness can be facilitated by the efforts of individual facilities and of professional organizations at the local, state, and national levels to promulgate practice guidelines for managing various problems encountered during rehabilitation. The developers of those guidelines typically take pains to ensure that the findings of credible outcomes studies are taken into account in guideline development.

A Qualification

The distinction that has been examined between program management–oriented and rehabilitation science–oriented outcomes studies is not a mutually exclusive one. Investigators may attempt to undertake studies that straddle the two categories. For instance, the rehabilitation scientist collecting her data in a particular facility may make special efforts to organize her findings so that they are relevant to the management questions of administrators in that facility. Clinical staff members who are conducting a study to dispel an administrator's qualms about continuing a treatment program may obtain findings that warrant being written up for journal publication. By and large, however, the two types of studies pose different requirements and meet different needs.

CONCLUSIONS

Approximately a decade has passed since publication of the last volume devoted wholly to outcomes research of relevance to medical rehabilitation (Fuhrer, 1987). During that period, both medical rehabilitation practices and research have changed at a dramatically accelerating rate. According to estimates cited by DeJong and Sutton (1995), medical rehabilitation is already a $15 billion–$20 billion a year industry that is expected to grow to more than $45 billion a year by 2000. Mirroring the turbulence in the health care industry at large, rehabilitation services are being reshaped, in large part because of payers' determination to reduce costs. Inpatient rehabilitation stays have been markedly curtailed and sites for delivering services have shifted increasingly from the hospital to skilled nursing facilities, a variety of outpatient settings, and the home. At the same time, providers have become keenly sensitized to payers' questions about evidence that their practices are effective and cost-justified, whatever the setting involved.

Also, significant strides have been made since the mid-1980s in shoring up the infrastructure of medical rehabilitation research. These developments have been propelled in large part by the steady maturation of the medical rehabilitation–related professions, especially by their commitment to strengthening the scientific foundation of their practices. Due in large measure to advocacy by practitioners of these professions, legislation was passed in 1990 establishing NCMRR as the focal point for medical rehabilitation research at the National Institutes of Health. Acting in concert with the longer-established federal agencies that support that research, NCMRR has emphasized investments in research training as a means of increasing research capacity. Some of the investigators being trained will commit their careers to drawing upon the exploding volume of knowledge in biologic, behavioral, and engineering sciences to develop the rehabilitation practices of tomorrow and to understand the underlying mechanisms of rehabilitation practices, both new and old. Others will work in clinical settings, and some of them, skilled in the concepts and techniques of outcomes research, will tackle the unknowns about rehabilitation practices that are discussed throughout this book.

Mobilizing this enlarged research capacity to meet the information demands of the practice arena is sure to hasten development of the evidence-based practice of medical rehabilitation. Consistent with the vision of evidence-based health care generally (Evidence-Based Medicine Working Group, 1992), this new practice paradigm presupposes the existence of a continually expanding and upgraded body of knowledge, fed by sound research, that is directly relevant to problems encountered in rehabilitation service settings on an everyday basis. It is a mode of practice in which the diagnosis and treatment of the health problems of people with disabilities are based on direct studies of those conditions rather than on speculative extrapolation from the pathophysiology of people generally. It is characterized as well by trained practitioners who are skilled in the appraisal of the research literature so that their own critical judgment can substitute for dependence on ostensible authorities. The beneficiaries of the evidence-based practice of medical rehabilitation will be patients, payers, and practitioners alike, who deserve the assurance of knowing that rehabilitation services are being progressively improved by dependable knowledge issuing from relevant research.

REFERENCES

Andrews, F., & Withey, S. (1976). *Social indicators of well-being: Americans' perceptions of life quality.* New York: Plenum Press.

Calman, K. (1984). Quality of life in cancer patients: An hypothesis. *Journal of Medical Ethics, 10,* 124–127.

Campbell, A., Converse, P., & Rodgers, W. (1976). *The quality of American life.* New York: Russell Sage Foundation.

DeJong, G., & Sutton, J. (1995). Rehab 2000: The evolution of medical rehabilitation in American health care. In P.K. Landrum, N.D. Schmidt, & A. McLean,

Jr. (Eds.), *Outcome oriented rehabilitation: Principles, strategies, and tools for effective program management* (pp. 3–42). Gaithersburg, MD: Aspen Publishers.

Diener, E. (1994). Assessing subjective well-being: Progress and opportunities. *Social Indicators Research, 31,* 103–157.

Evidence-Based Medicine Working Group. (1992). Evidence-based medicine: A new approach to teaching the practice of medicine. *Journal of the American Medical Association, 268,* 2420–2425.

Frisch, M. (1992). Clinical validation of the quality of life inventory: A measure of life satisfaction for use in treatment planning and outcome assessment. *Psychological Assessment, 4,* 92–101.

Fuhrer, M.J. (Ed.). (1987). *Rehabilitation outcomes research: Analysis and measurement.* Baltimore: Paul H. Brookes Publishing Co.

Fuhrer, M.J. (1995). Conference report: An agenda for medical rehabilitation outcomes research. *American Journal of Physical Medicine and Rehabilitation, 74,* 243–248; *Journal of Allied Health, 24,* 79–87; *Journal of Prosthetics and Orthotics, 71,* 35–39.

Gill, T.M., & Feinstein, A.R. (1994). A critical appraisal of the quality of quality-of-life measurements. *Journal of the American Medical Association, 272,* 619–626.

Johnston, M., & Keith, R. (1983). Cost-benefits of medical rehabilitation: Review and critique. *Archives of Physical Medicine and Rehabilitation, 64,* 147–154.

Kiresuk, T., & Sherman, R. (1968). Goal attainment scaling: A general method for evaluating comprehensive mental health programs. *Community Mental Health Journal, 4,* 443–453.

Laman, H., & Lankhorst, G. (1994). Subjective weighting of disability: An approach to quality of life assessment in rehabilitation. *Disability and Rehabilitation, 16,* 198–204.

Malec, J., Smigielski, J., & DePompolo, R. (1991). Goal attainment scaling and outcome measurement in postacute brain injury rehabilitation. *Archives of Physical Medicine and Rehabilitation, 72,* 138–143.

Nagi, S. (1976). An epidemiology of disability among adults in the United States. *Milbank Memorial Fund Quarterly, 54,* 439–467.

Peters, D. (1995). Human experience in disablement: The imperative of the ICIDH (International Classification of Impairments, Disabilities, and Handicaps). *Disability and Rehabilitation, 17,* 135–144.

Peters, D. (in press). Disablement observed, addressed, and experienced: Integrating subjective experience into disablement models. *Disability and Rehabilitation.*

World Health Organization. (1980). *International classification of impairments, disabilities, and handicaps.* Geneva, Switzerland: Author.

Index

Page numbers followed by "t" or "f" indicate tables or figures, respectively.